Advances in Experimental Medicine and Biology

Volume 899

More information about this series at http://www.springer.com/series/5584

Constantinos Koumenis
Lisa M. Coussens • Amato Giaccia
Ester Hammond
Editors

Tumor Microenvironment

Study Protocols

Springer

Editors
Constantinos Koumenis
Perelman School of Medicine
University of Pennsylvania
Philadelphia, PA, USA

Lisa M. Coussens
Cell & Developmental Biology
Oregon Health & Science University
Portland, OR, USA

Amato Giaccia
Department of Radiation Oncology
Stanford University School of Medicine
Stanford, CA, USA

Ester Hammond
Department of Oncology
University of Oxford
Oxford, Oxfordshire, UK

ISSN 0065-2598 ISSN 2214-8019 (electronic)
Advances in Experimental Medicine and Biology
ISBN 978-3-319-26664-0 ISBN 978-3-319-26666-4 (eBook)
DOI 10.1007/978-3-319-26666-4

Library of Congress Control Number: 2015959711

Printed on acid-free paper

This Springer imprint is published by Springer Nature
The registered company is Springer International Publishing AG Switzerland

Preface

It is universally accepted that the tumor microenvironment is extremely relevant to both the study of cancer biology and the search for improved therapies. However, it is also accepted that the study of biological mechanism in conditions which accurately mimic this environment is both technically challenging and highly specialized. At a recent tumor microenvironment meeting held in Mykonos, Greece, we decided that it would aid the field in general to publish detailed protocols, far exceeding the level of detail usually reported in papers. We hope that these prove useful and that we as a community can continue to share our collective expertise.

Philadelphia, PA, USA — Constantinos Koumenis
Portland, OR, USA — Lisa M. Coussens
Stanford, CA, USA — Amato Giaccia
Oxford, UK — Ester Hammond

Contents

Chapter 1
Staining Against Phospho-H2AX (γ-H2AX) as a Marker for DNA Damage and Genomic Instability in Cancer Tissues and Cells

Anika Nagelkerke and Paul N. Span

Abstract Phospho-H2AX or γ-H2AX- is a marker of DNA double-stranded breaks and can therefore be used to monitor DNA repair after, for example, irradiation. In addition, positive staining for phospho-H2AX may indicate genomic instability and telomere dysfunction in tumour cells and tissues. Here, we provide a protocol to perform immunostaining for phospho-H2AX on cells, cryosections and formalin-fixed, paraffin-embedded tissues. Crucial steps in the protocol and troubleshooting suggestions are indicated. We also provide suggestions on how to combine staining against γ-H2AX with stainings against components of the tumour microenvironment, such as hypoxia and blood vessels.

Keywords Histone 2A • DNA damage repair • Genomic instability • Telomere dysfunction • Immunohistochemistry • Immunofluorescence • Immunocytochemistry

1.1 Introduction

This protocol provides a procedure to stain cells for phospho-H2AX. H2AX is a modified version of the histone H2A. In the nucleus of cells, the DNA is wrapped around these and other histones, to ensure proper organisation of the DNA.

When DNA damage occurs, a complex cellular response is activated. This DNA damage response (DDR) involves the detection of the damaged site, the amplification of the signal through a cascade of protein kinases and the activation of a series of downstream effectors that promote cell cycle arrest, DNA repair or activation of apoptotic

A. Nagelkerke
Department of Molecular Materials, Institute for Molecules and Materials, Radboud University, Nijmegen, The Netherlands
e-mail: A.Nagelkerke@science.ru.nl

P.N. Span (✉)
Department of Radiation Oncology, RadboudUMC, Nijmegen, The Netherlands
e-mail: Paul.Span@Radboudumc.nl

C. Koumenis et al. (eds.), *Tumor Microenvironment*, Advances in Experimental Medicine and Biology 899, DOI 10.1007/978-3-319-26666-4_1

pathways [1]. An early event in the DDR is the phosphorylation of the histone H2AX at serine 139. This so-called γ-H2AX modification is dependent on the action of members from the phosphatidylinositol 3-kinase (PI3K)-like family of kinases, which includes ataxia telangiectasia-mutated (ATM), AT-related (ATR) and DNA-dependent protein kinase (DNA-PK) [2]. Depending on the type of lesions induced, different DNA repair mechanisms are activated. In eukaryotic cells, damaged bases and nucleotides are repaired by base excision repair (BER) and nucleotide excision repair (NER) pathways, respectively, while DSBs are repaired by two major mechanisms: homologous recombination (HR) and non-homologous end joining (NHEJ) [1].

Phospho-H2AX is a very robust marker of DNA double-stranded breaks, which can be stained for. This will visualise phospho-H2AX foci—bright dots—in the nucleus. These foci can be quantified by counting the number of positive cells or by counting the number of foci per nucleus. We have used this staining in the past to follow DNA damage repair kinetics, using phospho-H2AX as a marker [3]. We cultured cancer cells on coverslips, irradiated them with 2 Gy and fixed the cells after 0, 1, 3, 24 and 48 h. We stained for phospho-H2AX and analysed the number of positive cells. This allows quantification of the repair of DNA double-stranded breaks over time. As we were setting up this staining, we observed that cancer cells could exhibit unusual behaviour when it comes to the presence of phospho-H2AX in their nuclei. We noticed that even without being irradiated, cancer cells could display phospho-H2AX foci, a feature that is absent in normal, healthy cells [4, 5]. This positivity has been related to genomic instability and potentially to telomere erosion and dysfunction [6]. We therefore believe that this protocol is not only useful to monitor repair of DNA double-stranded breaks after DNA damage in a number of cell types (not limited to cancer cells), but can also provide a tool to study genomic instability. Combining staining against H2AX with stainings against microenvironmental parameters can provide spatial information on where DNA damage or genomic instability is most prevalent within the tumour microenvironment, for example relative to regions of hypoxia, blood vessels, necrotic tissue, etc.

This protocol contains details for fixed cells, cryo- and formalin-fixed paraffin-embedded (FFPE) sections. We also give an example on how a staining for multiple markers in combination with H2AX can be performed on cryosections, enabling analysis of phospho-H2AX expression in connection with the tumour microenvironment (hypoxic regions and proximity to blood vessels). Examples of the end results of our stainings are provided in Figs. 1.1 and 1.2.

1.2 Protocol

1.2.1 Materials Needed

1.2.1.1 General

- Staining dish and rack, and staining tray (see Fig. 1.3a, b)
- Tris-buffered saline (TBS, 10 mM Tris base, 150 mM NaCl, pH 7.4)

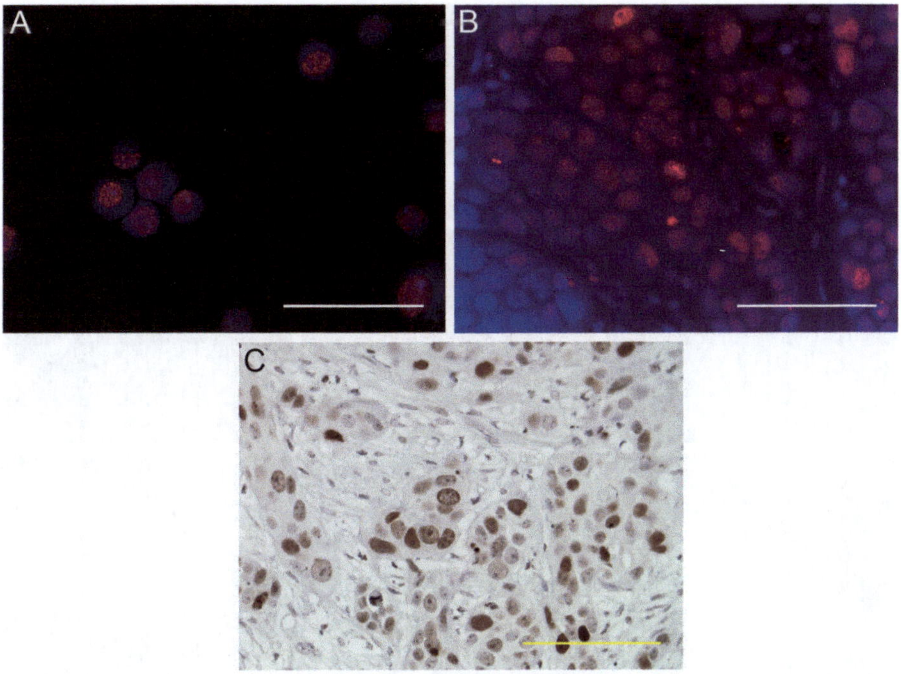

Fig. 1.1 Examples of phospho-H2AX stainings on fixed cells (**a**), frozen sections (**b**) and FFPE sections (**c**). The MDA-MB-231 breast cancer cells in (**a**) were irradiated with 2 Gy and fixed after 1 h. The SSCNij3 head and neck squamous cell carcinoma xenografts of (**b**) and (**c**) were irradiated with 10 Gy and harvested after 24 h. Scale bars equal 100 μm

- Bovine serum albumin (BSA, A7906, Sigma Aldrich, St. Louis, MO, USA)
- Triton X-100 (T8787, Sigma Aldrich, St. Louis, MO, USA)
- Rabbit-anti-phospho-H2AX (#2577, Cell Signaling Technology, Danvers, MA, USA)
- Super PAP-pen (00-8899, Life Technologies, Carlsbad, CA, USA)

1.2.1.2 For Fixed Cells and Cryosections

- Cy3-conjugated AffiniPure Fab fragment donkey-anti-rabbit (711-167-003, Jackson ImmunoResearch, West Grove, PA, USA) or equivalent
- Hoechst 33345 (B2261, Sigma Aldrich, St. Louis, MO, USA)
- Fluoromount W (21634.01, Serva, Heidelberg, Germany)

Optional:

- 9 F1 (undiluted supernatant from 9 F1 cells, which produce a monoclonal antibody to mouse endothelium)

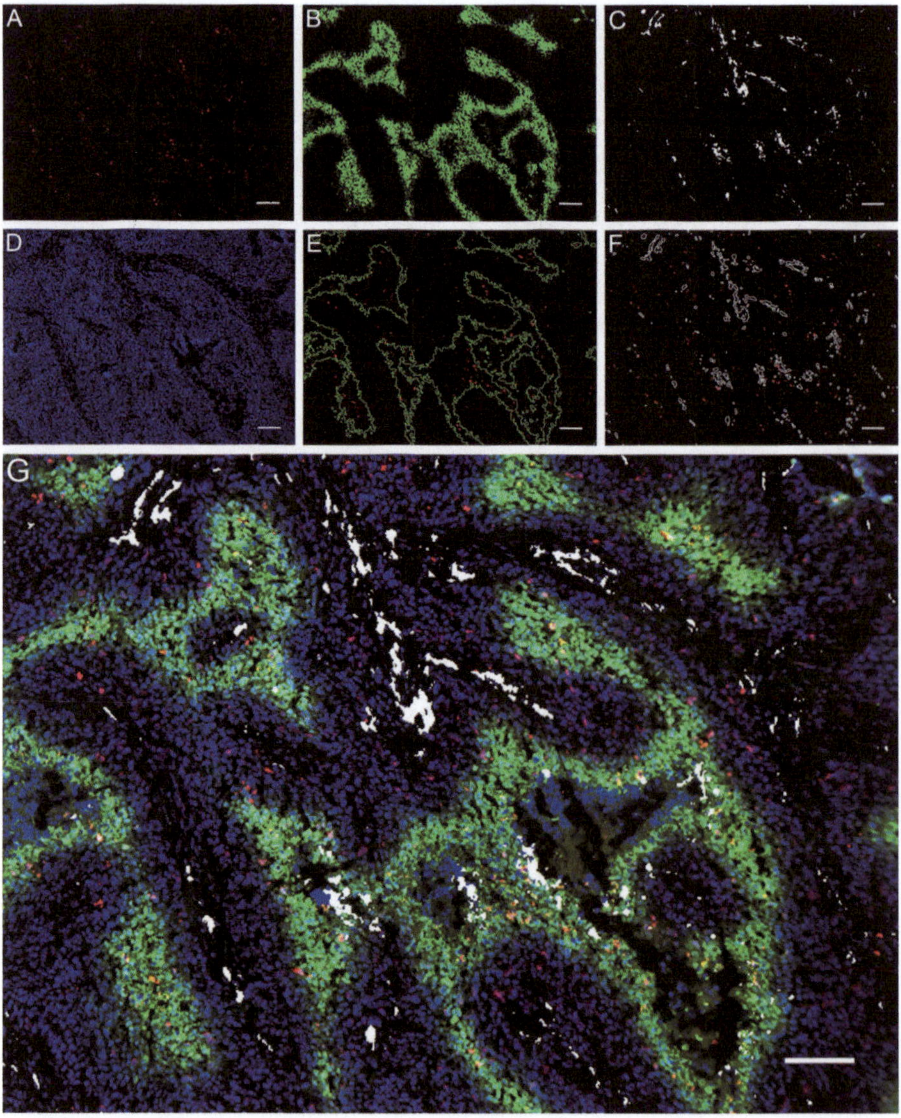

Fig. 1.2 Example of a phospho-H2AX staining (**a**) on a cryosection of a C38 colon carcinoma xenograft with endogenous expression of phospho-H2AX. Phospho-H2AX was combined with a staining against hypoxia with pimonidazole (**b**), blood vessels (**c**) and nuclei (**d**). (**e**) and (**f**) represent how phospho-H2AX is localised with respect to hypoxia and vasculature. A composite image is shown in (**g**). Scale bars equal 100 μm

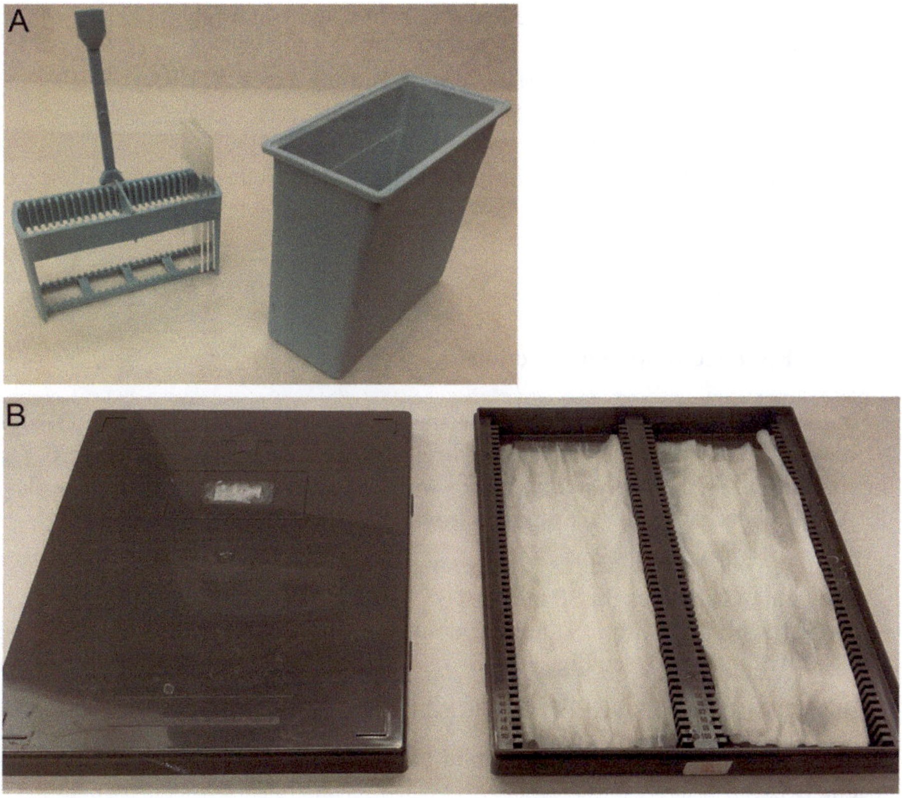

Fig. 1.3 Example of a staining dish and rack (**a**). All rinse steps are performed in these dishes. Example of a staining tray (**b**). All incubation steps are performed in this tray. Wet tissues are added to bottom of the tray to prevent evaporation

- Rabbit-anti-pimonidazole (a kind gift from J.A. Raleigh, also commercially available from Hypoxyprobe, Inc., Burlington, MA, USA)
- Alexa 647-conjugated chicken-anti-rat (A21472, Life Technologies)
- Alexa 488-conjugated donkey-anti-rabbit (A21206, Life Technologies)

1.2.1.3 For FFPE Sections

- Histosafe (Adamas Instruments BV, Leersum, The Netherlands)
- 70 %, 90 %, 96 %, 100 % EtOH
- Target retrieval solution pH 6.0 (S2369, DAKO, Copenhagen, Denmark)
- H_2O_2 (30 %, 76051800, Boom, Meppel, The Netherlands)
- Methanol
- Normal donkey serum (017-000-001, Jackson ImmunoResearch)

- Biotin SP-conjugated Affinipure Fab fragment donkey-anti-rabbit (711-067-003, Jackson ImmunoResearch)
- Vectastain ABC kit elite (PK-6100, Vector, Burlingame, CA, USA)
- DAB, peroxidase substrate kit (SK-4100, Vector)
- Hematoxylin (S3301, DAKO)
- Mounting medium (KP7275, Klinipath, Duiven, The Netherlands)

1.2.2 Procedure

1.2.2.1 Fixed Cells and Cryosections

To stain for phospho-H2AX in cells, we fix them in ice-cold (−20 °C) MetOH for 10 min at 4 °C. Cryosections can be fixed in cold (4 °C) acetone for 10 min at 4 °C. Do not fix cells cultured on polystyrene dishes with acetone, as acetone will destroy plastic. Allow the fixing agents to evaporate from your slides before continuing.

- Encircle your sections with a PAP-pen (see Fig. 1.4a).
- Rehydrate your slides for 30 min in TBS.
- Block for 30 min with 5 % normal donkey serum in TBS with 1 % BSA and 0.2 % Triton X-100 (see Fig. 1.4b).

  DO NOT RINSE; PROCEED TO PRIMARY ANTIBODY

- Incubate overnight at 4 °C with rabbit-anti-phospho-H2AX 1:500 in TBS with 1 % BSA.
- The following day, rinse your slides three times in TBS, and leave the last rinse for 30 min.
- Incubate for 1 h at room temperature with secondary antibody: Cy3-conjugated donkey-anti-rabbit 1:600 in TBS.
- Rinse your slides three times in TBS, and leave the last rinse for 30 min.
- Stain nuclei with Hoechst (1 mg/ml stock) 1:3000 in TBS for 5 min at room temperature.
- Mount slides with Fluoromount W.
- Let your slides dry at room temperature in the dark.
- You can check your slides under the microscope the next day.

1.2.2.2 Alternative Procedure to Analyse Multiple Markers on Cryosections

In this section we provide a protocol to stain against phospho-H2AX, whilst at the same time analysing hypoxia, through a staining against pimonidazole [7], vessels and all nuclei.

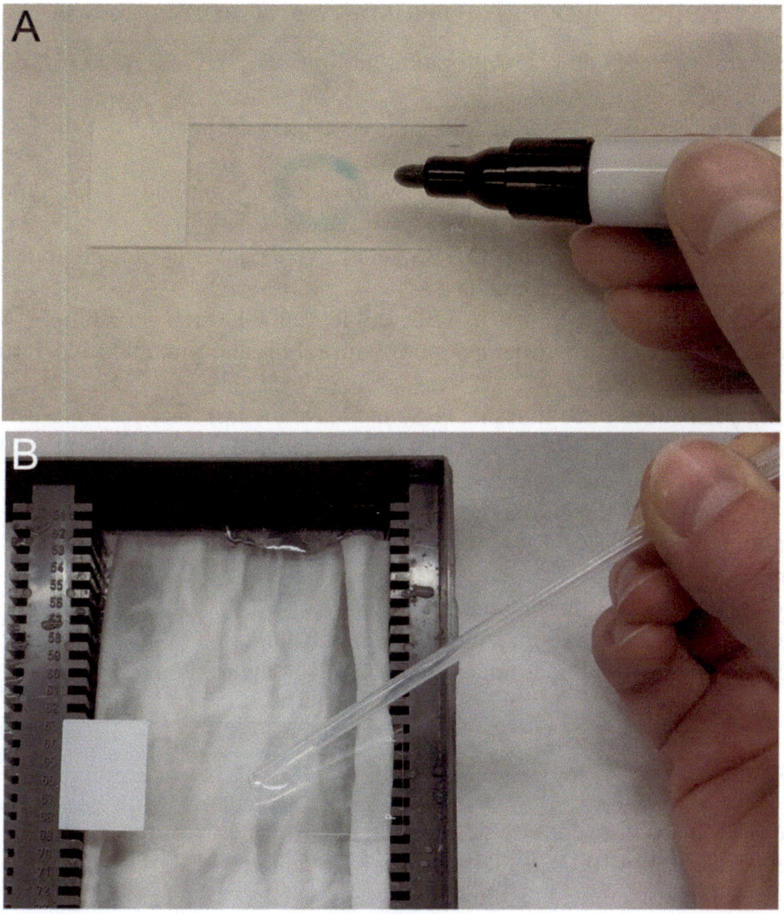

Fig. 1.4 Sections are encircled using a Super PAP-pen (**a**). This creates a hydrophobic ring, allowing liquid to be added to the sections. Super PAP-pen is suited for both immunofluorescence stainings and light microscopy stainings. Example of how sections are incubated with antibodies (**b**). The Super PAP-pen-encircled slides are placed in the staining tray. Liquid is added to the sections with a small Pasteur's pipette. The tray is closed and incubated at the indicated temperature for the indicated time

- Fix sections in cold (4 °C) acetone for 10 min at 4 °C.
- Allow to evaporate from slides before continuing.
- Encircle your sections with a PAP-pen.
- Rehydrate your slides for 30 min in TBS.
- Block for 30 min with 5 % normal donkey serum in TBS with 1 % BSA and 0.2 % Triton X-100.

DO NOT RINSE; PROCEED TO PRIMARY ANTIBODY

- Incubate overnight at 4 °C with rabbit-anti-phospho-H2AX 1:500 in TBS with 1 % BSA.
- The following day, rinse your slides three times in TBS, and leave the last rinse for 30 min.
- Incubate for 1 h at room temperature with secondary antibody: Cy3-conjugated donkey-anti-rabbit 1:600 in TBS.
- Rinse your slides three times in TBS, and leave the last rinse for 30 min.
- Incubate with 9 F1 for 45 min at 37 °C.
- Rinse your slides three times in TBS, and leave the last rinse for 30 min.
- Incubate for 1 h at room temperature with rabbit-anti-pimonidazole 1:1000 in TBS with 1 % BSA.
- Rinse your slides three times in TBS, and leave the last rinse for 30 min.
- Incubate for 1 h at 37 °C with Alexa 647-conjugated chicken-anti-rat 1:100 and Alexa 488-conjugated donkey-anti-rabbit 1:600 in TBS.
- Rinse your slides three times in TBS, and leave the last rinse for 30 min.
- Stain nuclei with Hoechst (1 mg/ml stock) 1:3000 in TBS for 5 min at room temperature.
- Mount slides with Fluoromount W.
- Let your slides dry at room temperature in the dark.
- You can check your slides under the microscope the next day.

1.2.2.3 FFPE Sections

- Deparaffinise your slides by submerging in Histosafe twice for 30 min.
- Rehydrate: 3 min 100 % EtOH (two times), 3 min 96 % EtOH (two times), 3 min 70 % EtOH (two times), 5 min dH_2O.
- Antigen retrieval: Boil slides for 30 min in target retrieval solution (pH 6.0, 10 mM).
- Allow the sections to cool down in this solution for 1 h.
- Rinse in TBS for 30 min (rinsing longer is not a problem).
- Block endogenous peroxidase: Submerge slides in 3 % H_2O_2 in MetOH for 10 min.
- Rinse in TBS for 10 min.
- Encircle your sections with a PAP-pen.
- Block for 30 min with 5 % normal donkey serum in TBS with 1 % BSA and 0.2 % Triton X-100.

DO NOT RINSE; PROCEED TO PRIMARY ANTIBODY

- Incubate overnight at 4 °C with rabbit-anti-phospho-H2AX 1:500 in TBS with 1 % BSA.
- The following day, rinse your slides three times in TBS, and leave the last rinse for 30 min.

- Incubate for 1 h at room temperature with secondary antibody: biotin-conjugated donkey-anti-rabbit 1:400 in TBS.
- Rinse your slides three times in TBS, and leave the last rinse for 30 min.
- Incubate for 30 min at room temperature with ABC-reagent in TBS.
- Rinse your slides three times in TBS, and leave the last rinse for 15 min.
- Rinse your slides three times in dH_2O, and leave the last rinse for 15 min.
- Incubate for approximately 15 min at room temperature with DAB* (Vector).
- Rinse your slides thoroughly with tap water; this will stop the DAB incubation.
- Counterstain the nuclei: incubate for 5 min in hematoxylin (DAKO).
- Rinse for approximately 10 min with running tap water.*
- Dehydrate sections: Dip in 70 % EtOH, dip in 90 % EtOH, dip in 96 % EtOH, dip in Histosafe, and keep in Histosafe for at least 30 min (leaving them longer is not a problem).
- Mount slides with KP mounting medium and let them dry at room temperature.
- You can check your slides under the microscope the next day.

*This incubation time is an approximation. Depending on the sections you are staining, the incubation time may differ. Check the developing staining intensity during your incubation (an inverted light microscope comes in handy) and stop when ready.

1.3 Troubleshooting

- High background staining, or even cytoplasmic staining for phospho-H2AX, which should be nuclear.

  Always include controls for all immunostainings you perform. Include a negative control, a section that you do *not* incubate with primary antibody. Instead, you incubate with TBS with 1 % BSA alone. The remainder of the staining is performed as described. This will allow you to determine the aspecific interactions your secondary antibody has with your material. You can also include a positive control, a section for which you are certain that phospho-H2AX is present. A section irradiated with a low dose is ideal for this purpose. If you believe that your staining on new material has failed for whatever reason, your positive control will indicate whether your staining was positive. In this protocol, we use TBS instead of phosphate-buffered saline (PBS) as we have found that rinsing with TBS instead of PBS gives better results, with less aspecific staining.
- Phospho-H2AX is especially suited for staining after low dosage of radiation. High dosage (>10 Gy) may lead to too much foci within one cell that cannot be distinguished: the entire cell will be stained.
- We choose to stain FFPE sections with DAB, not fluorescence. Fluorescence can be used on FFPE, but due to formalin fixing, FFPE sections may contain a lot of endogenous (auto)fluorescence, resulting in high background signals.

- Quantification in terms of the number of foci per nucleus may prove difficult, as the resolution of standard fluorescence microscopes is often too low. However, quantifying the number of positive cells, with positive being at least four foci per nucleus, will also provide useful data.

1.4 Conclusion

This protocol will enable you to perform phospho-H2AX staining on cells or tissues, to quantify DNA double-stranded breaks, their repair or genomic instability. Alternative protocols have been published. For example, Muslimovic et al. [8] reported on a flow cytometry-based method for use in non-fixed cells. Although this method might be faster, more quantitative and sensitive, it cannot be used in fixed or frozen cancer tissues. Western blotting usually requires a lot of tissue, which may not always be available. Also the latter techniques will not yield information on the location of damage within the tumour, which is important when investigating the tumour microenvironment.

References

1. Méndez-Acuña L, Di Tomaso MV, Palitti F, Martínez-López W. Histone post-translational modifications in DNA damage response. Cytogenet Genome Res. 2010;128:28–36.
2. van Attikum H, Gasser SM. The histone code at DNA breaks: a guide to repair? Nat Rev Mol Cell Biol. 2005;6:757–65.
3. Nagelkerke A, Bussink J, van der Kogel AJ, Sweep FC, Span PN. The PERK/ATF4/LAMP3-arm of the unfolded protein response affects radioresistance by interfering with the DNA damage response. Radiother Oncol. 2013;108:415–21.
4. Nagelkerke A, van Kuijk SJ, Sweep FC, Nagtegaal ID, Hoogerbrugge N, Martens JW, Timmermans MA, van Laarhoven HW, Bussink J, Span PN. Constitutive expression of γ-H2AX has prognostic relevance in triple negative breast cancer. Radiother Oncol. 2011; 101:39–45.
5. Sedelnikova OA, Bonner WM. GammaH2AX in cancer cells: a potential biomarker for cancer diagnostics, prediction and recurrence. Cell Cycle. 2006;5:2909–13.
6. Nagelkerke A, van Kuijk SJ, Martens JW, Sweep FC, Hoogerbrugge N, Bussink J, Span PN. Poor prognosis of constitutive ©-H2AX expressing triple negative breast cancers is associated with telomere length. Biomark Med. 2015;9(4):383–90.
7. Arteel GE, Thurman RG, Yates JM, Raleigh JA. Evidence that hypoxia markers detect oxygen gradients in liver: pimonidazole and retrograde perfusion of rat liver. Br J Cancer. 1995;72:889–95.
8. Muslimovic A, Ismail IH, Gao Y, Hammarsten O. An optimized method for measurement of gamma-H2AX in blood mononuclear and cultured cells. Nat Protoc. 2008;3:1187–93.

Chapter 2
Measuring DNA Replication in Hypoxic Conditions

Iosifina P. Foskolou, Deborah Biasoli, Monica M. Olcina, and Ester M. Hammond

Abstract It is imperative that dividing cells maintain replication fork integrity in order to prevent DNA damage and cell death. The investigation of DNA replication is of high importance as alterations in this process can lead to genomic instability, a known causative factor of tumor development. A simple, sensitive, and informative technique which enables the study of DNA replication, is the DNA fiber assay, an adaptation of which is described in this chapter. The DNA fiber method is a powerful tool, which allows the quantitative and qualitative analysis of DNA replication at the single molecule level. The sequential pulse labeling of live cells with two thymidine analogues and the subsequent detection with specific antibodies and fluorescence imaging allows direct examination of sites of DNA synthesis. In this chapter, we describe how this assay can be performed in conditions of low oxygen levels (hypoxia)—a physiologically relevant stress that occurs in most solid tumors. Moreover, we suggest ways on how to overcome the technical problems that arise while using the hypoxic chambers.

Keywords Hypoxia • DNA replication • DNA fiber assay

2.1 Introduction

DNA replication is one of the most important and well-regulated biological processes and enables the equal distribution of genetic information during cellular division. Eukaryotic cells start DNA replication in numerous regions (replication origins)

The authors disclose no potential conflicts of interest.

I.P. Foskolou • D. Biasoli • M.M. Olcina • E.M. Hammond (✉)
Cancer Research UK and Medical Research Council Oxford Institute for Radiation Oncology, Department of Oncology, University of Oxford, Old Road Campus Research Building, Oxford OX3 7DQ, UK
e-mail: iosifina.foskolou@oncology.ox.ac.uk; deborah.biasoli@oncology.ox.ac.uk; molcina@stanford.edu; ester.hammond@oncology.ox.ac.uk

C. Koumenis et al. (eds.), *Tumor Microenvironment*, Advances in Experimental Medicine and Biology 899, DOI 10.1007/978-3-319-26666-4_2

which are distributed along the chromosomes [1]. During the S-phase of the cell cycle, replication initiation proteins prepare the chromatin for the upcoming DNA replication and license the controlled firing of each replication origin [2]. Interestingly, not all replication origins fire during S-phase but instead most of them remain "silenced" during this process (dormant origins) and are usually activated when the major ones do not, for example, due to the presence of replication stress [3–8]. DNA replication is tightly monitored and cells need to ensure that the genome is duplicated efficiently and accurately in order to preserve genome stability [1, 9]. This fine control of DNA replication is of high importance since any defect in this biological process can result in DNA strand breaks and genomic instability, two well-known causative factors during tumor development [10].

Regions of low oxygen (hypoxia) occur in most solid tumors as a result of a high metabolic demand and an abnormally formed/inefficient tumor vasculature. The occurrence of hypoxic regions is an indicator of poor patient prognosis due to resistance to chemo- and radiotherapy as well as increased genomic instability, invasion, and metastatic potential [11–14]. Under severely hypoxic conditions (radiobiologic hypoxia) replication stress occurs, which is characterized by slow replication rates and the accumulation of stalled replication forks [15–18]. Moreover, hypoxia triggers the activation of DNA damage response (DDR) pathway including the ATR/ATM signaling without detectable DNA damage [19, 20]. Replication stress and the subsequent activation of the DDR pathway have been linked to the early stages of cancer development and have been proposed to act as a barrier to tumorigenesis [21, 22]. Hypoxia contributes to this pathway as hypoxic regions can be formed in preneoplastic lesions [21–23]. In order to study replication stress, accumulation of RPA foci and BrdU immunofluorescence can be used for the detection of single stranded DNA as well as the phosphorylation of common markers that are activated by the ATR pathway including γH2AX, Chk1 (Ser 345), and RPA (Ser 33) [24, 25]. Although these techniques are commonly used, they are limited and provide only indications of DNA replication stress. The most specific replication stress assay available to date is the direct measurement of DNA synthesis using the DNA fiber assay [26]. Here, we describe the adaptation of this sensitive microscopy-based method, to visualize DNA replication both in conditions of normal oxygen levels and in hypoxia.

The DNA fiber assay enables the study of DNA replication at a single molecule level [27–29]. In this technique, two different thymidine analogues are used sequentially in live cells and are incorporated into the nascent DNA. Subsequent staining of those analogues allows the visualization of the replication structures through the use of specific antibodies and fluorescence imaging (Fig. 2.1). A quantitative analysis can then be carried out by measuring the rate of movement of active replication forks as well as a qualitative analysis by classifying the status of the replication structures (stalled, ongoing, or new origins). The sensitivity and the wide range of information that can be extracted from this technique combined with its low cost makes it a powerful tool for the investigation of DNA replication in physiologically relevant conditions.

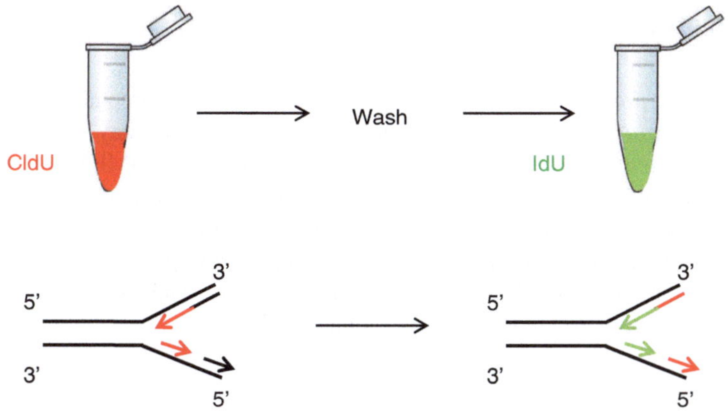

Fig. 2.1 Subsequent labeling of thymidine analogues (CldU and IdU) into the nascent DNA of live cells allows the visualization of the replication structures through the use of specific antibodies and fluorescence imaging

2.2 Solutions and Reagents

- Spreading Buffer (200 mM Tris–HCl, pH 7.4; 50 mM EDTA; 0.5 % SDS), once made stable for up to 6 months at room temperature.
- Fixation Buffer (Methanol/Acetic Acid 3:1), once made generally stable, keep at room temperature.
- Blocking Buffer (1 % BSA (Bovine Serum Albumin); 0.1 % Tween-20 diluted in 1× PBS), make fresh each time and keep at 4 °C.
- CldU (5-chloro-2′-deoxyuridine): Sigma-Aldrich UK (C6891-100MG). Stock solution 2.5 mM CldU diluted in culture media, once made stored at −20 °C for up to 2 months.
- IdU (5-iodo-2′ –deoxyuridine): Sigma-Aldrich UK (I7125-5G). Stock solution 2.5 mM IdU diluted in culture media, once made stored at −20 °C for up to 2 months.
- Rat anti-BrdU: Oxford Biotechnology (OBT0030). Dilute 1:500 in blocking buffer and keep on ice. Make fresh each time.
- Mouse anti-BrdU: Becton Dickinson Biosciences (347580; 7580). Dilute 1:500 in blocking buffer and keep on ice. Make fresh each time.
- Alexa Fluor 555-conjugated goat anti-rat IgG: Invitrogen (A21434). Dilute 1:500 in blocking buffer and keep on ice in the dark. Make fresh each time.
- Alexa Fluor 488-conjugated goat anti-mouse F(ab′)2 fragment: Invitrogen (A11017). Dilute 1:500 in blocking buffer and keep on ice in the dark. Make fresh each time.

Coverslip—Cover Glasses: Menzel Gläser 22 × 50 mm, Fisher Scientific UK Ltd (MNJ-350-070P)

Slides—Adhesion slides: SuperFrost® Plus 76 × 26 mm, Thermo Scientific (631-0447)

2.3 Protocol

The following protocol is optimized for the RKO human colorectal cancer cell line (available from ATCC). Cell density and time of incubation may vary in different cell lines and may need to be adjusted. Cells are cultured in DMEM culture media supplemented with 10 % FBS, in a standard humidified incubator at 37 °C and 5 % CO_2. For hypoxia treatment, a Bactron II anaerobic chamber (Shell Labs) was used. No oxygen is supplied to this chamber; however, a complete absence of oxygen cannot be guaranteed at all times due to potential leaks. The oxygen concentration at any time is estimated to be no higher than 0.1 %.

2.3.1 Day 1

2.3.1.1 Seeding

- Seed in each 5 cm^3 glass dish the number of cells needed to reach 50–60 % confluency on the following day. For RKO cells, 7×10^5 cells per glass dish are seeded. One dish per experimental condition is required
- Place the spreading buffer at 37 °C overnight
- Prepare CIdU (2.5 mM) and IdU (2.5 mM) stock solutions in the appropriate amount of culture media and store at −20 °C until use

Note: For experiments to be carried out in the anaerobic chamber, cells are plated on glass dishes to minimize the amount of potential oxygen being introduced into the chamber (since plastic absorbs and retains oxygen).

2.3.2 Day 2

2.3.2.1 Labeling

- Place CldU stock solution at 37 °C and IdU stock solution at 50 °C to thaw
- Prepare fresh working solutions (25 μM CldU and 250 μM IdU) by diluting the stock solutions in the appropriate amount of culture media. The CldU stock solution is diluted 1:100 to prepare the working solution, whereas the IdU stock solution is diluted 1:10

2.3.2.2 Normoxic Samples

- Aspirate media from cells
- Add 5 ml of the working solution containing CldU (25 μM) and incubate for 20 min at 21 % O_2 in a 37 °C incubator

- Wash once with media that does not contain any thymidine analogues
- Add 5 ml of the working solution containing IdU (250 μM) and incubate for 20 min at 21 % O_2 in a 37 °C incubator
- Wash once with 1× PBS and trypsinize cells
- Collect cells with 1 ml 1× PBS by pipetting (do not scrape—cells should remain intact)
- Centrifuge to spin cells down (950 × *g* for 6 min)
- Dilute cells to a concentration of 5×10^5 cells per ml and place them on ice
- Proceed straight to the spreading step

2.3.2.3 Hypoxic Samples

- Place the hypoxic samples in the chamber at the required oxygen tension
- *Note*: When labeling the hypoxic samples put the following in the pass box of the hypoxic chamber and let equilibrate for sufficient oxygen removal (at least 3 h)

  1. CldU and IdU working solutions
  2. Media that does not contain any thymidine analogues
  3. Spreading buffer
  4. Trypsin
  5. 1× PBS
  6. Tips for P-20 pipet
  7. 5 and 10 ml pipets
  8. Appropriate number of slides (at least three per condition)
  9. Apparatus that has the appropriate height (2 cm) to tilt the slides (a small carton/box is recommended)

- 3 h After passing the cells into the chamber replace the media with 5 ml of the working solution containing CldU (25 μM) and incubate for 2 h
- Wash once with media that does not contain any thymidine analogues
- Add 5 ml of the working solution containing IdU (250 μM) and incubate for 1 h
- Wash once with 1× PBS and trypsinize cells
- Collect cells with 1 ml 1× PBS by pipetting (do not scrape)
- Centrifuge to spin cells down (950 × *g* for 6 min)
- Dilute cells in half of the volume of 1× PBS used for normoxic samples
- Proceed straight to the spreading step

Note: The aforementioned labeling time for each thymidine analogue was optimized for our conditions. However, these times may need adjusting depending on the experimental procedure and the question to be addressed. The labeling time of each analogue is crucial and is taken into account under the analysis of the data so it is important to adjust appropriately, especially if different O_2 tensions are being used and/or drug treatments. For example, in the protocol described here, we have used shorter pulse labeling with the thymidine analogues in cells under normoxic conditions (20 min each) compared to the cells that are under hypoxic conditions

(2 h for CldU and 1 h IdU). This adjustment accounts for the fact that replication rates are much faster in the presence of O_2 due to the occurrence of replication stress under severely hypoxic conditions.

2.3.2.4 Spreading

- Spread each sample separately onto different slides (for each sample, use at least three slides and do not proceed with more than one sample at once since there will be insufficient time for the next steps)
- Pipet 2 μl of cell suspension at the top of each slide on each of the three slides (around 2000 cells) (Fig. 2.2)
- Wait 3–5 min for the drop of cell suspension to flatten (Fig. 2.3)
- Add 7 μl of spreading buffer and mix gently by stirring with a pipet tip (P-20)
- *Note*: While spreading use the P-20 pipet for pipetting both 2 μl of cells and 7 μl of spreading buffer and only the proposed slides. We have found that slides lacking a frosted section do not perform as well as those suggested here. While waiting for the drop to flatten, be careful not to let it dry. If the drop has flattened earlier than 3–5 min proceed straight to the next step.
- Incubate the slide at room temperature for 2 min
- Tilt the slides gently to an approximate angle of 30°–40° (Fig. 2.4)

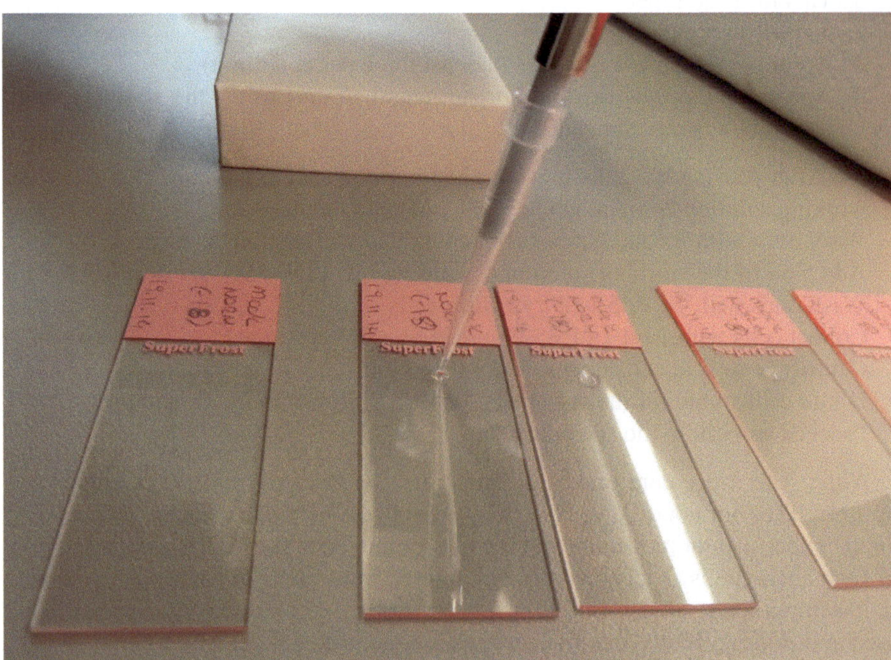

Fig. 2.2 Spreading procedure. Pipet 2 μl of the cell suspension at the top of each slide with a P-20 pipet

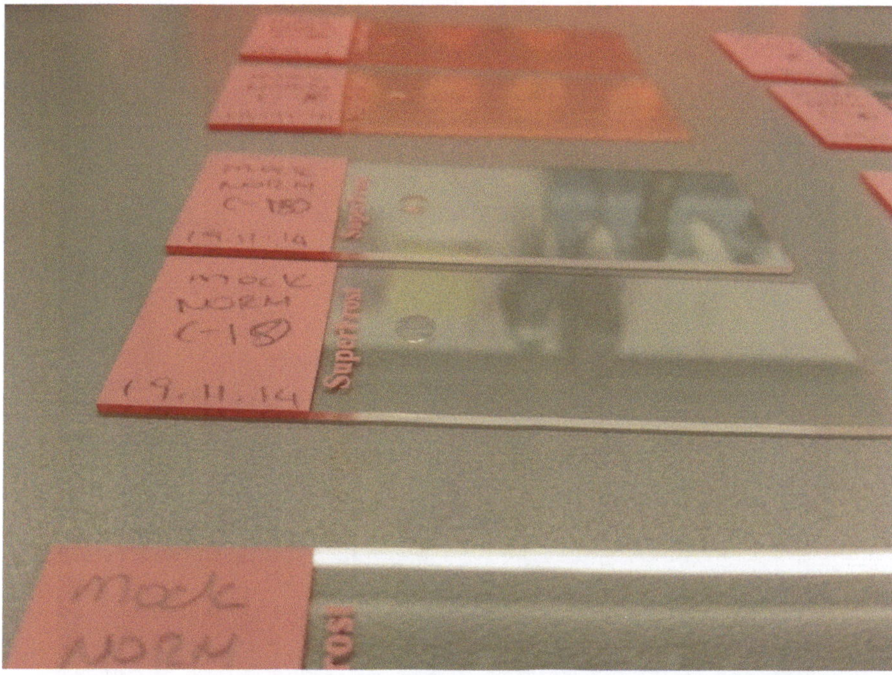

Fig. 2.3 Spreading procedure. Allow the drop of cell suspension for 3–5 min to flatten

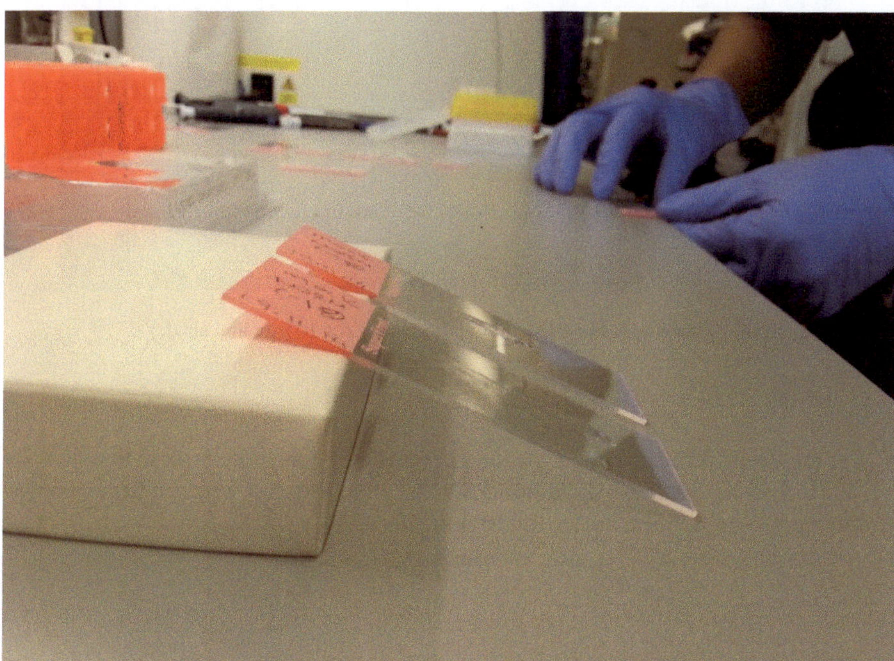

Fig. 2.4 Spreading procedure. Tilt the slides gently and let drops run down slowly to reach the bottom of the slide (approximately 20 s)

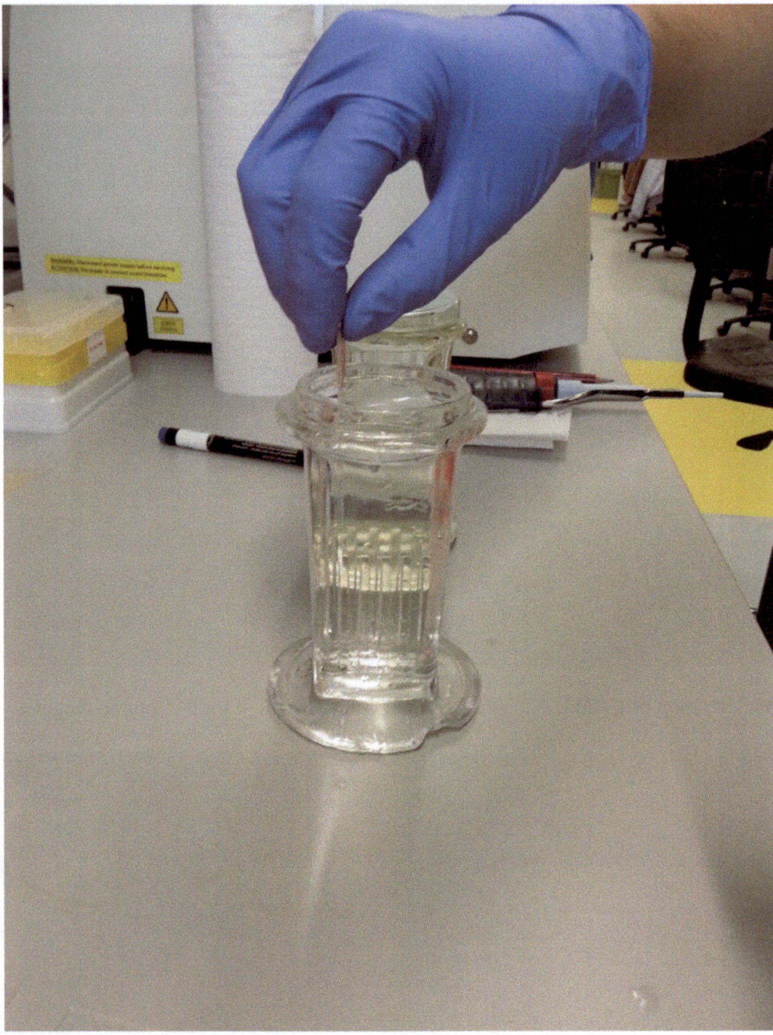

Fig. 2.5 Spreading procedure. Fix slides in fixation buffer for 10 min and air-dry

- Let the drops run down the slide slowly until they reach the bottom and air-dry
- While waiting for the drop to run down the slide proceed with the next sample
- Dip and fix in fixation buffer for 10 min (Fig. 2.5)
- Air-dry and store at 4 °C until staining

2.3.3 *Day 3*

2.3.3.1 Staining

- Wash the slides twice with deionized water for 5 min at RT
- Wash once with 2.5 M HCl for 5 min RT
- Discard the HCl
- Incubate with 2.5 M HCl for 80 min RT
- Discard the HCl and rinse twice with 1× PBS
- Wash twice with blocking buffer for 5 min each
- Discard the blocking buffer
- Incubate with blocking buffer for 1 h
- Add to each slide 150 μl of the primary antibodies diluted in blocking buffer (1:500 α-BrdU rat and 1:500 α-BrdU mouse) and cover with a coverslip
- Incubate at 37 °C for 1 h
- Wash three times with 1× PBS for 5 min each
- Incubate with 4 % PFA for 10 min (caution: do not incubate with PFA for more than 15 min)
- Wash three times with 1× PBS for 5 min each
- Incubate with blocking buffer for 1 min
- Discard the blocking buffer
- Incubate with blocking buffer for 5 min
- Discard the blocking buffer
- Incubate with blocking buffer for 25 min
- Discard the blocking buffer
- Add to each slide 150 μl of the secondary antibodies diluted in blocking buffer (1:500 α-rat 555 and 1:500 α-mouse 488) and cover with a coverslip
- Incubate at 37 °C for 1 h
- Rinse twice with 1× PBS
- Incubate with blocking buffer for 1 min
- Discard blocking buffer
- Incubate with blocking buffer for 5 min
- Discard blocking buffer
- Incubate with blocking buffer for 25 min
- Discard blocking buffer and rinse twice with 1× PBS
- Mount with mounting media (make sure the mounting media does not contain a nuclear dye such as DAPI, Hoechst, or Propidium Iodide) and cover with appropriate coverslip
- Store at 4 °C in the dark until imaging

2.3.4 Day 4

2.3.4.1 Imaging

Fibers are imaged using a LSM780 (Carl Zeiss Microscopy Ltd) confocal microscope and each image is converted in a TIF file for data analysis. While imaging try to focus on the green label, which is usually brighter when visualized with a ×60 lens. When the fibers are focused go to a field with single and well separated fibers and image with both labels. Avoid fields where you have too many fibers since this will complicate the subsequent quantification.

Note: Try to image the samples as soon as possible as fluorescence intensity decreases with time.

2.4 Analysis of the Data

Import the acquired images to a picture analysis program (e.g., ImageJ). For the qualitative analysis, count the percentage of fibers that have incorporated only the first label (stalled forks), both labels (ongoing forks) and only the second label (new origins) (Fig. 2.6). For the quantitative analysis, measure the length of the fiber tracts only of the ongoing forks and use the following formula to determine the replication rates ($V_{(\text{IdU kb/min})} = [(x \times 0.132\ \mu\text{m}) \times 2.59\ \text{kb}/\mu\text{m}]/t$ (min), where x = length of IdU in the program used). In general, the length of at least 100 fibers should be measured per condition and 100–200 replication structures should be counted. Each individual experiment should be repeated at least 3 times.

Note: For ImageJ software (NIH) the following settings are used

Qualitative analysis

1. Open TIF images with the ImageJ program
2. Go to Plugins from the toolbar and select Analyze
3. From Analyze select Cell Counter (Fig. 2.7)

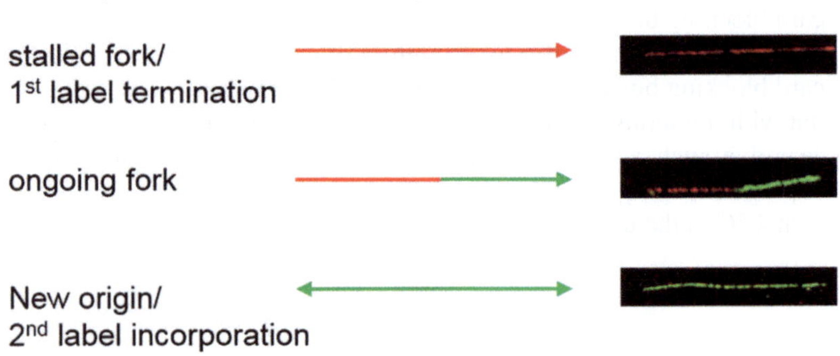

Fig. 2.6 Qualitative analysis of the data. Count the percentage of fibers that had incorporated only the first label (stalled forks), both labels (ongoing forks), or only the second label (new origins)

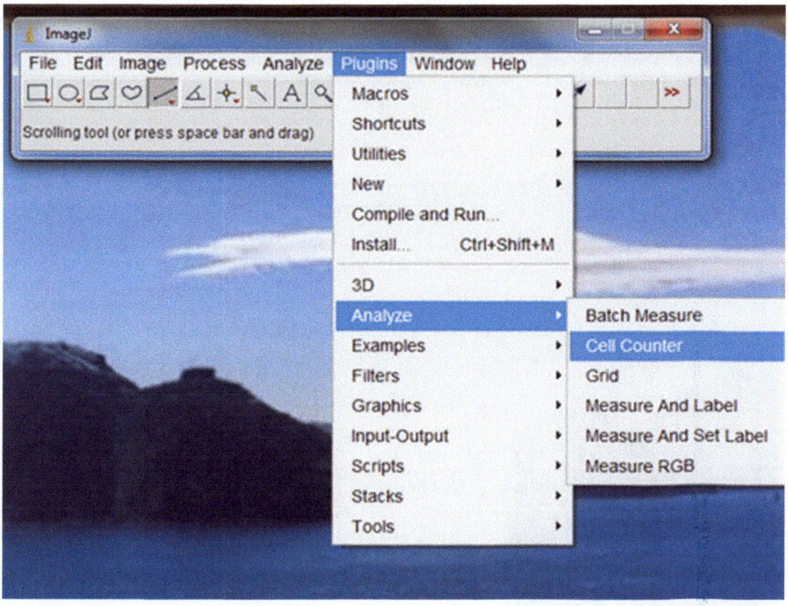

Fig. 2.7 Select the Cell Counter option from the ImageJ software (NIH) for the qualitative analysis of the data

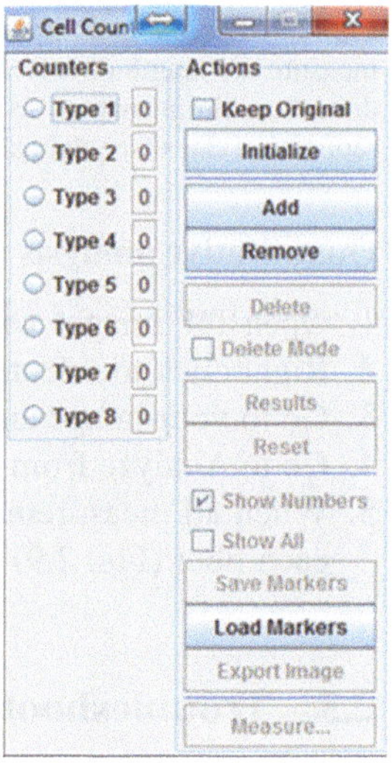

Fig. 2.8 Select from the Cell Counter window a different type to mark stalled forks, ongoing forks, or new origins and press Initialize to start counting

4. From Cell Counter use a different type (left column at the Cell Counter window) for stalled forks, ongoing forks, or new origins and press Initialize to start counting (Fig. 2.8)

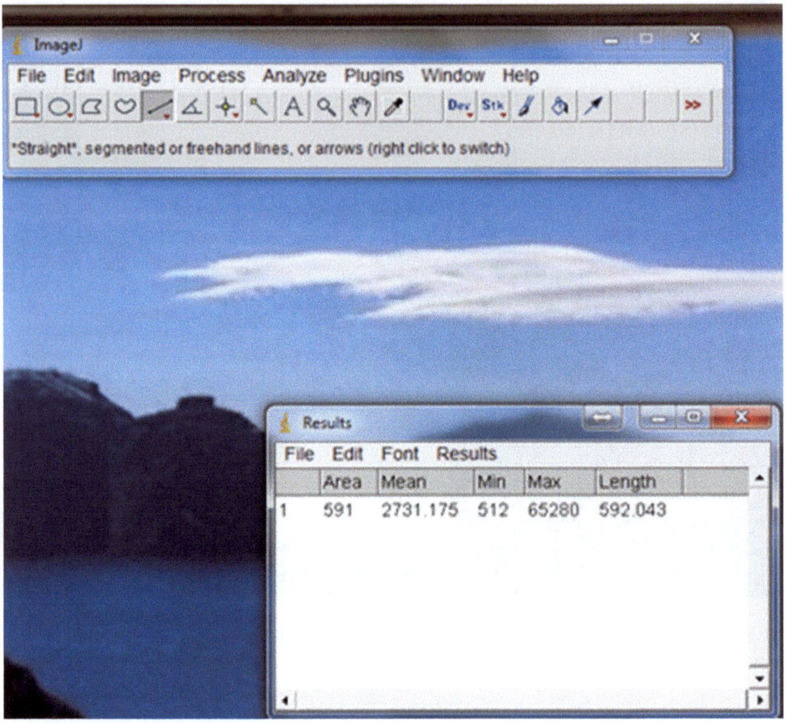

Fig. 2.9 For the quantitative analysis of the data, select the segmented line from the toolbar to measure the length of each fiber. When all measurements are completed use from the Results window the column named as Length (*right column*) to complete the formula that determines the replication rates (see data analysis)

Quantitative analysis

1. Open TIF images with the ImageJ program
2. Right click to select segmented line from toolbar
3. Go to your image and draw a line following each fiber
4. Go to Analyze from toolbar and select Measure
5. When all measurements are completed use from the Results table the length of each fiber (Fig. 2.9)

2.5 Troubleshooting

2.5.1 Unintentional Reoxygenation of Hypoxic Samples

Make sure that the media containing the thymidine analogues is well equilibrated before use in hypoxic chamber. Allow at least 2 h equilibration of the media in the pass box with the appropriate catalysts if required by the hypoxia chamber type.

2.5.2 Less DNA Fibers in Hypoxic Conditions

Usually it is difficult to count the amount of cells per sample in hypoxic conditions and this could result in less starting material in these conditions. Make sure that you spread two or three different concentrations per sample (usually 2× and/or 4× the amount you used for the normoxic samples).

2.6 Conclusion

The DNA fiber assay is a unique technique that allows most parameters that determine DNA synthesis during S-phase to be assessed individually, on the level of single replication forks as opposed to whole cell populations [30]. Previous genomic approaches that provide an overall replication profile of a cell population (such as FACS analysis with BrdU staining) are not sensitive enough for the investigation of DNA replication dynamics. In contrast, the DNA fiber technique presented here gives both quantitative and qualitative read-outs. Moreover, this technique enables the study of the changes to replication dynamics which may occur in response to different stresses and/or damaging agents. The investigation of the DNA replication process is indispensable not only for the further characterization of replication itself, but also to understand the alterations that occur in pathological conditions such as cancer. Hypoxic induction of DNA replication stress is characterized by an increased number of stalled replication forks and significantly reduced replication rates. The DNA fiber-labeling strategy is a great tool for the investigation of both the immediate and longer term changes to replication dynamics in these environments. A limitation of this technique though is the possibility of breakage of the DNA fibers while spreading them on a glass surface, which can lead to misinterpretation of the data. The need for controlling the orientation, density, and stretching of DNA fibers led to the development of the DNA combing technique, which has been successfully used to monitor DNA replication in a variety of organisms [26]. In this technique, DNA is stretched onto salinized slides with a constant stretching factor resulting in thousands of combed DNA molecules per slide, allowing detailed analysis of origin firing efficiency. The requirement for specific equipment (Combing System) for performing the aforementioned technique, however, limits its use in hypoxia due to technical problems (there is a possibility of reoxygenation of the samples if they have to be transferred outside of the chamber for the use of the equipment).

Acknowledgments We thank all members of the Hammond lab, past and present, for their assistance in the development of this protocol. DB and EMH are supported by Cancer Research UK (grant awarded to EMH). This work was supported by Cancer Research UK (CR-UK) grant number C38302/A12981, through a Cancer Research UK Oxford Centre Prize DPhil Studentship (awarded to IPF).

References

1. Branzei D, Foiani M. Maintaining genome stability at the replication fork. Nat Rev Mol Cell Biol. 2010;11:208–19.
2. Masai H, Matsumoto S, You Z, Yoshizawa-Sugata N, Oda M. Eukaryotic chromosome DNA replication: where, when, and how? Annu Rev Biochem. 2010;79:89–130.
3. Dershowitz A, Newlon CS. The effect on chromosome stability of deleting replication origins. Mol Cell Biol. 1993;13:391–8.
4. Ge XQ, Jackson DA, Blow JJ. Dormant origins licensed by excess Mcm2-7 are required for human cells to survive replicative stress. Genes Dev. 2007;21:3331–41.
5. Mcintosh D, Blow JJ. Dormant origins, the licensing checkpoint, and the response to replicative stresses. Cold Spring Harb Perspect Biol. 2012;4.
6. Schwob E. Flexibility and governance in eukaryotic DNA replication. Curr Opin Microbiol. 2004;7:680–90.
7. Woodward AM, Gohler T, Luciani MG, Oehlmann M, Ge X, Gartner A, Jackson DA, Blow JJ. Excess Mcm2-7 license dormant origins of replication that can be used under conditions of replicative stress. J Cell Biol. 2006;173:673–83.
8. Wyrick JJ, Aparicio JG, Chen T, Barnett JD, Jennings EG, Young RA, Bell SP, Aparicio OM. Genome-wide distribution of ORC and MCM proteins in S. cerevisiae: high-resolution mapping of replication origins. Science. 2001;294:2357–60.
9. Zeman MK, Cimprich KA. Causes and consequences of replication stress. Nat Cell Biol. 2014;16:2–9.
10. Halazonetis TD, Gorgoulis VG, Bartek J. An oncogene-induced DNA damage model for cancer development. Science. 2008;319:1352–5.
11. Brown JM, Giaccia AJ. The unique physiology of solid tumors: opportunities (and problems) for cancer therapy. Cancer Res. 1998;58:1408–16.
12. Erler JT, Bennewith KL, Nicolau M, Dornhofer N, Kong C, Le QT, Chi JT, Jeffrey SS, Giaccia AJ. Lysyl oxidase is essential for hypoxia-induced metastasis. Nature. 2006;440:1222–6.
13. Gray LH, Conger AD, Ebert M, Hornsey S, Scott OC. The concentration of oxygen dissolved in tissues at the time of irradiation as a factor in radiotherapy. Br J Radiol. 1953;26:638–48.
14. Hockel M, Vaupel P. Tumor hypoxia: definitions and current clinical, biologic, and molecular aspects. J Natl Cancer Inst. 2001;93:266–76.
15. Hammond EM, Dorie MJ, Giaccia AJ. Inhibition of ATR leads to increased sensitivity to hypoxia/reoxygenation. Cancer Res. 2004;64:6556–62.
16. Olcina MM, Foskolou IP, Anbalagan S, Senra JM, Pires IM, Jiang Y, Ryan AJ, Hammond EM. Replication stress and chromatin context link ATM activation to a role in DNA replication. Mol Cell. 2013;52:758–66.
17. Pires IM, Bencokova Z, Milani M, Folkes LK, Li JL, Stratford MR, Harris AL, Hammond EM. Effects of acute versus chronic hypoxia on DNA damage responses and genomic instability. Cancer Res. 2010;70:925–35.
18. Welford SM, Giaccia AJ. Hypoxia and senescence: the impact of oxygenation on tumor suppression. Mol Cancer Res. 2011;9:538–44.
19. Bencokova Z, Kaufmann MR, Pires IM, Lecane PS, Giaccia AJ, Hammond EM. ATM activation and signaling under hypoxic conditions. Mol Cell Biol. 2009;29:526–37.
20. Hammond EM, Denko NC, Dorie MJ, Abraham RT, Giaccia AJ. Hypoxia links ATR and p53 through replication arrest. Mol Cell Biol. 2002;22:1834–43.
21. Bartkova J, Horejsi Z, Koed K, Kramer A, Tort F, Zieger K, Guldberg P, Sehested M, Nesland JM, Lukas C, Orntoft T, Lukas J, Bartek J. DNA damage response as a candidate anti-cancer barrier in early human tumorigenesis. Nature. 2005;434:864–70.
22. Gorgoulis VG, Vassiliou LV, Karakaidos P, Zacharatos P, Kotsinas A, Liloglou T, Venere M, Ditullio Jr RA, Kastrinakis NG, Levy B, Kletsas D, Yoneta A, Herlyn M, Kittas C, Halazonetis TD. Activation of the DNA damage checkpoint and genomic instability in human precancerous lesions. Nature. 2005;434:907–13.

23. Hammond EM, Kaufmann MR, Giaccia AJ. Oxygen sensing and the DNA-damage response. Curr Opin Cell Biol. 2007;19:680–4.
24. Marechal A, Zou L. DNA damage sensing by the ATM and ATR kinases. Cold Spring Harb Perspect Biol. 2013;5.
25. Nam EA, Cortez D. ATR signalling: more than meeting at the fork. Biochem J. 2011;436:527–36.
26. Bianco JN, Poli J, Saksouk J, Bacal J, Silva MJ, Yoshida K, Lin YL, Tourriere H, Lengronne A, Pasero P. Analysis of DNA replication profiles in budding yeast and mammalian cells using DNA combing. Methods. 2012;57:149–57.
27. Jackson DA, Pombo A. Replicon clusters are stable units of chromosome structure: evidence that nuclear organization contributes to the efficient activation and propagation of S phase in human cells. J Cell Biol. 1998;140:1285–95.
28. Petes TD, Williamson DH. Fiber autoradiography of replicating yeast DNA. Exp Cell Res. 1975;95:103–10.
29. Takeuchi F, Hanaoka F, Goto M, Akaoka I, Hori T, Yamada M, Miyamoto T. Altered frequency of initiation sites of DNA replication in Werner's syndrome cells. Hum Genet. 1982;60:365–8.
30. Merrick CJ, Jackson D, Diffley JF. Visualization of altered replication dynamics after DNA damage in human cells. J Biol Chem. 2004;279:20067–75.

Chapter 3
Isolation of Proteins on Nascent DNA in Hypoxia and Reoxygenation Conditions

Monica M. Olcina, Amato J. Giaccia, and Ester M. Hammond

Abstract During S-phase both DNA replication and histone deposition must be co-ordinated at and around the replication fork. Replication stress can interfere with the fidelity of this process and can result in genomic instability. The study of proteins associated with DNA replication forks is important for a detailed understanding of DNA replication and chromatin assembly both under basal as well as replication stress conditions. iPOND (isolation of Proteins on Nascent DNA) allows the temporal study of proteins and protein modifications associated with replication forks in a variety of conditions, allowing the 'tracing' of protein association and histone deposition and maturation at active, stalled and damaged replication forks. Importantly, low oxygen (hypoxic) conditions, found in tumours, can result in replication stress. Here we describe the adaptation of the iPOND technique allowing the isolation of proteins and protein modifications specifically with replication forks undergoing hypoxia-induced replication stress. Furthermore, we describe the adaptation of this method for the study of factors associated with replication forks recovering from hypoxia-induced replication stress following periods of reoxygenation. These adaptations are important in order to study proteins associated with replication forks undergoing replication stress in physiologically relevant conditions.

Keywords DNA replication • Replication stress • iPOND • Hypoxia • Reoxygenation • Chromatin • Click chemistry • 5-Ethynyl-2′-deoxyuridine (EdU)

M.M. Olcina (✉)
CR-UK & MRC Oxford Institute for Radiation Oncology, Department of Oncology, University of Oxford, Oxford, UK

Department of Radiation Oncology, School of Medicine, Stanford University, Stanford, CA 94305, USA
e-mail: molcina@stanford.edu

A.J. Giaccia
Department of Radiation Oncology, School of Medicine, Stanford University, Stanford, CA 94305, USA

E.M. Hammond
CR-UK & MRC Oxford Institute for Radiation Oncology, Department of Oncology, University of Oxford, Oxford, UK

C. Koumenis et al. (eds.), *Tumor Microenvironment*, Advances in Experimental Medicine and Biology 899, DOI 10.1007/978-3-319-26666-4_3

3.1 Introduction

During DNA replication both DNA and the histones around which DNA is wrapped must be duplicated. To this end, the replisome is composed of factors typically associated with the replication machinery (such as helicases and DNA polymerases) as well as a variety of 'chromatin-associated factors'. The study of proteins associated with the replisome is important for a detailed understanding of a process so central to cell division [1].

Furthermore, replication is tightly controlled in order to prevent genomic instability. Fidelity of the process, however, can be compromised when replication occurs under conditions of stress, such as when nucleotide pools are depleted or when the replication machinery encounters an obstacle (such as the transcriptional machinery) [1]. Studying which proteins are associated with forks under conditions of replication stress is very relevant for the cancer field since cancer cells are frequently exposed to continuous replication stress. For instance, nucleotide depletion resulting from aberrant oncogene activation or low oxygen (hypoxic) conditions often encountered in tumours can result in replication stress [2–4]. Interestingly, the replication stress associated with severe hypoxia (<0.1 % O_2) has recently been found to be distinct from kinetically (and mechanistically) similar types of replication stress (such as replication stress induced by agents also leading to nucleotide pool depletion such as hydroxyurea) [2, 5, 6].

The iPOND technique (isolation of Proteins on Nascent DNA), originally described in 2011, has been central to the characterisation of the replisome and replisome-associated proteins, facilitating the detailed study of replication fork dynamics [7–9]. iPOND allows the spatial and temporal study of proteins and protein modifications associated with replication forks [7]. Importantly this technique enables such studies to be carried out in a variety of conditions, allowing the 'tracing' of protein association and histone deposition and maturation at active, stalled and damaged replication forks [10]. As a result of these advances, our understanding of the crosstalk between DNA replication, repair, histone deposition and epigenetic memory during DNA replication has been greatly enhanced [7–9].

In iPOND, nascent DNA is labelled with a nucleoside analogue of thymidine called 5-ethynyl-2′-deoxyuridine (EdU). EdU contains an alkyne group that can be covalently linked to biotin-azide by click chemistry (copper-catalysed cycloaddition). This allows single-step purification of the EdU-labelled DNA-protein complexes with streptavidin-coated beads. Following an elution step, proteins and their modifications can be analysed by immunoblotting or mass spectrometry [8].

Here we describe an adaptation of the iPOND technique that allows the isolation of proteins and protein modifications specifically with replication forks undergoing hypoxia-induced replication stress. Furthermore, we describe the adaptation of this method for the study of factors associated with replication forks recovering from hypoxia-induced replication stress following periods of reoxygenation. It is important to note that once cells are exposed to reoxygenation following acute periods (<8 h) of severe hypoxia (<0.1 % O_2) stalled replication forks may recover but will do so in a context of increased DNA damage caused by increased reactive oxygen species [2]. When normoxia, hypoxia and reoxygenation conditions are performed alongside, this protocol can provide valuable information regarding the differences in proteins (or complexes) associated with replication forks under these three different conditions (Figs. 3.1 and 3.2).

As part of the iPOND protocol, chase experiments, where EdU labelling is combined with increasing culture times without label (referred to as the chase period), can be carried out (Figs. 3.1 and 3.2). These experiments can provide a useful control when trying to validate whether a protein is strictly associated with active replication forks or whether it is simply carried alongside other chromatin components. Proteins truly associated with the replisome will not be detected in the chase sample. Furthermore, thymidine chase experiments can be used for studying the association of factors in relation to distance from the replication fork. This might be particularly relevant when studying processes such as histone deposition and maturation at elongating forks [1, 7].

3.2 Reagents

- EdU (5-ethynyl-2′-deoxyuridine) (Invitrogen, cat. No. E10187)
- Thymidine (Sigma, cat. no. T1895)
- 37 % (w/v) formaldehyde solution (Sigma, cat no. 1635)
- Phosphate Buffered Saline (PBS)
- Glycine (Fisher, cat. no. BP 381)
- Triton X-100 (Sigma, cat. No. T8787)
- Bovine serum albumin (BSA) (Sigma, cat. No. A7030)
- Dimethyl sulphoxide (DMSO)
- Copper (II) sulphate pentahydrate ($CuSO_4{\bullet}5H_2O$) (Fisher, cat. No. C489)
- (+) Sodium L-ascorbate (Sigma, cat. No. B10184)
- Sodium Dodecyl Sulphate (SDS) (Sigma, cat. No. L4390)
- Sodium Chloride (NaCl)
- Tris, pH 8.0 and pH 6.7
- Dithioerythritol (DTT) (Sigma, cat no. D-8255)

3.2.1 Reagent Setup

EdU: Dissolve EdU in DMSO for a final concentration of 10 mM. Aliquot and store at −20 °C protected from light. Stable for up to 1 year. Before use thaw at 37 °C. MW: 252.23.

Thymidine: Dissolve in water at a final concentration of 10 mM. Aliquot and store at −20 °C. Stable for up to 1 year. Use at a final concentration of 10 μM.

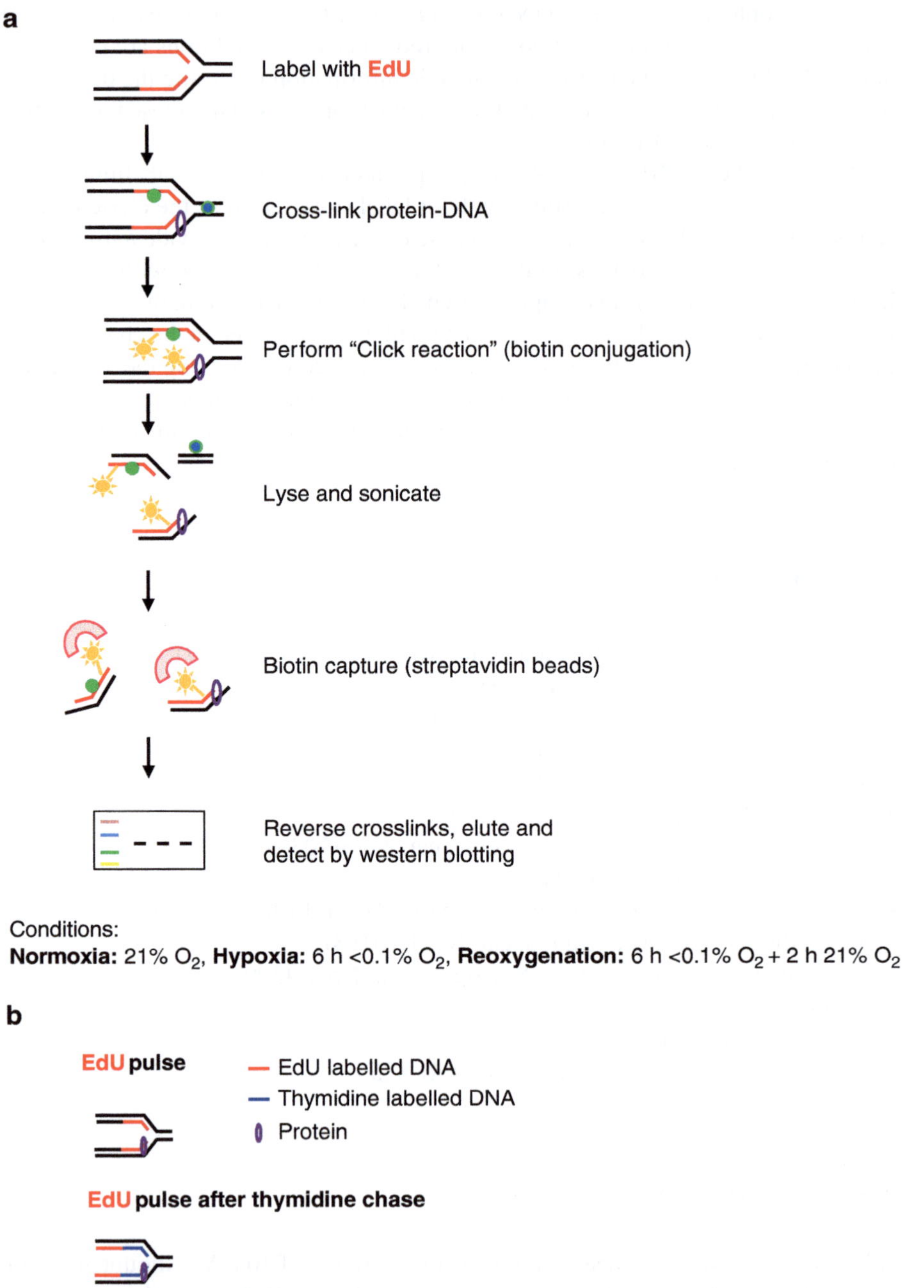

Fig. 3.1 Schematic representation of an overview of the iPOND experiment. (**a**) Schematic representation of the iPOND protocol performed under three different conditions: normoxia, hypoxia and reoxygenation. Adapted from [5, 8]. (**b**) Schematic representation of the thymidine chase experiment used to distinguish proteins specifically associated with the replication fork from non-specific chromatin binding factors. Thymidine chase displaces nascent EdU-labelled DNA away from the replication fork. Adapted from [5, 8]

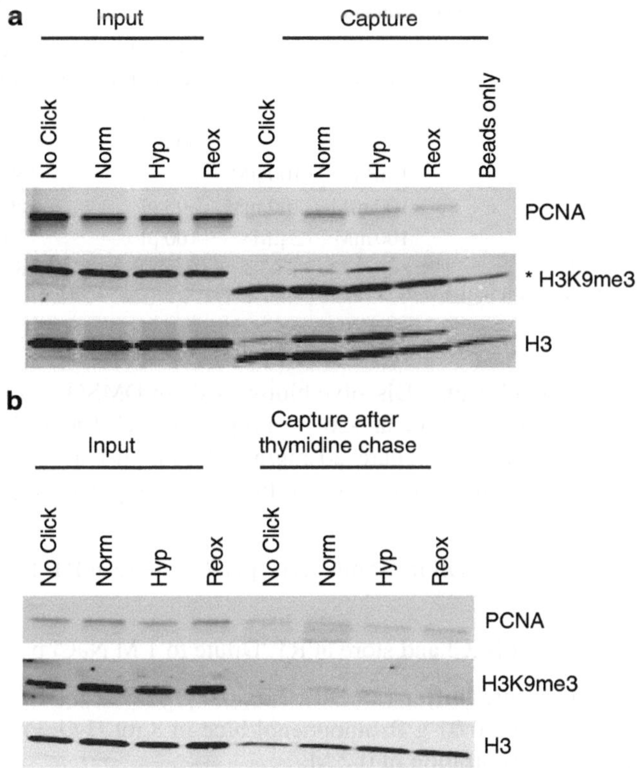

Fig. 3.2 Example of results that can be obtained when the iPOND protocol is used following exposure of cells to normoxia, hypoxia and reoxygenation. (**a**) iPOND was carried out following exposure of RKO cells to either Norm (21 % O_2), Hyp (6 h, <0.1 % O_2) or Reox (6 h, <0.1 % O_2 followed by 2 h of 21 % O_2). EdU labelling times: Norm (1 h), Hyp (6 h), Reox (2 h, during reoxygenation period). *Asterisk* denotes a non-specific band observed in all lanes at the end of the gel [5]. (**b**) Example of a thymidine chase experiment. iPOND was carried out following exposure of RKO cells to either Norm (21 % O_2), Hyp (6 h, <0.1 % O_2) or Reox (6 h, <0.1 % O_2 followed by 2 h of 21 % O_2). EdU labelling times: Norm (0.5 h), Hyp (3 h), Reox (1.5 h, during reoxygenation period). The chase into thymidine containing medium was performed for the last 30 min of each condition in Norm and Reox or for the last 3 h in Hyp. No click control represents a sample where the click reaction was carried out without biotin-azide [13]

1 % Formaldehyde/PBS: Dilute 37 % formaldehyde 1:37 with PBS (freshly prepared for each experiment). Keep at room temperature (RT) until cell fixation.

1.25 M Glycine: Prepare 1.25 M glycine stock solution. Store at RT. Use at 1:10 dilution for a final concentration of 0.125 M glycine.

Permeabilisation buffer: Make stock 20 % Triton X-100 and keep at RT. Dilute to 0.25 % Triton X-100 in PBS and store at 4 °C.

0.5 % BSA in PBS wash buffer. Prepare 0.5 % BSA in PBS. Filter and store at 4 °C.

Table 3.1 Click reaction cocktail components

Reagent	[Stock]	[Final]	Control reaction volume	Experimental reaction volume
1× PBS	–	–	3.9 ml	3.9 ml
DMSO	–	–	50 μl	–
Biotin-azide	1 mM	100 μM	–	50 μl
Sodium ascorbate	100 mM	100 mM	500 μl	500 μl
$CuSO_4$	100 mM	2 μM	100 μl	100 μl
Total volume (includes approximately 0.4 ml of cell pellet volume)			5 ml	5 ml

Click reaction stock solutions: Dissolve biotin-azide in DMSO to a final concentration of 1 mM. Aliquot and store at −20 °C. Prepare a stock 100 mM $CuSO_4$ solution in H_2O and store at RT. Prepare 20 mg/ml of sodium L-ascorbate (reducing agent) in H_2O and store on ice until needed. Prepare freshly and limit exposure to air (see also Table 3.1).

Lysis buffer: Prepare 1 % SDS in 50 mM Tris, pH 8.0. Store at RT. Prior to use add protease inhibitors.

Salt wash: Prepare 5 M NaCl and store at RT. Dilute to 1 M NaCl prior to use.

2× SDS Laemmli sample buffer (2× SB): Mix 0.4 g SDS, 2 ml 100 % Glycerol, 1.25 ml 1 M Tris 6.8 and 0.01 g Bromophenol blue in 8 ml H_2O. Prior to use add 1 M DTT to a final concentration of 0.2 M.

Note: For a full list of reagents and full instructions on crosslinking reversal and DNA fragment size analysis see full protocol [8].

Hypoxic chamber: For experiments where replication stress is desired a chamber that can be set <0.1 % O_2 (or at least <0.5 % O_2) is required.

Reoxygenation samples refer to conditions where cells have been placed in a hypoxic chamber for several hours before being returned to a standard tissue culture incubator (21 % O_2). See schematic for further details (Fig. 3.1).

3.3 Method

- **Cell culture preparation—Timing 1–10 days**

1. Each sample requires at least 1×10^8 cells at the time of EdU pulse. The required number of cells may vary depending on the application and cell type. For iPOND in hypoxia, RKO colorectal cancer cells have been used successfully. Other cell lines (including HEK293T, HCT116, U2OS and mouse embryonic fibroblasts and have been used in the original iPOND protocol) [1, 8].

   NOTE: Theoretically any cell that can incorporate EdU during DNA replication can be used in this protocol.

2. Use typically 8–10 × 150 mm dishes per condition for RKO cells: Plate 6–7 × 10^6 cells per dish 1 day before EdU pulse. Ideally plate 1 day before EdU incubation to ensure cells are growing optimally. Always remember that you need a no click control in addition to your experimental samples

   CRITICAL STEP: Need to include one extra dish for counting the cell number in step 3.

   Cells must be in log phase of growth and cannot be overgrown. It is useful to monitor appropriate incubator temperature and CO_2 content; otherwise EdU incorporation will not be maximal.

   (If performing chases, media may need to be equilibrated to 37 °C and appropriate CO_2 content overnight.)

   Ideally cells should be plated in glass dishes for experiments performed <0.1 % O_2. If this is not feasible the incubation times under hypoxic conditions may need to be prolonged to account for delayed replication stress in the presence of residual oxygen present in plastic dishes.
3. On the day of EdU incorporation: determine the cell number in the extra dish of cells. The number will be used to calculate the amount of the reagents for each sample in step 29.
4. Plan out times to pulse (chase), fix, quench, collect and wash samples.

   CRITICAL STEP: Stagger samples ensuring that each sample is treated equally throughout all steps.
5. EdU incorporation: Add 23 μl of the 10 mM EdU stock into 23 ml of cell culture media in each dish to achieve a final EdU concentration of 10 μM. (Or alternatively make aliquots of 23 ml of media with 23 μl EdU mix in falcons, replace media and add these 23 ml of media to each dish. This is sometimes more convenient for the reoxygenation samples or if you are doing chase experiments).

   If not performing chase experiments proceed to formaldehyde crosslink once EdU incorporation time has ended.

For normoxic samples: Return to the incubator for the desired pulse time (typically 1 h, this may need to be optimised to ensure equal EdU incorporation between different conditions).

For hypoxic samples: Add EdU and immediately place cells into the hypoxic chamber (typically for 6 h).

For reoxygenation samples: Place dishes in the hypoxic chamber and add EdU at the time of reoxygenation (typically as soon as they come out of the chamber and for 2 h).

6. **To perform thymidine chase or addition of drug**: Remove plates from incubator and decant media.
7. Carefully wash cells with 5 ml of chase media (pre-equilibrated).
8. Add 20 ml of chase media containing 10 μM thymidine or desired concentration of desired drug. Return to the incubator for the desired length of time. It is important that these steps are performed as fast as possible to prevent pH and temperature changes in the media that can affect replication rates:

For this experiment typically, **Normoxia** = 30 min thymidine chase, **Hypoxia** = 3 h EdU3 h thymidine chase, **Reoxygenation** = 30 min chase at the end of the reoxygenation timecourse.

NOTE: To allow the experiment to be feasible a decreased number of dishes (e.g. 4 × 150 mm dishes) may need to be used for thymidine chase experiment controls in order to allow the experimental samples and control samples to all fit into the chamber at once. This may limit the strength of the signal achieved at the end of the experiment.

- **Formaldehyde crosslinking and collection of cells—Timing 1 h/time point**

9. Decant media after EdU pulse and or chase.
10. Immediately fix cells on the dish by adding 10 ml of 1 % Formaldehyde in PBS (made fresh) and incubate for 20 min at RT. Rock gently at the start and then leave them to incubate.
11. Quench crosslinking by adding 1 ml of 1.25 M glycine.
12. Remove glycine and add 5 ml of PBS + Protease inhibitor cocktail (Pi) per plate.
13. Rock/wash plate for 5 min.
14. Collect samples by scrapping and transfer to a 50 ml falcon tube. Note the volume. The same volume will be used for the PBS washes.
15. Centrifuge for 5 min at 900 × *g* 4 °C.
16. Decant supernatant.
17. Wash pellets 1× with PBS and centrifuge for 5 min at 900 × *g* 4 °C. Vortex to resuspend pellets in PBS.
18. After last wash decant PBS.

PAUSE POINT—Samples can be flash frozen and stored at −80 °C for several weeks.

- **Cell permeabilisation—Timing 1 h**
- *TIP: For permeabilisation, click reaction and lysis, prepare the necessary buffers before/during permeabilisation (see Table* 3.1 *for full* click reaction cocktail components):

  - *Permeabilisation buffer: 125 μl of Triton X-100 in 50 ml PBS*
  - *0.5 % BSA in PBS*
  - *PBS + Pi*
  - *Copper sulphate: 0.025 g in 1 ml*
  - *(+) Sodium* 1 *-ascorbate: 0.06 g in 3 ml (make this as close to the end as possible)*
  - *Thaw rest of the reagents for click reaction.*

19. Resuspend cells in permeabilisation buffer at a concentration of 1×10^7 cells/ml
20. Incubate cells at RT for 30 min.
21. Spin down for 5 min at 900 × *g*, 4 °C.
22. Carefully decant supernatant.

23. Wash cells 1× with cold 0.5 % BSA in PBS.

    CRITICAL STEP: BSA prevents cell pellet from detaching from wall of 50 ml falcon tube.
24. Centrifuge 5 min at 900 × *g*, 4 °C and decant supernatant.
25. Wash cells 1× with PBS.
26. Spin down 5 min at 900 × *g* 4 °C.
27. Decant supernatant and place pellets on ice while finishing click reaction cocktail preparation.

- **Click reaction—Timing 2 h**

28. Thaw an aliquot of stock biotin-azide by placing on 37 °C heat block or incubator
29. To calculate click reaction volumes follow Table 3.1 (actual volumes should be adjusted based on the cell number measured per sample (step 3)):

    NOTE: Two click reaction cocktails should be prepared: one for the control (no click) and one for the experimental samples (this one should contain biotin-azide).
30. Combine click reaction cocktail ingredients on ice (in a falcon before adding to the pellets) in the order listed in Table 3.1.
31. Resuspend cell pellets in click reaction cocktail by vortexing and transfer to 15 ml falcon.
32. Rotate reaction at RT for 1–2 h protected from light.
33. Centrifuge samples 5 min at 900 × *g*, 4 °C and decant supernatant.
34. Wash cells 1× with cold 0.5 % BSA in PBS using the same volume as used in click reaction for one sample.
35. Centrifuge samples 5 min at 900 × *g*, 4 °C and decant supernatant.
36. Wash cells 1× with PBS using the same volume as used in click reaction for one sample.
37. Decant PBS and invert tubes on paper towel to facilitate removal of all PBS.

PAUSE POINT—The samples can be flash frozen and stored at −80 °C for a few days.

- **Cell lysis and sonication—Timing 1 h**

38. Add Pi to lysis buffer before use and place on ice. (Make extra since this buffer will also be required to wash beads at capture stage.)
39. Resuspend samples at a concentration of 1.5×10^7 cells per 100 μl of lysis buffer and transfer to 1.5 ml Eppendorfs on ice. If a sonication control is necessary, take 5 μl of each sample before sonication.
40. Sonicate cells using a microtip sonicator:

    – Pulse 15 s constant pulse, 40 s pause at 13–16 W (or standard settings (10–20 %).
    – Repeat pulse 1× for every 200 μl of cell lysate.
    – Total pulse 4–5 min per sample.

- **CRITICAL STEP**: Lysate should appear clear/opaque after sonication and not cloudy. Cloudiness is an indicator of improper ratio of SDS to protein in lysate or insufficient sonication (see Table 3.2 for troubleshooting).
- Prevent overheating during sonication by placing samples on ice.

41. Centrifuge samples for 10 min at 16,100 × *g*, RT.
    CRITICAL STEP: Lysates should appear clear after sonication. The presence of white precipitate on top of the lysate indicates insufficient lysate clearing (see Table 3.2 for troubleshooting).
42. Note the lysate volume (LV).
43. Take 5 μl of sonication control at this step if DNA fragment size analysis is desired.
44. Dilute lysate 1:1 (v/v) with cold PBS containing Pi.
    CRITICAL STEP: Samples have been diluted to contain 0.5 % SDS, 25 mM Tris because biotin capture appears to be less efficient in lysates containing 1 % SDS.
45. Note the final capture volume (FCV).
46. Remove 15 μl of lysate as the sample input and place on ice. Add 2× SB in 1:1 (v/v) and freeze at −80 °C.

Table 3.2 Potential problems, reasons and solutions are highlighted to facilitate troubleshooting

Problem	Possible reason	Solution
Limited cell recovery	Insufficient pelleting during centrifugation	Increase time and speed of centrifugation. Add BSA to wash solution
Cloudy cell lysate following sonication	SDS-protein complexes have precipitated from solution or samples were not sonicated sufficiently (resulting in incomplete lysis)	Increase sonication times ensuring minimal sample foaming. Appropriate volumes of lysis buffer must be used
White precipitate after biotin capture centrifugation	Following sonication, cell membrane lipids failed to be properly pelleted	Lysate should be clear following sonication and centrifugation. If white precipitate is observed, centrifuge lysate again to ensure clearing
Control (no click) sample has high background	Non-specific binding to streptavidin beads	Include pre-clearing step. Increase the number of washes
Low control proteins signal	Limited EdU incorporation	Increase cell numbers to ensure optimal growth conditions. May need to increase EdU labelling times or duration of hypoxic treatment depending on oxygen concentrations used
Detection of protein of interest is low in input samples	Formaldehyde crosslinking may hinder epitope detection or antibody used is of poor quality	Optimise immunoblotting and potentially consider increasing boiling time for full formaldehyde crosslinking reversal

47. Pre-clear samples with protein A agarose beads to remove non-specific background for 1 h (wash beads as described below first). After pre-clearing remove 15 μl as pre-clearing input samples. This step is not essential but it may help when high background is detected in the no click control (see Table 3.2 for troubleshooting).

- **Biotin capture of biotin-tagged nascent DNA and associated proteins—Timing 16–20 h**

48. Incubate each sample with streptavidin-agarose beads at a concentration of 100 μl bead slurry (50 μl packed volume) per 1×10^8 cells.
49. Wash beads for all samples together by centrifuging bead slurry at $1800 \times g$ for 1 min, RT.
50. Carefully aspirate storage buffer off beads.
51. Wash beads 2× with 1:1 (v/v) of lysis buffer containing Pi.
52. Wash beads 1× with 1:1 (v/v) of PBS containing Pi.
53. Resuspend beads 1× with 1:1 (v/v) of PBS containing Pi.
54. Add equal volume of beads to each sample using pipet tip that is cut at the end.
55. Rotate biotin captures in cold room for 16–20 h.

- **Elution of proteins bound to nascent DNA—Timing 1–4 h**

56. Take down captures after 16–20 h of capture.
57. Centrifuge the streptavidin-agarose beads with captured DNA and associated proteins for 3 min at $1800 \times g$ RT.
58. Carefully aspirate most of the supernatant
    CRITICAL STEP: Supernatant should be light blue/clear with no precipitate (see Table 3.2 for troubleshooting).
59. Wash beads with 1 ml of cold lysis buffer (no additives needed).
60. Rotate at RT for 5 min.
61. Centrifuge for 1 min at $1800 \times g$ RT.
62. Wash 1× with 1 ml of NaCl.
63. Rotate and pellet beads as in steps 60–61.
64. Repeat Lysis Buffer washes (steps 59–61) × 2.
65. After last wash, aspirate all of the supernatant. Protein-DNA complexes isolated on beads are the Capture sample.
66. To elute proteins bound to nascent DNA, add 2× SB to packed beads 1:1 (v/v of packed beads. E.g. 100 μl SB: 100 μl packed beads—typically use 50 μl packed beads/1×10^8 cells).
67. Incubate capture and input samples for 25 min at 95 °C.
68. Centrifuge for 1 min at $1800 \times g$ RT. The supernatant is ready to use in standard SDS-PAGE and immunoblotting procedures.

- **Analysis of proteins using western blotting**

69. Prepare standard SDS-PAGE gels in order to analyse both the proteins of interest and positive control (typically a known replication protein and a histone). Generally each sample from (1×10^8 cells) can provide enough

samples to be analysed in two to three immunoblots. It is important to note that depending on the proteins to be analysed and the antibody quality different amounts of proteins may be required.

Both the input and the iPOND purified samples should be examined concurrently. Typically load 2 μl of input and 20 μl of capture samples.

70. Perform standard electrophoresis, transfer, and immunoblotting using desired antibodies.
71. Mass spectrometry analysis can also be performed at this stage. Native iPOND (performed without formaldehyde crosslinking as described in [8]) facilitates mass spectrometry analysis.

3.4 Concluding Remarks

The protocol described above is an adaptation of the original iPOND technique that can be feasibly carried out under hypoxic conditions. Importantly, this protocol can be used to study both proteins associated with the replication forks undergoing hypoxia-induced replication stress and those associated with forks undergoing replication stress recovery following periods of reoxygenation (Figs. 3.1 and 3.2) [5]. This protocol can be combined with the use of drugs or can be carried out in cell lines containing mutations or deletions in genes of interest providing an easy way to interrogate the role of different factors in the recruitment of proteins to or around the replication fork under hypoxia/reoxygenation conditions.

Limitations to this protocol include the length and the high number of cells required. Modifications to the original iPOND protocol, however, have now been described that shorten the protocol by combining the cell lysis and nuclei harvesting steps. This reduces the number of washes resulting in improved yields due to reduced sample loss. Formaldehyde crosslinking is also omitted in this protocol, a modification that may facilitate mass spectrometry analysis [11].

This protocol also does not provide resolution at the single replication fork level; rather the data obtained should be interpreted as an average representation of replication forks present in that particular sample [8]. However, the original iPOND protocol and the adaptation described here provide important spatial and temporal information regarding the association of proteins bound directly or indirectly to DNA at or around replication forks. It is important to note that the level of spatial and temporal information that can be obtained by this method primarily depends on the EdU labelling time and the DNA synthesis rates under varying conditions. Under hypoxic conditions significantly different from those described in this protocol, EdU labelling times might need to be altered in order to account for changes in DNA replication rates under different conditions. The ultimate experimental goal will also determine the most appropriate EdU labelling times. Shorter times are recommended when studying proteins specifically associated with the replisome (or at the replication fork) whilst longer labelling periods should be used for the identification of proteins involved in chromatin deposition or maturation [5, 8].

While other established protocols such as chromatin fractionation and chromatin immunoprecipitation allow DNA-protein complex purification and could potentially be used to isolate complexes present at the replication fork, these techniques cannot provide information about the spatial location of a particular protein (or its modifications) in the genome with respect to replication. Such spatial information may be obtained by the use of certain imaging techniques such as super-resolution immunofluorescence or proximity ligation assays; however, these techniques require specific antibodies and are, therefore, not suitable for the identification of novel unknown replication associated factors [1].

Coupling iPOND to unbiased approaches such as LC-MS/MS allows the use of this powerful technique in the identification of novel players at active, stalled or damaged replication forks [12]. It would be interesting to carry out the iPOND in hypoxia/reoxygenation protocol coupled to LC-MS/MS in order to isolate novel factors associated with the replication fork under conditions of hypoxia-induced replication stress as well as during reoxygenation. Given that hypoxia-induced replication stress is different from replication stress induced by other agents typically used in the study of DNA replication (such as hydroxyurea), it is important to have the necessary tools to study factors associated with replication forks under these conditions [6].

Acknowledgements We are very grateful to Bianca Sirbu and David Cortez for help and advice on the iPOND procedure when we were adapting it for use under hypoxia and reoxygenation conditions. This work was supported by a Cancer Research UK grant (awarded to E.M.H.) and an MRC Centenary award (awarded to M.M.O.).

References

1. Dungrawala H, Cortez D. Purification of proteins on newly synthesized DNA using iPOND. Methods Mol Biol. 2015;1228:123–31.
2. Pires IM, et al. Effects of acute versus chronic hypoxia on DNA damage responses and genomic instability. Cancer Res. 2010;70(3):925–35.
3. Bester AC, et al. Nucleotide deficiency promotes genomic instability in early stages of cancer development. Cell. 2011;145(3):435–46.
4. Hammond EM, et al. The meaning, measurement and modification of hypoxia in the laboratory and the clinic. Clin Oncol (R Coll Radiol). 2014;26(5):277–88.
5. Olcina MM, et al. Replication stress and chromatin context link ATM activation to a role in DNA replication. Mol Cell. 2013;52(5):758–66.
6. Hammond EM, Green SL, Giaccia AJ. Comparison of hypoxia-induced replication arrest with hydroxyurea and aphidicolin-induced arrest. Mutat Res. 2003;532(1–2):205–13.
7. Sirbu BM, et al. Analysis of protein dynamics at active, stalled, and collapsed replication forks. Genes Dev. 2011;25(12):1320–7.
8. Sirbu BM, Couch FB, Cortez D. Monitoring the spatiotemporal dynamics of proteins at replication forks and in assembled chromatin using isolation of proteins on nascent DNA. Nat Protoc. 2012;7(3):594–605.
9. Lopez-Contreras AJ, et al. A proteomic characterization of factors enriched at nascent DNA molecules. Cell Rep. 2013;3(4):1105–16.

10. Cortez D. Preventing replication fork collapse to maintain genome integrity. DNA Repair (Amst). 2015;32:149–57.
11. Leung KH, Abou El Hassan M, Bremner R. A rapid and efficient method to purify proteins at replication forks under native conditions. Biotechniques. 2013;55(4):204–6.
12. Sirbu BM, et al. Identification of proteins at active, stalled, and collapsed replication forks using isolation of proteins on nascent DNA (iPOND) coupled with mass spectrometry. J Biol Chem. 2013;288(44):31458–67.
13. Olcina del MM. Hypoxia-induced chromatin changes and ATM signalling. 2014, DPhil. University of Oxford.

Chapter 4
In Vivo Interrogation of the Hypoxic Transcriptome of Solid Tumors: Optimizing Hypoxic Probe Labeling with Laser Capture Microdissection for Isolation of High-Quality RNA for Deep Sequencing Analysis

Lauren K. Brady, Vladimir Popov, and Constantinos Koumenis

Abstract Global gene expression analysis is a powerful method for identifying biological networks and regulatory mechanisms that govern cellular or tissue-level responses to physiologic stress. In the context of tumor biology, differential gene expression studies have provided information about the growth, aggressiveness, prognosis, and therapeutic response of tumors in patients. Scientists are using these valuable data to investigate pathways that can be targeted therapeutically with the goal of improving patient outcome. RNA sequencing enables nucleotide resolution of expression of whole transcriptomes, but arrives with a new set of challenges surrounding the management and analysis of large datasets. This chapter aims to review technical advancements to current methods for isolating high-quality RNA for sequencing studies directly from hypoxic tissues and introduces select widely used applications for gene expression analyses of next-generation sequencing data.

Keywords RNA sequencing • Hypoxia • Gene expression • Tumor microenvironment • Laser capture microdissection

L.K. Brady
Department of Radiation Oncology, Perelman School of Medicine, University of Pennsylvania, Philadelphia, PA 19104, USA

Cellular and Molecular Biology Graduate Group, Perelman School of Medicine, University of Pennsylvania, Philadelphia, PA 19104, USA

V. Popov • C. Koumenis (✉)
Department of Radiation Oncology, Perelman School of Medicine, University of Pennsylvania, Philadelphia, PA 19104, USA
e-mail: Costas.Koumenis@uphs.upenn.edu

C. Koumenis et al. (eds.), *Tumor Microenvironment*, Advances in Experimental Medicine and Biology 899, DOI 10.1007/978-3-319-26666-4_4

4.1 Introduction

Hypoxia, a state of reduced cellular oxygen, influences cellular survival, growth, and metabolism by triggering widespread changes in gene expression [1]. While transient hypoxia occurs from an imbalance between oxygen supply and consumption in normal tissues and during development, hypoxia (acute or chronic) is a key feature of solid tumors that contributes to therapeutic resistance and positively correlates with tumor aggressiveness. FDA-approved bioreductive dyes, such as EF5, have made it possible to investigate the level of hypoxia in patients as a marker to both predict tumor growth in addition to tumor treatment resistance and identify hypoxia in tumor patients affected by several different cancers, including head and neck, breast, and prostate [2]. The current scope of hypoxia research is expanding to also include genome-wide expression data to identify key hypoxia-responsive genes and pathways that correlate with patient prognosis with the ultimate goal that some of these genes or pathways may be targeted to augment patient response to therapy. Preliminary microarray studies in samples from head and neck cancer patients have reported that expression patterns of specific gene isoforms may correspond to the level of hypoxia and predict patient survival [3]. In addition, major signaling pathways known to be overactive in cancer which impact cell growth, survival, and angiogenesis also impact expression and processing of mRNA isoforms [4]. There is an immediate need for analyzing next-generation sequencing of hypoxic tumors to investigate in greater detail how expression of individual mRNA isoforms correlates with patient outcome. This chapter will highlight select ongoing and developing research probing the molecular changes that occur following hypoxia-induced changes in gene expression and some of the latest advancements to enhance study of the molecular basis of hypoxic tumors.

4.2 Tumor Hypoxia and Resistance to Therapy

Solid tumors often contain poor vasculature and decreased blood supply to distal regions, creating separate, oxygen-poor microenvironments within the tumor tissue. There are several solid tumors that are considered more hypoxic than others, such as glioblastoma multiforme, head and neck carcinomas, breast, cervix, and prostate cancers [5–7]. Hypoxic tumors exhibit resistance to radiation therapy and some chemotherapies due to the lack of sufficient oxygen essential for the formation of free radicals necessary to cause DNA damage [8]. Low oxygen levels and associated tissue acidity also decrease cellular uptake of chemotherapies and result in reduced drug delivery to tumors [8]. Acute hypoxia, which may last only minutes to hours, refers to fluctuation in oxygen supply due to inadequate blood flow and may only affect parts of the tumor [9]. Chronic hypoxia accounts for the majority of hypoxia found in tumors. This largely occurs due to limitations in oxygen diffusion, often caused by networks of irregular vessels and increased distances between vessels in tumors compared to normal tissues [10, 11].

Moreover, development of blood vessels is tightly regulated by the expression of pro-angiogenic factors (i.e., VEGF) and anti-angiogenic factors (i.e., thrombospondin), which respond to demand for oxygen and nutrients. Expression of these and other angiogenic-related factors is regulated by HIF-1 [12]. The network and structure of blood vessels are often disrupted in tumors due to overexpression of pro-angiogenic factors and increased cellular growth rates in tumors. Uncovering a deeper knowledge of which genes and isoforms are differentially expressed in hypoxic regions of tumors will provide a better understanding of how pathways that impact resistance to therapy, such as angiogenesis, are regulated.

4.3 Regulation of Gene Expression in Hypoxic Tumors

Many of the biological changes that occur in hypoxic tumors are a result of vast differences in gene expression profiles between hypoxic and normoxic tissues. Hypoxia-responsive genes have historically been studied in relation to the major *H*ypoxia *I*nducible transcription *F*actors (HIFs). HIF-1 is a heterodimeric protein which includes an oxygen-responsive alpha subunit and constitutively active beta subunit. Under normoxic conditions, HIF-1 is constantly synthesized and degraded [13]. In the presence of normal oxygen concentrations, HIF-1 is hydroxylated on proline residues, where it interacts with von Hippel-Lindau factor (VHL), becomes ubiquitinated, and is eventually degraded via the proteasome. Hydroxylation also prevents co-factor binding to HIF-1a, further inhibiting its transcription regulatory function. Decreased oxygen prevents this process, which results in stabilized HIF-1 protein [13, 14]. These conditions permit HIF-1a proteins to heterodimerize with a beta subunit and induce transcription of target genes involved in glucose metabolism, cell survival, and cell migration [15].

Some well-known examples of HIF-1a transcriptional targets are vascular endothelial growth factors (VEGF) involved in angiogenesis, GLUT1, also known as SLC2A, glucose transporter involved in glycolysis, and carbonic anhydrase IX (CA9), which is a regulator of cellular pH [16]. Expression of these and other HIF-1a regulated proteins also correlates with the metastatic potential of tumors and therapeutic resistance [17]. Recently, it has been described that hypoxia not only alters total gene expression levels of these targets, but HIFs may play a role in influencing alternative splicing of several of these target genes, including ADM and CA9 [18, 19]. It remains unclear what the biological consequences of altered splicing in hypoxic tumors may be and what HIF-independent factors regulate splicing in the hypoxic tumor microenvironment. Additional work in our group and others is currently investigating the impact of hypoxia on splicing and expression of mRNA isoforms in tumors.

4.4 Identifying and Isolating Hypoxic Tissue for Molecular Studies

Even though regulation of mRNA and miRNA has been extensively studied in vitro [20, 21], in vivo analysis of hypoxic tumors was limited due to small quantities of poor-quality RNA when isolated from immunohistochemical samples using traditional methods. Although in vitro hypoxic conditions can represent oxygen levels in tumors, these conditions do not take into the account many other factors present in the tumor microenvironment that contribute to physiologic stress like low nutrient levels, low pH, infiltrating immune cells, and necrotic tissue, or, more critically, the interplay between these factors and the effect on gene expression. A prime example of this is lactic acidosis, which when it co-occurs with hypoxia, results in reduced stabilization of HIF-1 and counteracts the usual induction of hypoxia-responsive genes. This occurs in part due to lactic acidosis stimulating the Unfolded Protein Response (UPR) as well as an inflammatory response [22].

Studying changes in gene expression due to stresses that arise in the tumor microenvironment, such as hypoxia or acidosis, can be simplified by utilizing in vitro systems. However, it is crucial to pair these studies with the respective in vivo models in order to gain a more complete understanding of the basic biology of the tumor microenvironment. As a result, there is an immediate need for improved methods to isolate DNA and RNA from tumor samples. To achieve this goal, our group developed an approach utilizing a combination of EF5 staining, laser capture microdissection (LCM), and modification to traditional RNA purification methods to specifically isolate high-quality RNA from hypoxic and normoxic regions for gene expression studies [23].

4.4.1 *Chemical-Based Imaging of Hypoxic Tissues Using Oxygen-Sensitive Dyes*

Imaging techniques utilizing oxygen-sensitive molecules followed by immunofluorescence staining offer the advantage as being a safe and noninvasive method for identifying hypoxia in patient tumors. For example, a patient may undergo injection of a bioreductive dye several hours prior to a surgery for tumor resection, after which the removed tissue can be studied using antibodies against the bioreductive dyes followed by microscopy analysis.

While there are several different chemical classes that when metabolized under low oxygen levels can be used as markers for identifying tumor hypoxia, we will focus on two 2-nitroimidazole molecules: EF5 and pimonidazole. EF5 is a fluorinated derivative of etanidazole that is reduced in regions of hypoxia where it covalently binds to adjacent proteins and DNA. This stable binding makes EF5 ideal for use as ^{18}F-EF5 for PET scans in patients or animals, or allows for subsequent staining with anti-EF5 antibodies conjugated to fluorochromes, such as Cy3 or Cy5, for downstream microscopy-based applications at the bench [24]. Another bioreductive dye, pimonidazole, represents a widely used choice for detection of hypoxic tissue in both lab and clinic. Pimonidazole binds to thiol-containing proteins (present in hypoxic cells) by forming protein adducts in areas of low oxygen. Pimonidazole is also highly water soluble, chemically stable, exhibits low toxicity, and is taken up efficiently by tumors [25]. Oxygen levels can be quantified using either of these molecules by comparison with a series of in vitro standards, or through relative analysis by staining of nontumorous tissue. However, pimonidazole binding also depends on pH [26] while EF5 does not and is also a lipophilic molecule, which offers the advantage of increased biodistribution compared to other hypoxia markers [24].

The use of these molecules has enabled the collection of clinical data to strengthen the finding that hypoxic tumors are indeed correlated with poor prognosis. In addition, these methods allow safe and precise staining of hypoxic tissues, which in combination with the relatively novel technology of laser capture microdissection (LCM) has very recently allowed for the optimization and development of downstream methods for excising enough intact RNA for gene expression analysis.

4.4.2 Laser Capture Microdissection (LCM)

LCM is a relatively novel technology that allows isolation of homogenous sample from a heterogeneous population. Originally developed at NIH by Lance Liotta and Emmert-Buck, the laser microdissection system allows rapid one-step selection and isolation of tissue from a heterogeneous sample under direct microscopic visualization [27]. Moreover, technology advancements have demonstrated a successful single-cell capture from different types of tissue sections, including immunostained cells [28].

There are two, general classes of laser capture microdissections systems: infrared (IR LCM) and ultraviolet (UV-LCM). The platform on either system can be manual or robotic [29, 30] and consists of inverted microscope, infrared laser diode, laser control unit, a controlled microscope stage with vacuum for slice immobilization, a CCD camera, and viewing monitor. Even though both IR and UV offer certain advantages, there seems to be overall preference for UV-LCM. In addition to being faster and more precise during sample collection, the quality of the sample (even at single-cell level) can be used for the extraction of nucleic acids and PCR-based analyses [30].

4.4.3 RNA Extraction for Subsequent Genomic Analysis

Marotta et al. were the first to publish on the use of UV-LCM to extract high-grade RNA from specific hypoxic and normoxic tumor sections for subsequent microarray analysis. Specifically, 9L gliosarcoma cells were used to establish tumors in a rodent model. At the experimental endpoint, animals were anesthetized and the bioreductive dye, EF5, was injected through tail vain at the concentration 30–80 mg/kg 1–2 h before tumor excision [23]. Tumors were embedded into either low melting agarose or OCT and stored at −80 °C. In order to maintain the integrity of the RNA, the tissue samples must be kept free of RNAses and DNAses, which degrade the nucleic acids. Activity of these enzymes can be partially inhibited by taking several additional measures during the preparation of tissue slides, including limiting humidity and by preparing samples at a low temperature. One tumor sample will be sectioned onto several membrane slides at a thickness of 10 μm tissue slices using a cryostat at −20 °C. Slides are processed in the same orientation to enable collection of several dissections per slide and eventual pooling of material collected from slides derived from the same tumor sample. To ensure optimal conditions, after tissues have been sectioned onto membrane slides and during the antibody staining protocol, slides are washed thoroughly and then dehydrated with ethanol. In addition, during incubation periods, slides are stored in 50-ml conical tubes containing desiccant pellets and kept on ice or in a 4 °C cold room throughout the experiment.

Once slides have been stained with a secondary antibody containing fluorochrome, laser capture microdissection can be performed. Microdissection is carried out on areas of the tumor with the strongest EF5 (or other appropriate marker of hypoxia) signal to collect hypoxic samples. To avoid necrotic tissue, which will also exhibit a strong EF5 signal due to lack of oxygen, slides must also be stained with a nuclear stain, such as Hoescht, to enable researchers to distinguish hypoxic cells (with intact nuclei) from anoxic/necrotic cells (with fragmented nuclei). Areas of the same tumor that display little to no signal from the secondary antibody are collected as paired normoxic controls (see Fig. 4.1a–c for overview; [23]). All material collected by LCM is immediately frozen on dry-ice pellets and stored at −80 °C until RNA extraction.

4.4.4 Assessment of Sample Quality

Pooled samples from LCM can then be processed using a user-preferred RNA isolation protocol. Phenol-chloroform based methods are still the standard for yielding the highest-quality material. Standard protocols for preparing cDNA libraries for RNA sequencing recommend a minimum of 0.1 μg high-quality RNA to begin, but specialized

Fig. 4.1 (continued) sequenced and the sequences are aligned to a reference genome. (**f**) Data visualized against a RefSeq transcript model, using the IGV browser with a sashimi view to plot sequencing reads and count reads that span particular exon junctions. (**g**) Advanced applications are used to measure expression differences at alternatively spliced exons. (**h**) Differential expression analysis can be interpreted by using software to carry out network analyses. This network of actin motility genes that changed expression in hypoxic vs. normoxic tumors was generated through the use of QIAGEN's Ingenuity Pathway Analysis (IPA®,QIAGEN Redwood City, www.qiagen.com/ingenuity)

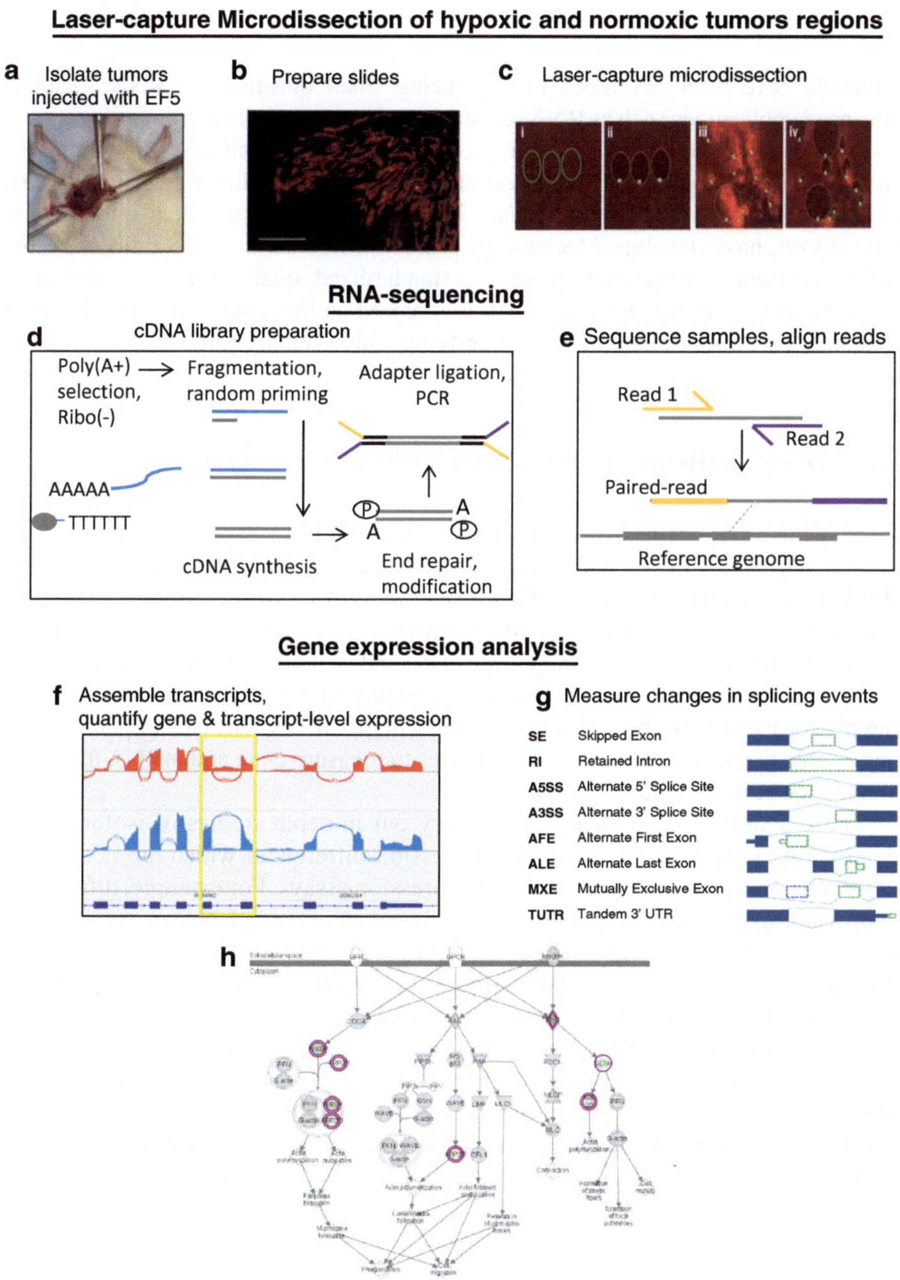

Fig. 4.1 Experimental overview for in vivo labeling paired with LCM for RNA sequencing of hypoxic tumors. (**a**) Representative image of injection of EF5 into an animal model of tumor hypoxia. After tumor is excised, (**b**) membrane slides are prepared with antibodies against EF5 to visualize areas of hypoxia, stained in *red*. (**c**) Laser capture microdissection (LCM) can then be used to remove normoxic ((*i*) pre-LCM, (*ii*) post-LCM) and hypoxic ((*iii*) pre-LCM, (*iv*) post-LCM) tissue. Panels **a**–**c** modified from [23]. Following RNA extraction, cDNA libraries are prepared (**d**) using mRNA depleted of rRNAs and annealed with primers specific for the sequencing platform. (**e**) Libraries are

protocols have been developed to sequencing small quantities of RNA, enabling advanced applications such as RNA sequencing of material isolated from a single cell.

Traditionally, the purity and quality of RNA has been evaluated by imaging the signal of RNA samples processed on ethidium-bromide stained agarose gels and comparing the ratio of 28S to 18S rRNA. More advanced systems, such as the Agilent bioanalyzer, have developed technology which utilizes the 28S:18S ratio and other additional sample measures to produce a standardized, quality score reported as an RNA Integrity Number (RIN) [31]. RNA is scored on the scale from 1 to 10, with 1 as a measure of poor-quality and 10 signifying a high-quality sample.

4.5 Deep Sequencing for Transcriptomic Analysis

Prior to the arrival of next-generation sequencing, mRNA expression studies were carried out using Sanger sequencing of cDNAs/EST (expressed sequence tags). While EST sequencing can offer base-pair resolution, it is low-throughput and not practical for global analyses. Microarrays can measure expression nearly transcriptome-wide, but rely on hybridization and will not provide nucleotide-level resolution. Next-generation sequencers, distinguished as non-Sanger DNA sequencing platforms, achieve high-throughput sequencing of DNA strands in parallel [32] and enable users to sequence cDNA libraries to measure gene and mRNA transcript abundance at base-pair resolution.

These data provide information to carry out in-depth studies of isoform-level expression as well as allele-specific expression differences which are not always detectable on a global scale using other expression assays. For example, differential expression of miRNAs, alternative splicing, and changes in RNA processing have historically been observed to occur in certain cancers, but now widespread high-throughput analyses of RNA expression at nucleotide resolution are allowing for deeper investigation into these areas on a global scale.

With any technique, RNA-seq arrives with intrinsic challenges, some of which arise due to limitations in representation of transcriptome, quality and amount of starting material, etc. Several highly discussed advantages and disadvantages to RNA-seq will be reviewed in this chapter, with special focus on how these aspects impact the study of complex biological systems, such as expression profiling of tumor models.

4.6 Library Preparation/Study Design Tips

The varying technologies available for sequencing RNA samples and the differing techniques for preparing cDNA libraries for sequencing can play a large role in the profile, quality, and how representative of your biological samples the data are. There are numerous nuances to the design and preparation phases of planning an RNA sequencing study and a few of these are highlighted in the sections to follow.

4.6.1 Brief Review of Commonly Used Sequencing Technologies

Ion Torrent and Roche/454 are two examples of system that apply pyrosequencing technologies. Roche's 454 was the first commercially available next-generation sequencer. These systems can offer the advantage of long, paired-end reads with average read lengths exceeding 2500 base pairs [33]. The disadvantages include a high error rate, especially at homopolymers, which can make quantifying long regions of repeat bases challenging and inaccurate.

Alternatively, sequencing by synthesis methods, such as those offered by Illumina platforms, can provide sequencing data with a less than 5 % error rate. Reads are shorter than the previously mentioned systems, but are now approaching near 300 base pairs. However a sequencing capacity of several hundred million reads per lane, low error rate, and the ability to deliver data in a relatively short period (1–2 days) have made Illumina a leading competitor for DNA, RNA, and CHIP-sequencing applications. Read length is in part limited by a bridge amplification step. Briefly, cDNA library material with adapter primers ligated to the ends is denatured to a single strand and allowed to attach to the flow cell containing sequences complementary to the adapters (for complete details, see review by Quail et al. [34]). The bridge amplification will occur to create small clusters of each molecule to be sequenced. If these clusters are formed too close together, it will be problematic to capture high-quality fluorescent images and is one factor which determines of how many high-quality reads can be sequenced.

Additional technologies include third-generation sequencing platforms, such as PacBio's SMRT sequencing. This technology employs loading of cDNA onto circularized templates for sequencing which allows for advanced applications, such as long-read sequencing of full-length cDNA libraries. This method is advantageous for studies like identification and verification of transcript variants and spliceforms, as long reads can span across alternatively spliced exon-intron junctions and provide another technology for verification of these events. However, relative quantification of these studies can be a challenge, due to several reasons including biases in the size of cDNAs that are successfully loaded onto circularized templates during library preparation.

4.6.2 User Tips for Study Design and Sample Preparation

Since RNA sequencing is a time- and resource-expensive undertaking, it is critical to spend sufficient time during the planning and design phases of the project. Studies investigating the expression of rare transcript variants or aiming to capture reads at a particular exon-junction may consider deep sequencing whereas research detailing broad gene expression changes across several experimental variables or time-points may be better suited for multiplexing several samples into one sequencing lane. For example, one Illumina sequencing lane can produce several hundred million reads, which is most times more than adequate for a single sample, as detecting additional transcripts becomes saturated around 200 million reads [35]. Sequencing multiple samples per lane is possible by adding index or barcode sequences to adapter primers. This helps to reduce the cost of the experiments and may reduce technical variability across samples as well. For those seeking greater statistical power for identifying differentially expressed events, it is recommended to pool samples and sequence more replicates rather than deeply sequencing only one sample as there is a greater reduction in the background noise of RNA-seq data as increasing replicates are sequenced compared to sequencing a single sample more deeply to achieve more reads [36].

Commercially available kits and reagents for preparing strand-specific libraries can be more costly, but will yield more information that will increase both the accuracy of alignment and confidence in assigning reads to gene models (discussed in more detail later in this chapter). In addition, these data can be used to investigate less-understood levels of gene expression regulation, such as anti-sense transcription, which require directional information.

Methods to enrich for certain species of RNA can be as simple as using oligo-dT primers during the reverse transcription step in preparing the cDNA libraries to capture polyadenylated mRNAs (which comprise 3–5 % of total RNA). Similarly, there are reagents available for the depletion of ribosomal RNAs, which can account for as much as 80 % of the total RNA material in the cell [37] (Fig. 4.1d, e). More complex enrichment strategies including adding hybridization steps with probes to select for certain genes based on sequence complementarity. Targeted sequence approaches are ideal for those interested in detecting a specific subset of genes or events. These strategies have been applied to examine changes in expression of specific groups of genes, gene fusion events, and even base-pair level changes such as RNA editing sites [38, 39].

4.7 Analysis of RNA Sequencing Data

Regardless of which technology and instrument is used to sequence cDNA libraries, the instruments produce raw image files which must be converted sequencing reads which are ultimately formatted as FASTA files. For example, Illumina platforms must compile raw images as clusters, which are then converted to sequence reads; 454/Ion Torrent technologies are converted from flowgrams to FASTQ files (reviewed in [34]). PacBio systems decode video images as FASTQ. FASTQ files contain the sequencing results and also additional information about the quality of the sequencing data [40]. FASTQ uses Phred-scaled base qualities.

Now it is common to obtain several hundred million sequencing reads per sample, which will yield a large raw data file. After acquiring sequencing data, there are three major analysis steps to produce quantitative gene/transcript expression data: (a) quality control, (b) alignment and assembly, and (c) quantification. Downstream applications then combine statistical analyses with additional computational methods such as over-representation analysis and clustering to interpret the biological meaning of the expression data. Several of these programs commonly used to aid in generating biological hypotheses from differential expression data will be highlighted later in this chapter.

4.7.1 Quality Control

Data can be filtered such that only high-quality reads within a given threshold of quality scores are included for processing. Moreover, reads that correspond to the adapter primer sequences or sequences added for barcoding samples must be used to sort samples accordingly and then trimmed. These types of data mining and processing steps can be achieved using a number of publicly available/open-source platforms such as sickle or scythe (Table 4.1). Programs such as Fastqc enable users to process and visualize a quality profile of the data with various histogram and graph interfaces (bioinformatics.babraham.ac.uk/projects/fastqc). The open-source tool Galaxy provides a user-friendly interface for several steps of data processing, including the FASTQ Groomer and trimmomatic features for the quality control steps described above (see usegalaxy.org for more information).

4.7.2 Alignment and Transcript Assembly

Depending on the scientific question to be addressed with the RNA-seq data, there are two primary methods of aligning the sequencing reads: *genome-guided* approaches begin by aligning sequencing reads to a previously annotated reference genome and then assembling transcripts from spliced alignments while *genome-independent* methods begin by using RNA-seq reads to first assemble transcripts de novo and then align these independently assembled transcripts to the genome. Popular genome-guided aligners include STAR, BWA, and bowtie (see Table 4.1 for additional examples). A few of these also allow for building transcript models via a genome-independent approach, such as Trinity (Table 4.1). Traditional genome-guided approaches are the standard for global gene expression studies and those preferring evidence-based gene models. Ab initio gene prediction may be more useful for specialized applications such as identifying rare spliceforms and small RNA species or gene fusion events.

Reference genomes are available for download as convenient, annotated BED files from websites such as the UCSC Genome Browser webpage. Commonly used reference genomes are those from ENSEMBL (curated by the European Molecular Biology Laboratory, European Bioinformatics Institute and Welcome Trust Sanger Institute), UCSC Gene Tracks (University of California Santa Cruz), and RefSeq (maintained by the National Center for Biotechnology Information) [41]. All of the

Table 4.1 A highlight of leading publically available resources to facilitate analysis of RNA sequencing data

Analysis stage	Resource	Applications	References
Quality control/file processing	Fastqc	Overview quality profile of high-throughput sequencing data, QC processing tools	http://www.bioinformatics.babraham.ac.uk/projects/fastqc/
	Bedtools	File merging, counting, and sorting	http://bedtools.readthedocs.org/en/latest/
Alignment/assembly	TopHat	Assembles reads to a reference genome	[43]
	Trinity	De novo transcript assembly	(Grabherr et al. 2011)
	GSNAP	Fast assembler for short reads	[45]
	BWA	Burrows-Wheeler Aligner's Smith-Watermann method for fast alignment, long-read capabilities (reads >100 base pairs)	(Li and Durbin 2010)
	MapSplice	Alignment of spliced junctions without using canonical models	[44]
	Bowtie	Fast, short-read aligner	(Langmead and Salzberg 2012)
	STAR	"Superfast" aligner	(Dobin et al. 2013)
Quantification/statistical analyses	Cufflinks, Cuffdiff	Uses TopHat output to build transcript models with or without a reference model; quantification, normalization, and differential expression analysis	[46–48]
	MISO	"Mixture of isoforms" approach to analyze differential expression of mRNA isoforms and alternative splice events	[49]
	edgeR	R package in Bioconductor for statistical analyses of gene expression data	(Robinson et al. 2010)

reference genomes offered from these platforms are evidence based, but differ in how they use and filter available data to construct the references.

There are many programs available for either genome-guided or independent methods of alignment, which differ according to the time to process samples, the computing memory required for running the programs, and the performance/accuracy of the aligner (as reviewed in [42]). In addition to using a reference annotation to guide the alignment of reads, more advanced options specific for mRNA data are offered from splice-aware short-read aligners, which instruct intron-aware or split-read alignments and are available from numerous programs such as TopHat, STAR, GSNAP, MapSplice, and GSTRUCT [43–45]. Many of the developers for these alignment programs also offer packages for de novo transcript assembly, some of which include Cufflinks, Augustus, mGene, and Oases/Trinity (Table 4.1).

It is important to note that there are additional types of quality control processing after the alignment step. Additional post-processing steps may be necessary depending on the nature of the data and the scientific questions being addressed. Some examples include removing duplicate reads (PCR/optical reads), recalibrating base scores, adjusting replicates, and cleaning-up alignments at SNPs/indels. Programs available for these types of post-processing control steps include GATK, SMRA, and BEDtools.

4.7.3 Data Visualization

For many downstream applications, aligned FASTA files must be converted to other file types such as SAM or BAM (text and binary-based sequence alignment format). The most commonly used software for this conversion is samtools (samtools.sourceforge.net). Sorted SAM files can be visualized using programs such as the Integrative Genomics Viewer (broadinstitute.org/igv/) (Fig. 4.1f), Artemis, Apollo, and JBROWSE which will plot aligned reads against reference gene models. Reference gene models can be imported from numerous sources such as GenBank, GFF3, GTF, and EMBL.

4.7.4 Quantification

After reads are aligned and gene and transcript models have been assembled, quantification of gene expression values can be carried out using software complementary to many of aligner and data processing packages listed above. Popular options include Cufflinks, MISO, RSEM, and eXpress. Expression of RNA-seq data is often reported as the normalized figure, RPKM or FPKM. The reads (or read fragments) per kilobase of transcript per million mapped reads normalize to account for both gene length and the number of uniquely mapped reads so that comparison can be made across different samples (as well as different genes). One caveat to this approach is that since there are a finite number of RNA-seq reads per sample, there may be a bias for highly expressed genes, which consume a large number of these limited reads. To address this issue, mRNA expression can alternately be reported as counts per million (CPM) or transcripts per million (TPM). Regardless of how the total expression values are reported, it is best to carry out differential abundance statistics using effective read counts. Frequently used programs for statistical analyses of differential expression include Cuffdiff, MISO, edgeR, DESeq, and DEXseq (Table 4.1).

Cufflinks can be used for gene-level as well as transcript-level quantification. In addition, there are options to use annotated transcript models for analysis or to assemble transcripts de novo. The Cuffdiff suite of this software package offers a splicing and gene structure analysis which measures differential expression across different events such as alternate transcription start sites, spliced exons, and changes in untranslated regions [46–48]. Likewise, MISO offers multiple options for measuring changes in isoform expression (see Fig. 4.1g) such as a whole transcript-level analysis as well as an exon-level method which calculates changes in events such as alternatively spliced exons, introns, and differences in usage of splice sites [49].

4.8 Biological Interpretation of Gene Expression Data

RNA sequencing can yield an overwhelming amount of data. Working with any large dataset will present numerous challenges, including where to begin with sorting results, characterizing biologically meaningful trends in the data, and generating hypotheses for additional functional studies. Many researchers find methods such as over-representation analyses, clustering, and pathway-based correlations useful in interpreting the biological significance of differentially expressed genes. In this section, we will present a brief overview of commonly used systems for analysis and categorization of differential gene expression data.

4.8.1 Over-representation Analysis

To determine if a particular family or biologically related subset of genes is enriched in experimental samples compared to controls, several over-representation methods are available. These methods essentially identify groups of genes that are collectively enriched in the whole set of expressed genes. Functional annotation of genes and identifying enrichment can be carried out by many programs including the preferred programs GSEA (gene set enrichment analysis), http://amigo.geneontology.org, and GOrilla. These methods are beneficial for identifying biologically meaningful trends in the data which otherwise may have been overlooked. For example, a handful of genes with a modest expression change (i.e., fold change differences $|1.3|$) may not appear to have a large impact until one realizes all of these genes are functioning in the same pathway. While this type of analysis helps to recognize biological trends in differentially expressed genes, it is important to be aware of several caveats. These programs do not rely on the absolute amount of fold change in expression and therefore do not rely on statistical thresholds either. However, these methods are useful for identifying general trends and patterns in groups of changes that are differentially expressed, for example induction of DNA repair genes in irradiated samples.

4.8.2 Pathway-Based Analysis

Programs such as DAVID, KEGG, REACTOME, MSigDB, and cytoscope are capable of integrating fields from several curated databases to build a pathway-centered scheme from user data. Other advanced features build networks with links that share evidence-backed information such as the type of relationship between genes or gene hubs, direct and indirect interactions, shared upstream regulators such as common transcription factors, and links to the complementary/supporting PubMed publications. One such program is the Ingenuity Pathway Analysis platform, which is available to users who purchase a license. For example, a comparative RNA-seq analysis of hypoxic and normoxic areas of tumors confirmed a network of genes involved in actin mobility is differentially expressed (Fig. 4.1h, Brady et al. unpublished observation). Like all computational correlative analyses, limitations exist, including pathway cross-talk which may produce false positives.

4.9 Future of RNA Sequencing: Technical Developments and Custom Applications

Technological advances have allowed for the cost and time to carry out each RNA sequencing experiment to continually decrease. This is particularly advantageous for time-sensitive experiments, such as sequencing patients to guide treatment practices in the use of targeted therapies, which is now becoming possible due to such advances. In addition, instruments are equipped with user-friendly devices such as touch screens which allow real-time visualization of sequencing runs and offer options of connecting with technical support via internet access. As instruments become easier to use and smaller, the goal is to see more "bench-top" sequencers which allow researchers to carry out their own experiments on their own schedules rather than spend time waiting in a cue of users at a core facility. The sample preparation techniques are also advancing to enable researchers to sequence samples using very little starting material and even enable sequencing the RNA from a single cell. Moreover, it may soon be possible to directly sequence RNA molecules on a high-throughput scale, which will avoid the need for PCR amplification steps.

Many labs are developing their own custom protocols to target specific species of RNA or isolate RNA precisely during a certain step of regulation. Examples include CAGE-seq (*c*ap *a*nalysis of *g*ene *e*xpression) to map transcription start sites at 5′ ends of genes [50], global run-on sequencing (GRO-seq) of nascent transcripts exiting the RNA polymerases [51] (Core et al. 2008), and more recently the updated version precision run-on sequencing (PRO-seq) and ribosomal profiling of nucleosome-protected regions of RNA [52].

Our custom LCM-RNA-seq approach has captured previously uncovered layers of regulation to mRNA levels. This method has allowed us to detect widespread changes in RNA processing such as differences in splicing and UTR lengths, and has led to the discovery of hypoxia-induced isoforms with different functional impacts compared with those expressed at basal normoxic conditions. The additional layers of biological information that are uncovered by deeply sequencing tumor RNA will help to advance the current understanding of the hypoxic microenvironment and reveal new mechanisms of gene expression regulation.

References

1. Koumenis C, Maxwell PH. Low oxygen stimulates the intellect. Symposium on hypoxia and development, physiology and disease. EMBO Rep. 2006;7(7):679–84.
2. Komar G, Lehtiö K, Seppänen M, Eskola O, Levola H, Lindholm P, Sipilä H, Seppälä J, Grénman R, Solin O, Minn H. Prognostic value of tumour blood flow, [18F]EF5 and [18F] FDG PET/CT imaging in patients with head and neck cancer treated with radiochemotherapy. Eur J Nucl Med Mol Imaging. 2014;41:2042–50.
3. Moller-Levet CS, Betts GNJ, Harris AL, Homer JJ, West CML, Miller CJ. Exon array analysis of head and neck cancers identifies a hypoxia related splice variant of LAMA3 associated with a poor prognosis. PLoS Comput Biol. 2009;5(11):1–13.
4. Oltean S, Bates DO. Hallmarks of alternative splicing in cancer. Oncogene. 2013;33(46):5311–8.
5. Brizel DM, Scully SP, Harrelson JM, Layfield LJ, Bean JM, Prosnitz LR, Dewhirst MW. Tumor oxygenation predicts for the likelihood of distant metastases in human soft tissue sarcoma. Cancer Res. 1996;56(5):941–3.
6. Nordsmark M, Overgaard M, Overgaard J. Pretreatment oxygenation predicts radiation response in advanced squamous cell carcinoma of the head and neck. Radiother Oncol. 1996;41(1):31–9.
7. Rampling R, Cruickshank G, Lewis AD, Fitzsimmons SA, Workman P. Direct measurement of pO2 distribution and bioreductive enzymes in human malignant brain tumors. Int J Radiat Oncol Biol Phys. 1994;29(3):427–31.
8. Vaupel P, Mayer A, Höckel M. Tumor hypoxia and malignant progression. In: Chandan KS, Gregg LS, editors. Methods in enzymology, vol. 381. New York: Academic; 2004. p. 335–54.
9. Rofstad EK, Gaustad JV, Egeland TA, Mathiesen B, Galappathi K. Tumors exposed to acute cyclic hypoxic stress show enhanced angiogenesis, perfusion and metastatic dissemination. Int J Cancer. 2010;127(7):1535–46.
10. Maftei CA, Bayer C, Shi K, Astner ST, Vaupel P. Quantitative assessment of hypoxia subtypes in microcirculatory supply units of malignant tumors using (immuno-)fluorescence techniques. Strahlenther Onkol. 2011;187(4):260–6.
11. Vaupel P, Mayer A. Hypoxia in tumors: pathogenesis-related classification, characterization of hypoxia subtypes, and associated biological and clinical implications. Adv Exp Med Biol. 2014;812:19–24.

12. Laderoute KR, Alarcon RM, Brody MD, Calaoagan JM, Chen EY, Knapp AM, Yun Z, Denko NC, Giaccia AJ. Opposing effects of hypoxia on expression of the angiogenic inhibitor thrombospondin 1 and the angiogenic inducer vascular endothelial growth factor. Clin Cancer Res. 2000;6(7):2941–50.
13. Semenza GL. Hydroxylation of HIF-1: oxygen sensing at the molecular level. Physiology (Bethesda). 2004;19:176–82.
14. Tatum JL, Kelloff GJ, Gillies RJ, Arbeit JM, Brown JM, Chao KS, Chapman JD, Eckelman WC, Fyles AW, Giaccia AJ, Hill RP, Koch CJ, Krishna MC, Krohn KA, Lewis JS, Mason RP, Melillo G, Padhani AR, Powis G, Rajendran JG, Reba R, Robinson SP, Semenza GL, Swartz HM, Vaupel P, Yang D, Croft B, Hoffman J, Liu G, Stone H, Sullivan D. Hypoxia: importance in tumor biology, noninvasive measurement by imaging, and value of its measurement in the management of cancer therapy. Int J Radiat Biol. 2006;82(10):699–757.
15. Weinmann M, Belka C, Guner D, Goecke B, Muller I, Bamberg M, Jendrossek V. Array-based comparative gene expression analysis of tumor cells with increased apoptosis resistance after hypoxic selection. Oncogene. 2005;24(38):5914–22.
16. Pawlus MR, Wang L, Hu CJ. STAT3 and HIF1[alpha] cooperatively activate HIF1 target genes in MDA-MB-231 and RCC4 cells. Oncogene. 2014;33(13):1670–9.
17. Bristow RG, Hill RP. Hypoxia and metabolism. Hypoxia, DNA repair and genetic instability. Nat Rev Cancer. 2008;8(3):180–92.
18. Sena JA, Wang L, Heasley LE, Hu C-J. Hypoxia regulates alternative splicing of HIF and non-HIF target genes. Mol Cancer Res. 2014;12:1233–43.
19. Sena JA, Wang L, Pawlus MR, Hu C-J. HIFs enhance the transcriptional activation and splicing of adrenomedullin. Mol Cancer Res. 2014;12(5):728–41.
20. Denko N, Wernke-Dollries K, Johnson AB, Hammond E, Chiang CM, Barton MC. Hypoxia actively represses transcription by inducing negative cofactor 2 (Dr1/DrAP1) and blocking preinitiation complex assembly. J Biol Chem. 2003;278(8):5744–9.
21. Denko NC, Fontana LA, Hudson KM, Sutphin PD, Raychaudhuri S, Altman R, Giaccia AJ. Investigating hypoxic tumor physiology through gene expression patterns. Oncogene. 2003;22(37):5907–14.
22. Tang X, Lucas JE, Chen JL, LaMonte G, Wu J, Wang MC, Koumenis C, Chi JT. Functional interaction between responses to lactic acidosis and hypoxia regulates genomic transcriptional outputs. Cancer Res. 2012;72(2):491–502.
23. Marotta D, Karar J, Jenkins WT, Kumanova M, Jenkins KW, Tobias JW, Baldwin D, Hatzigeorgiou A, Alexiou P, Evans SM, Alarcon R, Maity A, Koch C, Koumenis C. In vivo profiling of hypoxic gene expression in gliomas using the hypoxia marker EF5 and laser-capture microdissection. Cancer Res. 2011;71(3):779–89.
24. Koch CJ, Hahn SM, Rockwell Jr K, Covey JM, McKenna WG, Evans SM. Pharmacokinetics of EF5 [2-(2-nitro-1-H-imidazol-1-yl)-N-(2,2,3,3,3-pentafluoropropyl) acetamide] in human patients: implications for hypoxia measurements in vivo by 2-nitroimidazoles. Cancer Chemother Pharmacol. 2001;48(3):177–87.
25. Gross MW, Karbach U, Groebe K, Franko AJ, Mueller-Klieser W. Calibration of misonidazole labeling by simultaneous measurement of oxygen tension and labeling density in multicellular spheroids. Int J Cancer. 1995;61(4):567–73.
26. Vordermark D, Brown JM. Endogenous markers of tumor hypoxia predictors of clinical radiation resistance? Strahlenther Onkol. 2003;179(12):801–11.
27. Emmert-Buck MR, Bonner RF, Smith PD, Chuaqui RF, Zhuang Z, Goldstein SR, Weiss RA, Liotta LA. Laser capture microdissection. Science. 1996;274(5289):998–1001.
28. Suarez-Quian CA, Goldstein SR, Pohida T, Smith PD, Peterson JI, Wellner E, Ghany M, Bonner RF. Laser capture microdissection of single cells from complex tissues. Biotechniques. 1999;26(2):328–35.
29. Liu A. Laser capture microdissection in the tissue biorepository. J Biomol Tech. 2010;21(3):120–5.
30. Vandewoestyne M, Goossens K, Burvenich C, Van Soom A, Peelman L, Deforce D. Laser capture microdissection: should an ultraviolet or infrared laser be used? Anal Biochem. 2013;439(2):88–98.

31. Schroeder A, Mueller O, Stocker S, Salowsky R, Leiber M, Gassmann M, Lightfoot S, Menzel W, Granzow M, Ragg T. The RIN: an RNA integrity number for assigning integrity values to RNA measurements. BMC Mol Biol. 2006;7:3.
32. Ozsolak F, Milos PM. RNA sequencing: advances, challenges and opportunities. Nat Rev Genet. 2011;12(2):87–98.
33. Au KF, Underwood JG, Lee L, Wong WH. Improving PacBio long read accuracy by short read alignment. PLoS One. 2012;7(10):e46679.
34. Quail MA, Smith M, Coupland P, Otto TD, Harris SR, Connor TR, Bertoni A, Swerdlow HP, Gu Y. A tale of three next generation sequencing platforms: comparison of Ion Torrent, Pacific Biosciences and Illumina MiSeq sequencers. BMC Genomics. 2012;13:341.
35. Toung JM, Morley M, Li M, Cheung VG. RNA-sequence analysis of human B-cells. Genome Res. 2011;21(6):991–8.
36. Liu Y, Zhou J, White KP. RNA-seq differential expression studies: more sequence or more replication? Bioinformatics. 2014;30(3):301–4.
37. Alberts B, Johnson A, Lewis J, et al. Molecular biology of the cell. 4th ed. New York: Garland Science; 2002.
38. Levin JZ, Berger MF, Adiconis X, Rogov P, Melnikov A, Fennell T, Nusbaum C, Garraway LA, Gnirke A. Targeted next-generation sequencing of a cancer transcriptome enhances detection of sequence variants and novel fusion transcripts. Genome Biol. 2009;10(10):R115.
39. Li JB, Levanon EY, Yoon J-K, Aach J, LeProust E, Zhang K, Gao Y, Church GM. Genome-wide identification of human RNA editing sites by parallel DNA capturing and sequencing. Science (New York, NY). 2009;324(5931):1210–3.
40. Cock PJ, Fields CJ, Goto N, Heuer ML, Rice PM. The Sanger FASTQ file format for sequences with quality scores, and the Solexa/Illumina FASTQ variants. Nucleic Acids Res. 2010;38(6):1767–71.
41. Pruitt KD, Tatusova T, Maglott DR. NCBI Reference Sequence (RefSeq): a curated non-redundant sequence database of genomes, transcripts and proteins. Nucleic Acids Res. 2005;33(Database issue):D501–4.
42. Soneson C, Delorenzi M. A comparison of methods for differential expression analysis of RNA-seq data. BMC Bioinformatics. 2013;14(91).
43. Trapnell C, Pachter L, Salzberg SL. TopHat: discovering splice junctions with RNA-Seq. Bioinformatics. 2009;25(9):1105–11.
44. Wang K, Singh D, Zeng Z, Coleman SJ, Huang Y, Savich GL, He X, Mieczkowski P, Grimm SA, Perou CM, MacLeod JN, Chiang DY, Prins JF, Liu J. MapSplice: accurate mapping of RNA-seq reads for splice junction discovery. Nucleic Acids Res. 2010;38(18):e178.
45. Wu TD, Nacu S. Fast and SNP-tolerant detection of complex variants and splicing in short reads. Bioinformatics. 2010;26(7):873–81.
46. Trapnell C, Hendrickson DG, Sauvageau M, Goff L, Rinn JL, Pachter L. Differential analysis of gene regulation at transcript resolution with RNA-seq. Nat Biotechnol. 2013;31(1):46–53.
47. Trapnell C, Roberts A, Goff L, Pertea G, Kim D, Kelley DR, Pimentel H, Salzberg SL, Rinn JL, Pachter L. Differential gene and transcript expression analysis of RNA-seq experiments with TopHat and Cufflinks. Nat Protoc. 2012;7(3):562–78.
48. Trapnell C, Williams BA, Pertea G, Mortazavi A, Kwan G, van Baren MJ, Salzberg SL, Wold BJ, Pachter L. Transcript assembly and quantification by RNA-Seq reveals unannotated transcripts and isoform switching during cell differentiation. Nat Biotechnol. 2010;28(5):511–5.
49. Katz Y, Wang ET, Airoldi EM, Burge CB. Analysis and design of RNA sequencing experiments for identifying isoform regulation. Nat Methods. 2010;7(12):1009–15.
50. Shiraki T, Kondo S, Katayama S, Waki K, Kasukawa T, Kawaji H, Kodzius R, Watahiki A, Nakamura M, Arakawa T, Fukuda S, Sasaki D, Podhajska A, Harbers M, Kawai J, Carninci P, Hayashizaki Y. Cap analysis gene expression for high-throughput analysis of transcriptional starting point and identification of promoter usage. Proc Natl Acad Sci U S A. 2003;100(26):15776–81.
51. Churchman LS, Weissman JS. Nascent transcript sequencing visualizes transcription at nucleotide resolution. Nature. 2011;469(7330):368–73.
52. Ingolia NT, Lareau LF, Weissman JS. Ribosome profiling of mouse embryonic stem cells reveals the complexity and dynamics of mammalian proteomes. Cell. 2011;147(4):789–802.

Chapter 5
Gas Chromatography Coupled to Mass Spectrometry (GC–MS) to Study Metabolism in Cultured Cells

Fiona Grimm, Louise Fets, and Dimitrios Anastasiou

Abstract Cancer cells exhibit characteristic patterns of metabolic behaviour that can be exploited for therapeutic purposes. Conditions found within the tumour microenvironment, such as hypoxia and selective nutrient availability, are known to influence the metabolism of cancer and stromal cells. Understanding cancer metabolism requires the use of analytical methods that allow detection and quantification of many metabolites simultaneously. Gas chromatography–mass spectrometry (GC–MS) is a versatile method to quantify metabolite abundance and, in combination with stable isotope labelled compounds, can yield important insights into the activity of metabolic pathways in cancer cells. This chapter provides an overview of the use of GC–MS for metabolic analysis of adherent cancer cells with an emphasis on the technical background that should be taken into consideration when designing and executing GC–MS-based metabolomics experiments.

Keywords Cancer metabolism • Metabolomics • Stable isotopes • Cancer • Cell lines • GC–MS • Gas chromatography • Mass spectrometry • Chemical derivatisation

5.1 Introduction

Metabolism is fundamental for the function of all cells. Metabolic reaction sequences allow cells to convert nutrients from their environment into energy or use them in processes that support cellular functions [1]. Consequently, metabolic aberrations have been linked to various diseases including cancer [2]. Metabolic changes in cancer may, in part, reflect the particular physiological state of cancer cells, such as increased proliferation. However, increasing evidence suggests that major oncogenic pathways lead to convergent changes in metabolism that are essential for

F. Grimm • L. Fets • D. Anastasiou (✉)
Cancer Metabolism Laboratory, The Francis Crick Institute, Mill Hill,
The Ridgeway, London, NW7 1AA, UK
e-mail: fiona.grimm@crick.ac.uk; louise.fets@crick.ac.uk; dimitrios.anastasiou@crick.ac.uk

C. Koumenis et al. (eds.), *Tumor Microenvironment*, Advances in Experimental Medicine and Biology 899, DOI 10.1007/978-3-319-26666-4_5

cancer development and, in some tumours, mutations of metabolic enzymes alone can drive tumorigenesis [3].

Altered metabolism in cancer cells can impact various aspects of tumorigenesis, including enhanced proliferation, survival under stress and metastasis [3–6]. Conditions found within the tumour microenvironment, such as hypoxia and limitation of some nutrients, are known to influence metabolism in both cell-autonomous and non-cell-autonomous manners [7–12]. Understanding how metabolism is altered in cancer promises to yield fundamental insights into its role in tumorigenesis and, importantly, given that metabolic processes are largely catalysed by enzymes, which are amenable to manipulation by small molecules, metabolic pathways are likely to prove a rich source of potential therapeutic targets [13, 14]. Devising rational interventions to interfere with cancer metabolism necessitates the need for appropriate analytical methods that give a broad systematic overview of metabolic pathways.

Unlike other classes of biomolecules, such as proteins and ribonucleic acids, which have relatively similar properties within the class, metabolites have vastly divergent physicochemical characteristics. Therefore, diverse analytical protocols are warranted in order to extract and measure many metabolite classes from biological samples simultaneously [15–19]. This is particularly important when sample material is scarce and maximum information from each sample is desirable. Furthermore, information-rich datasets in combination with computational modelling (systems biology) can provide powerful novel insights that cannot be readily obtained from small-scale analyses of metabolites [20–22]. To this end, several analytical methods are currently being employed, each with its own advantages and disadvantages. *Metabolomics* is a term broadly used to describe experiments where the amounts of a large number of metabolites from a single sample are measured. Metabolomics experiments can provide the researcher with a snapshot of cellular metabolism and can give insight into how metabolite amounts change between different conditions (e.g. following treatment with a drug or after knockdown of a protein).

Recent technological advances in mass spectrometry have yielded relatively affordable instruments with increased sensitivity and resolution that are suitable for metabolomics [23, 24]. Mass spectrometry is used to determine the molecular mass of analytes and, in combination with analyte fragmentation, can provide structural information that aids the identification of small molecules in a sample. Given the complexity of biological material, mass spectrometry is often coupled to chromatography to reduce sample complexity. Gas chromatography coupled to mass spectrometry (GC–MS) has been used to study various classes of metabolites [25, 26]. Compared to other methods, GC–MS is more labour intensive, as it requires the derivatisation of analytes to allow their separation in the gas chromatography column (see Sect. 5.2.4); however, it provides a method to measure reliably several classes of metabolically important biomolecules, such as organic acids, amino acids and fatty acids in a robust and economical manner.

Unless a metabolite can be produced and consumed exclusively through a specific process, changes in metabolite concentrations alone are not always informative about the activity through a metabolic pathway. Stable isotope labelled compounds can be used to study metabolic pathway activity or *flux* [27]. In this approach, select atoms in a molecule that is used as a precursor for metabolism can be replaced with heavier, stable isotopes (e.g. ^{13}C, ^{15}N, ^{2}H). The fate of these atoms through intermediates in a metabolic pathway can be traced by the characteristic mass shift measured in the mass spectrometer. Quantitation of the rate by which these atoms are enriched in particular intermediates in a pathway can yield information about flux through this pathway [28, 29]. Whether stable isotope labelling data can be interpreted in a qualitative or quantitative manner is not only determined by the experimental question, but also by the experimental design. This discussion is outside of the scope of this chapter; however, more information can be found in [28, 30].

GC–MS metabolomics protocols encompass several steps, each of which can affect data quality and, ultimately, the success of the experiment. Furthermore, each of these steps often needs to be tailored to the specific experimental question to be addressed. Understanding the technical principles underlying each step and how a GC–MS instrument operates are essential for experimental design and troubleshooting potential problems. This chapter is intended to provide an overview of the technical background required when designing GC–MS metabolomics experiments, with researchers that employ this technique for the first time in mind.

5.2 Sample Preparation

5.2.1 Culture and Treatment of Cells for Metabolomics Experiments

5.2.1.1 Cell Numbers and Splitting

Similarly to other medium- and high-throughput methods, detection of the maximum possible number of metabolites from a single sample analysis is desirable. The ability to detect a broad range of metabolites with varying abundances relies considerably on instrument sensitivity and dynamic range. For cultured cancer cells, availability of material is not typically considered limiting as cell cultures can be scaled up as needed. However, both the sensitivity of different GC–MS instruments and the biomass content between cell lines may vary considerably, therefore, it is necessary to determine empirically the number of cells required for each sample. Determining an optimal cell number will allow the detection of a maximum number of features while generating the minimum number of saturated peaks (see Sect. 5.3.4.3). Table 5.1 gives examples of the approximate numbers of cells that work well for a number of different cell lines. Importantly, cells should be split at least 24 h prior to the experiment, in order to minimise disturbances to metabolism caused by cell splitting.

Table 5.1 Indicative numbers of cultured cell lines that yield amounts of metabolites suitable for one GC–MS sample analysis

Cell line	Cell type	Cell number
MCF7	Human breast adenocarcinoma	0.5×10^6
MCF10A	Human breast fibrocystic disease	0.6×10^6
HCC1569	Human breast metaplastic carcinoma	0.8×10^6
H1299	Human non-small cell lung carcinoma	0.3×10^6

5.2.1.2 Medium Composition and Medium Change Prior to Experiment

Medium composition is a critical determinant of cellular metabolism and should therefore be carefully adapted to suit the experimental question addressed. Concentrations of major media components, such as carbohydrates and amino acids, have been historically optimised to maximise cell proliferation, in particular taking into consideration that regular medium replenishment to maintain constant nutrient concentrations is impractical. However, excessively high nutrient concentrations (such as 10–25 mM glucose found in common media formulations) are likely to influence metabolism and should be adapted to reflect concentrations likely to be experienced by cells under physiological conditions.

Furthermore, medium should be replaced with fresh medium 24 h and again 1–2 h before cells are harvested or the experimental treatment is started. If pre-treatment of cells with a test drug is the aim of the experiment, pre-treatment can also be combined with these media changes. Following exposure to cells for 1–2 days, which is typical during routine cell culture, nutrients and growth factors in the medium are progressively depleted, while metabolic by-products (e.g. lactate) accumulate. Due to the continuous exchange of components between the medium and cells, such changes in medium composition may not be predictable or reproducible, but are likely to establish a metabolic state different to that of cells with fresh medium. This will be reflected in the metabolic profiles of cells harvested without prior medium change. Furthermore, metabolic and signalling changes can be induced when media are replaced. When the experimental design necessitates media change anyway (e.g. to add a stable isotope-labelled compound or a drug whose effects are to be tested), the additional media change prior to the actual treatment is still recommended as it ensures that any fluctuations in metabolism are less likely to stem from the shift from old to fresh medium, because the treatment medium composition is closer to the fresh culture medium.

When using stable isotope-labelled metabolites as precursors to assay the activity of a particular metabolic pathway, it is also necessary to think about the dilution of the labelled compound by the cognate unlabelled molecule from serum. Although it is simple to correct for a partially labelled metabolite precursor, if the relative contribution of this metabolite through a pathway of interest is low, higher precursor labelling increases the likelihood of detecting labelled derivative metabolites. These problems can be overcome by dialysing the serum before adding it to media. A molecular weight cut-off (MWCO) of 3500 is recommended as higher cut-offs may lead to growth factors being dialysed out, which can affect cell physiology and proliferation. Consideration should also be given on how media components could affect labelling of intracellular metabolites—for example, the presence of pyruvate in the media is likely to dilute any ^{13}C-glucose-derived label in intracellular glucose-derived pyruvate and downstream pathways such as TCA intermediates.

5.2.1.3 Number of Technical Replicates

Due to the many stages involved in metabolomics experiments, there are several steps at which variability can be introduced as a result of sample losses, degradation or a failed instrument run. Some metabolites are more susceptible to degradation than others so, dependent on which metabolites are of interest, more or fewer technical replicates are necessary to ensure confidence in the data. Power analysis after a pilot experiment should be used to decide on a suitable number of technical replicates. As an indication, five replicates typically provide reliable measurements across a large number of metabolites and can be used as a starting point when embarking on a new project.

5.2.1.4 Unlabelled Control Samples (Only Relevant for Tracer Experiments)

Heavy isotopes used for labelling can be found in nature to a greater or lesser extent, with ^{13}C-carbon accounting for approximately 1 % of all carbon atoms. In order to fully interpret ^{13}C-labelling data, the relative contribution of naturally occuring isotopes to the abundance of synthetic isotope-labelled ions should be corrected for, or 'stripped', from raw numbers. Taking into account the molecular formula of the fragment being examined (plus that of any derivatising agent, see Sect. 5.2.4), this can (and should) be calculated theoretically [31]. However, a replicate experiment where the tracer compound is replaced with unlabelled compound can also be used for this purpose. This approach should further be applied to confirm how well the stripping algorithm works. Detection of residual isotope-containing metabolite ions after stripping in samples without tracer may be indicative of the presence of a contaminating ion, precluding the use of this fragment for quantification, or that the fragment has been misidentified and the calculated/predicted molecular formula is incorrect (for more information on ion quantification from isotopically labelled samples see Sect. 5.4.2.3).

5.2.2 Harvesting Cells and Media Samples

How cells are harvested at the end of the experiment can have a major impact on the results obtained. A major consideration is that the time between cells being removed from the incubator and quenching of metabolism should be as minimal as practically possible. Other key points that warrant particular attention are discussed below.

5.2.2.1 Media Samples

Consumption and release of metabolites from and into the media, respectively, during the course of the experiment can provide a lot of information on cellular function [32]. Accurate pipetting of media volumes when added to cells is essential for meaningful measurements of metabolite concentrations in media. In the case of adherent cells, media samples are easy to obtain and can be analysed along with intracellular samples on the GC–MS. As soon as samples are removed from the incubator, they should be rapidly pipetted into pre-prepared microfuge tubes prior to further handling of the cells. These media samples can then be stored directly at −80 °C.

5.2.2.2 Cell Washing

Prior to metabolite extraction, the medium must be completely removed from the culture dish. Since media contain several metabolites also found in cells at high concentrations, even a small amount of medium left on the plate after aspiration can cause large errors in the quantitation of intracellular metabolite concentrations. By washing with phosphate-buffered saline (PBS), contaminating metabolites are removed and measurement accuracy is improved. However, it is important to consider how cellular metabolism could be affected by this washing step. Cells can respond extremely quickly to changes in their environment, potentially causing metabolome alterations [33]. Therefore, it might be more appropriate not to wash cells and instead to aspirate residual media and directly quench cellular metabolism, provided that media components do not interfere with the measurements at the heart of the experimental question.

Another issue to consider is whether to wash cells with ice-cold or room temperature PBS. Although rapid cooling of the plate will slow metabolism and therefore minimise physiological changes during harvesting, cold shock may also lead to metabolic artefacts. Again, this is something that should be evaluated on a case-by-case basis, with the nature of the experimental question in mind.

In all cases, it is important to remove the medium and complete the washing step as quickly as possible to minimise the potential issues described above. By pouring, instead of pipetting, the medium from the plate and pouring on PBS, it is possible to wash a plate twice within a few seconds, with only residual PBS requiring aspiration. This method works well for adherent cells, however, for cell lines that attach loosely on the plate and are susceptible to being washed off the plate, the washing steps have to be performed more carefully.

When performing large experiments, cell culture plates should be harvested in small batches of four to six plates, ideally in randomised order to eliminate experimental bias. By harvesting replicates of the same sample class in a randomised order, variability in these experimental steps will be spread evenly across all sample classes. This is particularly important in isotope labelling experiments and experiments with relatively short time points.

5.2.2.3 Quenching

To stop metabolism rapidly and completely, it is necessary to quench cells [34]. In mammalian cell cultures, this is typically achieved using extreme cold, such as liquid nitrogen [35] or by carrying out the extraction steps on dry ice (with pre-cooled extraction solvents). However, high temperature conditions for rapid quenching have been described in metabolomics experiments using yeast or bacterial cultures, e.g. by addition of hot ethanol [36]. Quenching metabolism by snap-freezing in liquid nitrogen immediately after washing followed by placing plates on dry ice during addition of pre-cooled methanol works effectively. At this point, particularly if many batches of plates require washing and quenching, plates can be stored at −80 °C until all batches have been processed.

5.2.3 Extraction of Metabolites and Sample Storage

5.2.3.1 Extraction Buffer Composition and Temperature

Given the vast diversity of intracellular metabolites, different solvents and protocols may be appropriate, dependent on the experimental question. Even when aiming for an extraction method that gives the best overview of cellular metabolism, there are a plethora of extraction options. Buffers based on a mixture of methanol, water and chloroform are widely used and allow consistent extraction and separation of a broad range of both polar and apolar metabolites.

5.2.3.2 Metabolite Extraction and Phase Separation

Cells can be removed from the plate, by scraping with a rubber-tipped cell scraper. Trypsinisation is not recommended, as it requires time and leads to significant metabolite leakage [37]. By scraping with chilled methanol and on a bed of dry ice, the extraction begins at the same time as the cells are quenched. Typically, 4.5 parts methanol are added to the plate, cells are scraped and transferred to a microfuge tube that contains 1 part chloroform. Methanol extraction is repeated with the same volume (4.5 parts equivalent) to ensure quantitative removal of the cells from the plate. For a 6-cm dish, a total final volume of 1.8 ml works well (2 × 810 μl methanol + 180 μl chloroform); however, this should be adjusted proportionally to the size of the plate used. Samples are then sonicated in a cooled water bath (3 × 8 min) to fully break up any large protein aggregates and improve extraction efficiency, and stored overnight at 4 °C. Precipitated cell debris is then pelleted by centrifugation (18–20,000 × *g*, 10 min, 4 °C), and supernatant can be stored at −80 °C. The final ratio of 9:1 (v/v) methanol/chloroform used here has been shown to be effective in the extraction of a broad range of metabolites [35], but is not biphasic, and therefore polar and apolar metabolites are still combined. To allow phase separation, samples are dried down under a nitrogen stream or in a vacuum concentrator. They can then be resuspended in 1:3:3 (v/v) chloroform/methanol/water, to partition polar metabolites into the upper, aqueous phase and apolar metabolites into the lower, organic phase.

5.2.3.3 Internal Standards

The use of an internal standard can be helpful for both relative and absolute quantification of metabolites. Spiking biological samples with a known amount of internal standard can be used to correct for losses during sample preparation. As with extraction conditions, there is no one perfect internal standard, and ideally, one should use a reference compound of a similar chemical nature to the metabolites of interest. It is essential that the metabolite standard itself is not present in the biological sample, therefore unnatural metabolites, such as *nor*-leucine, *nor*-valine or isotopically labelled essential amino acids (e.g. valine) are good options. For general applications, *scyllo*-inositol (1 mM stock in water, stored at −20 °C, used at 1 nmol per sample), a stereoisomer of inositol, can be used. *Scyllo*-inositol separates well chromatographically from endogenous *myo*-inositol in samples, and also has a good *relative molar response factor* (see Sect. 5.4.2.2). Before using the internal standard the first time, it is important to verify that it cannot be detected in the samples of interest. For example, while *scyllo*-inositol is undetectable in breast cancer cell lines, it has previously been detected in human brain samples [38] and would not be an appropriate internal standard for metabolomic analysis of this tissue.

For analysis of apolar samples, it is necessary to use a separate, apolar standard compound. Again, preliminary analysis of which metabolites are present in any given sample type is vital, but for breast cancer cell lines, lauric acid containing a ^{13}C-labelled carbon at position 1 is useful (10 mM stock in chloroform, stored at −80 °C, used at 20 nmol per sample).

To obtain absolute quantification of a metabolite by GC–MS, its amount should be compared to a known amount of a reference compound that has been added to the analyte sample and has identical chemical and physical characteristics but a different mass so that is it distinguishable from the analyte itself, i.e. an isotopically labelled metabolite standard. This accounts, among others, for extraction, derivatisation and ionisation efficiency, which vary between compounds dependent on which functional groups are present (see Sect. 5.4.2 for further details). Practically, this is not always feasible for metabolomics experiments with very complex samples, but can be addressed (when doing unlabelled experiments) by the full labelling of the entire metabolome of yeast, for example with ^{13}C, and using this as an internal standard [39].

5.2.4 Sample Derivatisation

Gas chromatography requires analytes to be in the gaseous phase when they enter the chromatography column (see Sect. 5.3.1.2). Since many of the most sought after metabolites are highly polar, they show poor volatility and the high temperatures required for them to vaporise can lead to thermal instability. It is therefore necessary to derivatise metabolites with compounds that reduce polarity and improve volatility. The most commonly used derivatisation technique is silylation, and this will be discussed further in the section below.

5.2.4.1 Sample Drying

During *silylation*, active hydrogens in –NH, –OH and –SH groups are replaced with a trimethylsilyl group (discussed further in Sect. 5.2.4.3). This reaction is very sensitive to water, which can significantly reduce reaction yield, so complete drying of the sample before derivatisation is vital.

To minimise the amount of derivatisation agent, the samples are typically dried down in conical glass vial inserts using a vacuum evaporator (1500 rpm, 40 °C, 3–4 h). The conical inserts also facilitate efficient sample aspiration by the autosampler injection syringe (see Sect. 5.3.1.1). Samples should not be kept at high temperatures for any longer than necessary to avoid sample decomposition. Once dry, vials are washed twice with 40 μl of methanol to remove any traces of aqueous solvent.

5.2.4.2 Oximation

Many polar metabolites have low thermal stability and low volatility. The first step in the derivatisation process, therefore, is the reaction of the dried metabolites with methoxyamine HCl in pyridine. This results in the *oximation* of most carbonyl groups. Addition of the methoxime group allows a resonance structure to be formed that displaces electron density onto the N-bound carbon, which therefore reduces its reactive potential (see Fig. 5.1).

As well as increasing stability of metabolites, oximation can also reduce the complexity of the sample. For example, monosaccharides exist in both linear and cyclic forms. The cyclic forms tend to predominate, and multiple stereoisomers can be formed. D-glucose, for example, can exist as α-D-glucopyranose, β-D-glucopyranose, α-D-glucofuranose or β-D-glucofuranose, therefore potentially giving rise to four distinct chromatographic peaks. Only the linear form contains a carbonyl group, which can be converted to an oxime that, in turn, prevents sugar cyclisation. Methoximation, therefore, results in the accumulation of all glucose molecules into

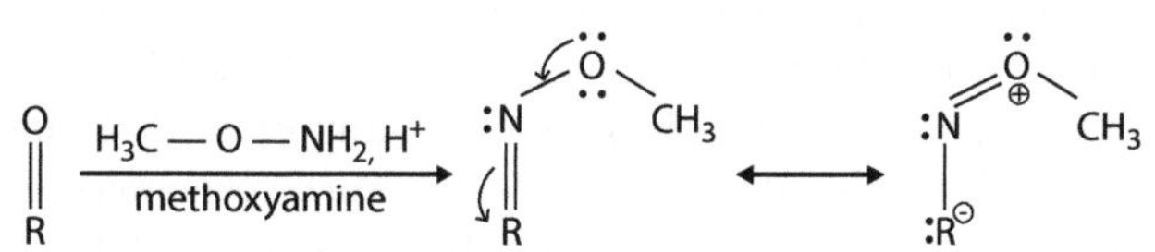

Fig. 5.1 Methoximation. Mechanism of methoximation of aldehyde and ketone groups, and demonstration of how resonance structure provides stabilisation

the linear form, reducing complexity by resulting in just two glucose peaks due to two methoxime stereoisomers [40].

To set up the oximation reaction, samples are resuspended in 20 μl of 20 mg/ml methoxyamine-HCl in pyridine (a full list of reagents can be found in Sect. 5.5.2) and briefly mixed by vortexing before allowing the reaction to continue overnight at room temperature to ensure that it has reached completion. It should be noted that methoxyamine is used rather than hydroxylamine, since the latter would lead to the formation of an additional alcohol group that could subsequently be silylated. Using methoxyamine, only native activated hydrogens are silylated in the second step of derivatisation [41].

5.2.4.3 Silylation

To increase volatility of metabolites, polar groups can be modified by the addition of a protecting group, thereby minimising dipole–dipole interactions. The most commonly used derivatisation method in GC–MS involves the addition of a silyl group to active hydrogens in groups such as –OH, –NH and –SH, a process known as *silylation*. Under the umbrella of silylation, there are many reagent choices, which have varying silyl donor power and add slightly different protecting groups. A comprehensive review of these reagents can be found in Zaikan and Halket's "A Handbook of Derivatives for Mass Spectrometry" [41].

Within this plethora of silylation reagents, the two most commonly used protecting groups are trimethylsilyl (TMS) and *tert*-butyldimethylsilyl (TBDMS). Derivatives containing these protecting groups can be generated using *N*,*O*-bis(trimethylsilyl)trifluoroacetamide (BSTFA) + 1 % trimethylchlorosilane (TMCS, used as a catalyst) or *N*-methyl-*N*-(*tert*-butyldimethylsilyl)trifluoroacetamide (MTBSTFA) + 1 % *tert*-butyldimethylchlorosilane (TBDMCS as a catalyst) respectively (see Fig. 5.2 for details). Both types of derivatisation agents react with a range of functional groups, albeit with varying efficiency. TBDMS derivatives have been shown to be generally more stable against hydrolysis, however, due to the significantly bulkier functional group, TBDMS is less efficient in the derivatisation of more sterically hindered active hydrogens, such as tertiary alcohols or axial groups in sugar rings [41]. Like in other aspects of metabolomics, selection of the most suitable reagent is ultimately dependent on the experimental question and the specific metabolites of interest. In general, TMS derivatisation gives a good coverage of acids, amino acids, alcohols and sugars and is stable for at least 24 h, making it amenable to long sample queues (see Sect. 5.3.2).

To derivatise, 20 μl of BSTFA + 1 % TCMS are added to the methoximated samples, and briefly mixed by vortexing. The reaction proceeds for 1 h at room temperature, during which blanks are run on the GC–MS (see Sect. 5.3.2). All silyl derivatives are susceptible to hydrolysis, so it is important that vials are capped tightly (using a lid with a self-sealing septum, which can be penetrated by the injection needle) as rapidly as possible after addition of the silylating agent.

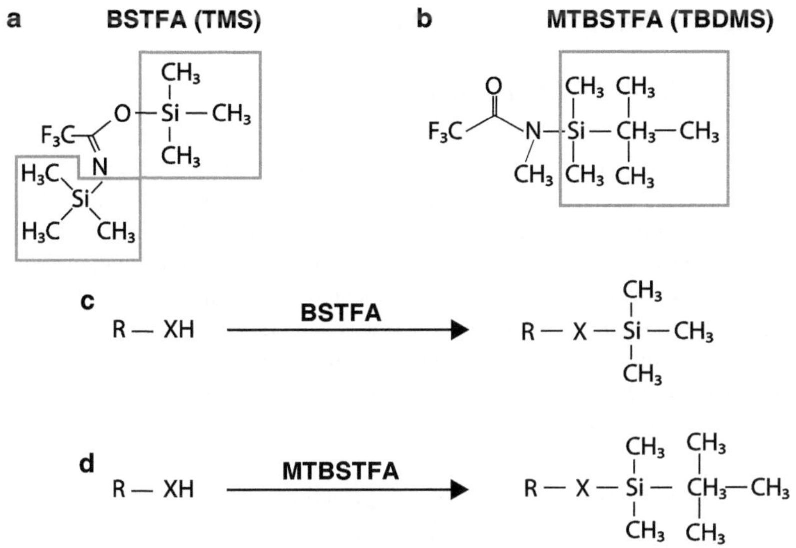

Fig. 5.2 Silylation. (**a**) Structure of BSTFA with TMS groups highlighted in *grey boxes*. (**b**) Structure of MTBSTFA with TBDMS groups highlighted in *grey boxes*. (**c**) Derivatisation of an active hydrogen (X refers to either N, O or S) with BSTFA. (**d**) Derivatisation of an active hydrogen (X refers to either N, O or S) with MTBSTFA

5.2.4.4 Lipids

Analysis of lipids is a very large field within itself, with dedicated protocols for each of the steps described above, dependent on which classes of lipids are studied. It is possible, however, to get some basic insights into the fatty acid content of cellular lipids by using biphasic extraction (Sect. 5.2.3.2) and analysis of the organic phase, where lipids partition. Volatile methyl-ester derivatives of fatty acids from the apolar fraction can be obtained by a trans-esterification reaction using a reagent such as Meth-Prep II (Fisher Scientific). With this method, information on fatty acid chain length, saturation and isotopic labelling can be obtained, although information about the class of the lipid (triglyceride, phospholipid, cholesterol ester, etc.) before trans-esterification is lost. In combination with solid phase extraction to separate lipid classes prior to trans-esterification, it is possible to elucidate fatty acid content for each of these lipid classes separately [42].

To derivatise, the apolar fraction is dried down and subsequently resuspended in 25 μl of 2:1 (v/v) chloroform–methanol. After addition of 7 μl of Meth-Prep II reagent, samples are vortexed briefly and left at room temperature for an hour before analysis by GC–MS.

5.3 Sample Analysis by GC–MS

5.3.1 The GC–MS Instrument

The basic structure of a GC–MS instrument is outlined as a schematic shown in Fig. 5.3. Samples are aspirated from their respective vials and injected into the instrument by the autosampler (automatic liquid sampler, ALS). In the injector, analytes are vaporised and then swept onto the capillary gas chromatography (GC) column by the carrier gas. The column is located in a temperature-controlled oven and connected to the mass spectrometer (mass selective detector, MSD). After elution from the column, analytes are ionised in the ion source by electrospray ionisation (EI) and the resulting fragment ions are subsequently separated according to their mass-to-charge ratio (*m/z*) by a single quadrupole mass filter. An electron

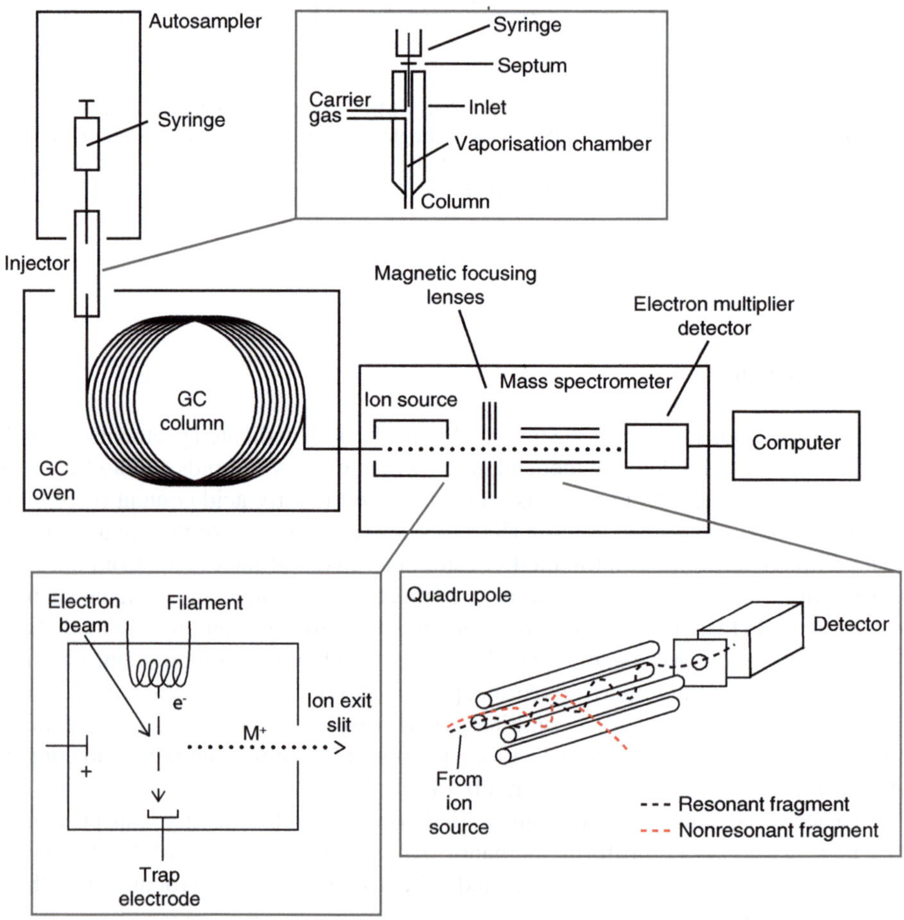

Fig. 5.3 Schematic overview of a typical GC–MS instrument configuration

multiplier detector (EMD) detects ion fragments that reach the detector and ion counts are stored and analysed in a connected computer.

Various manufacturers produce GC–MS instruments. For the purposes of this chapter, our discussion will be based on the use of an Agilent GC–MS instrument (components listed in Sect. 5.5.3.) and associated software; however, the general principles are applicable to a wide range of GC–MS instruments and data analysis packages.

5.3.1.1 Sample Injection

The sample is aspirated from the vial into the ALS syringe and injected into the GC injection port (inlet) through a self-sealing, replaceable septum. Pre-programmed ALS syringe washes before and after injection of samples ensure minimal sample carry-over (recommended washes—hexane: 3 × 8 μl pre-injection and 6 × 8 μl post-injection, methanol: 3 × 8 μl post-injection). A constant septum purge flow (3 ml/min, helium carrier gas) sweeps across the bottom of the septum and the top of the inlet to prevent septum bleed from entering the GC column and instead discards it through a purge vent. Once in the inlet, the liquid sample is immediately vaporised and swept onto the column by mixing with the carrier gas. To achieve complete vaporisation and to ensure all components reach the MS without condensing, the inlet temperature needs to be above the boiling point of the least volatile component to be analysed. Since very high temperatures can cause thermal decomposition, the inlet temperature needs to be optimised in order to maximise vaporisation and to minimise decomposition.

The injector contains a replaceable glass tube (liner), which is chemically inert and reduces the interaction (i.e. absorption or decomposition) of the injected compounds with the metal inlet. In addition, it contains deactivated glass wool, which traps non-volatile compounds and prevents them from entering the GC column, thereby extending the column lifetime and reducing contamination. It also has a taper, which is important to funnel the analyte gas onto the column entrance to reduce their residence time in the hot inlet and prevent chemical decomposition. Residence time is a function of the liner volume and total flow rate through the inlet (total flow rate will be discussed in Sect. 5.3.1.2). Therefore, inlet liner volume and diameter are other important parameters to consider for the sample residence time in the inlet [43].

Typically, 8 μl of sample are aspirated into the ALS syringe and 1–2 μl are injected at a dispense rate of 1 μl/s in splitless mode, at an inlet temperature of 270 °C. Typical inlet volumes are ~1 ml (for the instrument used in our lab: internal diameter 4 mm, volume 900 μl), so a maximum injection volume of 2 μl should not be exceeded due to expansion of the solvent during vaporisation. If the volume of the vaporised sample exceeds the inlet volume, backflash occurs and part of the sample will escape through the top of the inlet or contaminate the carrier gas line. Backflash should therefore be avoided as it can lead to poor reproducibility. 0.5 min after injection the inlet is purged with carrier gas (40 ml/min) to a split vent to remove residual sample in the inlet and minimise sample carry-over.

A split valve connected to the inlet controls how much of the sample volume is allowed to reach the column. The preferred method of sample introduction for the analysis of trace components is injection in splitless mode, where nearly the entire sample volume is injected onto the column [43]. Splitless injection results in high sensitivity and a low detection limit but can also lead to column overloading and detector saturation if the sample is too concentrated. If this is the case, diluting the final sample, or using less starting material for sample preparation, are recommended. How overloaded peaks and detector saturation can be recognised will be discussed in Sect. 5.3.4. A detailed discussion on issues related to sample injection can be found in [44].

5.3.1.2 Chromatography Column and Factors Influencing Metabolite Separation

Chromatographic separation of the injected compounds occurs as a result of differential interaction of compounds with the stationary phase of the GC column [45]. The stationary phase is a porous material with a large surface area for interactions with compounds in the sample. Analytes are carried through the column by a chemically inert gas (carrier gas) that plays the role of the mobile phase. Helium is most commonly used as carrier because of its low viscosity, which aids good chromatographic separation.

Most stationary phases consist of high molecular weight, thermally stable polymers. Polysiloxanes, which are liquid polymers, are among the most commonly used materials of this type because of their stability, robustness and versatility. We typically use a relatively low polarity DB-5ms column, packed with phenyl arylene polymer, which is equivalent to a commonly used (5 %-Phenyl)-methylpolysiloxane phase but exhibits lower column bleed. This is because the arylene polymer is stronger and stiffer, due to the incorporation of a phenyl group into the polysiloxane backbone, leading to less degradation at higher temperatures and greater inertness. Column bleed is the background continuously generated by the column through elution of stationary phase degradation products. Its intensity increases at higher temperatures and a typical bleed profile can be obtained by running a blank sample (see Sect. 5.3.4.1 and Fig. 5.4a).

The degree of chromatographic separation is dependent on various parameters, including column material and diameter, column length, column temperature and temperature gradient length. Longer columns generally achieve higher chromatographic resolution. Another critical factor affecting peak resolution is the flow rate of the mobile phase, which needs to be slow enough to allow sufficient time for interaction of the analytes with the stationary phase. Column temperature influences both the flow rate of the carrier gas and the degree analytes exist in gas phase. At high column temperatures, analytes with low boiling temperatures spend more time in gas phase, thereby interacting for less time with the stationary phase leading to their rapid elution with poor resolution. Conversely, low column temperatures lead to prolonged retention of analytes with high boiling points. Consequently, precise control

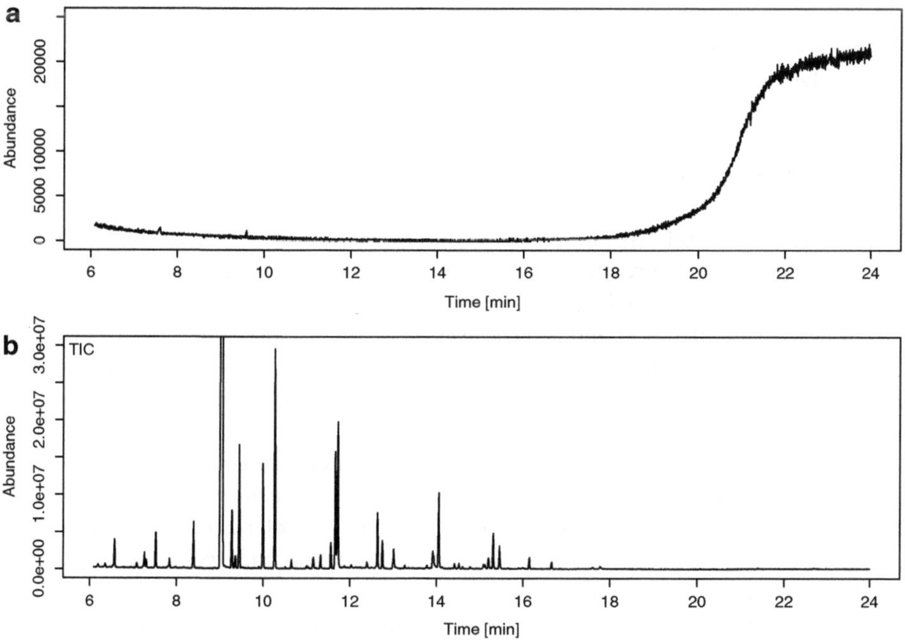

Fig. 5.4 Examples of total ion current chromatograms (TICs). (**a**) Example TIC of a hexane blank to illustrate the column bleed profile. Typical column bleed profiles show a flat baseline at lower temperatures, which rises between 19 and 21 min, corresponding to temperatures between 282.5 and 320 °C, starting at ~40 °C below the upper temperature limit of the column. The background levels continue to rise until upper temperature of 320 °C is reached at 21 min followed by a flat baseline. Times and temperatures are specific to the method routinely used in our lab (see Sect. 5.3.2) and therefore only indicative as they may vary between instruments and labs. (**b**) Example TIC of a polar metabolite cell extract. 0.4×10^6 MCF7 breast cancer cells were harvested 24 h after seeding, polar metabolites were extracted using H_2O:MeOH:$CHCl_3$ (1:3:1) containing 1 nmol of the internal standard *scyllo*-inositol, and subjected to methoximation and TMS derivatisation prior to analysis by GC–MS

of column temperature is important for reproducible chromatography. To this end, the chromatography column is located within a temperature-controlled oven that allows a gradual increase ("ramping") of the column temperature during the chromatography run. Temperature ramping allows the gradual separation of compounds with increasing boiling points at good resolution. This is particularly important for efficient separation of complex metabolite mixes extracted from cells that have a broad range of boiling points. As the ideal flow rate is directly related to the rate of temperature ramping (with faster ramping rates generally requiring higher flow rates), the carrier gas flow rate has to be adjusted in line with column temperature. For a 30 m column, the typical flow rate is set to 0.9 ml/min but is automatically adjusted by the operating software to shorter column lengths after routine column trimming (see Sect. 5.3.4.1). During the cooling down period after a run, the post-run flow rate is set to 1.5 ml/min at a column oven temperature of 70 °C to prevent accumulation of moisture.

In order to maximise column lifetime, it is crucial to reduce contamination by using an appropriate injection port liner (see Sect. 5.3.1.1) and by adding a bake-out step at the end of every run to elute high-boiling point contaminants (see Sect. 5.3.2.2).

5.3.1.3 Ionisation and Separation by *m*/*z*

The GC column outlet is connected to the ion source by a transfer line, which is heated to 280 °C to prevent the eluting compounds from condensing. Gaseous compounds eluting from the GC column first have to be ionised before they can be separated by the MS. Soft and hard ionisation methods exist, which result in low or high degrees of ion fragmentation, respectively. A broadly used ionisation method is Electron Impact (EI) ionisation. EI takes place at the ion source and involves the collision of the eluted neutral molecules with electrons emitted from a heated filament (230 °C, 70 eV), leading to the loss of an electron from the analyte. The resulting charged species, which is referred to as the *molecular ion*, is unstable and breaks down to produce smaller fragment ions via predictable chemical rearrangement pathways. As a result, a characteristic fragment ion fingerprint is produced for each compound, which is used for metabolite identification (see Sect. 5.4.1). Electron Impact (EI) is a hard ionisation technique, which means that the resulting mass spectrum will mainly contain fragment ions and the molecular ion will usually not be visible. Milder ionisation methods, such as chemical ionisation (CI), can be used if detection of the molecular ion is warranted.

Following ionisation, the resulting ions are pushed away from the source and through ion-focussing lenses into the mass analyser by the positive voltage on a repeller electrode. The mass analyser separates ions according to their mass-to-charge ratio (*m*/*z*). Quadrupole mass analysers, consisting of four oppositely charged rod electrodes, scan through the specified mass range (in our standard method: 50–565 *m*/*z*) by applying radio frequencies that stabilise the trajectory of a specific *m*/*z* value (resonant fragments). Quadrupoles are commonly used mass analysers because they are inexpensive and easy to use, while having relatively low maintenance requirements, high sensitivity and a fast scan rate. In addition, they only require a moderate vacuum, which is why it is feasible to connect them to a GC. Compared to other mass analysers, however, they have limited mass resolution and mass range.

In addition to scan mode, mass analysers can also be used in a targeted mode known as SIM (single ion monitoring). In SIM mode, the mass analyser measures only specified *m*/*z* values, while all other ions are not scanned for. Consequently, a greater amount of the selected ion can reach the detector per scan, thereby affording SIM measurements higher sensitivity and a lower detection limit for the specified ions at the expense of losing information for other ions. SIM mode is therefore only recommended for follow-up experiments where only specific ions of interest need to be measured with higher sensitivity.

5.3.1.4 Ion Detection

Ion detection involves the conversion of ions that reach the detector into electrons (electric current) and the processing of the resulting signal. An electron multiplier detector (EMD) additionally amplifies the electronic signal to increase signal intensity. The degree of signal amplification (gain) is controlled by the voltage that is applied to the first dynode of the EM (electron multiplier voltage, EMV). The sensitivity of the detector decreases over time due to accumulation of contamination and the EMV setting therefore has to be gradually increased to reach the same signal intensities (see Sect. 5.3.1.4) [46].

5.3.2 GC–MS Analysis of Samples

5.3.2.1 Preparing the Instrument for a Sample Run: Performance Checks, Tuning and Calibration

Instrument performance checks immediately prior to sample runs, in conjunction with regular long-term instrument maintenance, are essential to obtain high quality GC–MS data. Detailed instructions can usually be found in the manufacturer's manuals, but several important points will be highlighted in this section.

The inlet liner needs to be changed on a regular basis since it becomes contaminated with non-volatile compounds over time. Its lifetime depends on instrument usage and the complexity of sample matrices, but it should be changed at least once per month. The same is true for injection port septa, which are worn out by repeated injections. Standard septa last between 100 and 200 injections until their self-sealing capacity is lost but septa with longer life times are available (see Sect. 5.3.1.1). Leaky septa will lead to sample loss and negatively affect sensitivity.

Before every use, the MS has to be *calibrated* and *tuned* [47]. Both of these adjustments are done automatically and simultaneously during execution of an auto-tune programme, which needs to run daily or before the start of every sample queue. Before starting the auto-tune programme, the MS must be at an acceptable vacuum and vials containing solvents for needle washes (usually hexane and methanol) need to be refilled. In addition, helium gas levels in the gas cylinder need to be checked and replaced before the cylinder is completely empty.

Calibration is the adjustment of the quadrupole frequency so that each point on the *m*/*z* axis of the spectrum corresponds to the expected mass fragment from a calibration compound. PFTBA (perfluoro-*tert*-butylamine) is a volatile liquid typically used for calibration, which fragments into characteristic ions (mainly $m/z = 69$, 219 and 302).

Tuning, on the other hand, ensures that the fragments generated from the calibration compound have the expected relative signal intensities by adjusting the repeller, ion focusing lens and electron multiplier voltages. For PFTBA, the ratio of *m*/*z* 69:219:302 ion peaks should, ideally, be 1:4:10. After execution of the auto-tune programme, the user should additionally check for gas leaks in the tune report. Gas leaks are typically caused by worn-out septa or loose column nuts and can be stopped by septum replacement and column nut tightening before a blank sample and re-tuning.

In summary, parameters to monitor in the MSD auto-tune report and common fixes are:

Gas leaks—Replace septa and tighten column nuts if gas leaks of >5 % are detected. Prolonged oxygen exposure is a major cause of column damage.

Rising repeller voltage—Clean the ion source.

Unusually high EMV needed to detect calibration peaks—Possibly indicative of detector contamination or damage. Operating the detector at very high levels of gain should be avoided to extend EM lifetime.

5.3.2.2 The GC Chromatography Method

The GC chromatography method is specified in a method file (file extension .M in the case of Agilent software). The method file contains all necessary instrument settings for sample injection, chromatography, ionisation, separation and detection as well as communication between the instrument parts to ensure exact timing.

A mixture of analytes with different retention times can be resolved by gas chromatography into, ideally, non-overlapping peaks by gradually raising (ramping) the GC oven temperature, resulting in a linear temperature gradient. Slower temperature ramping usually achieves better resolution but causes longer analysis times. In our experience, a useful trade-off between peak resolution and sample throughput (as explained in Sect. 5.3.1.2) is afforded by a 24-min gradient consisting of four distinct chromatography steps:

Initial hold—After loading the sample onto the column, the GC oven is held at the starting temperature of 70 °C for 2 min to equilibrate the system. The starting temperature needs to be above the boiling point of the sample solvent but below the boiling point of the analyte mix.

Ramp 1—The GC oven temperature rises from 70 to 295 °C between minutes 2–20 at 12.5 °C/min. During this time, analytes are moved along the column by the carrier gas and sequentially elute from the column. This part of the chromatogram contains most metabolite peaks.

Ramp 2—The GC oven temperature rises from 295 to 320 °C between minutes 20–21 at 25 °C/min. Only few, highly polar metabolites will elute from the column at such high temperatures.

Final hold/column bake out—The temperature is held at 320 °C for 3 min to 'clean' the column. This step reduces sample carry-over into the next run. The bake out temperature needs to be above the boiling point of least volatile sample components to completely clean the column. However, the temperature should not be high enough to cause thermal column damage.

5.3.2.3 Sample Queue Design

At the beginning of each sample queue, the GC column needs to be conditioned until a stable baseline is reached. Every sample queue should therefore start with one to two hexane blanks, followed by quality control (QC) or standard mixes that contain metabolites of interest, to equilibrate the column. Hexane blanks should also be scheduled after every five to seven samples throughout the queue.

To be able to identify metabolites with a high level of confidence, pure standard metabolites need to be analysed for comparison with the biological samples. Initially, standards should be run individually and at different concentrations, which also aids with determining the limit of detection for each metabolite by the instrument. After determining optimal concentration for each standard, they can be combined into *standard mixes*, to generate non-overlapping chromatography peaks. If metabolites of interest overlap, several standard mixes should be prepared. The standard mix(es) should be analysed multiple times per queue, for example at the beginning and at the end (and, depending on the length of the queue, in the middle) to control for sample/derivatisation stability. Samples can also be mixed (pooled) together and used as QC samples throughout the queue, but since GC–MS chromatograms are normally very reproducible this is not always necessary. If, however, the user wishes to include QC samples, the QC sample mix should be divided into separate vials and each vial used only once per injection. This is because multiple penetrations of the septum on the sample vial cap by the syringe will lead to deterioration and incomplete sealing of the cap septum. This can lead to rapid evaporation of the solvent through the damaged vial cap, which will affect metabolite concentrations in the QC sample.

To minimise the effect of variations in instrument performance, such as decreasing sensitivity over time due to contamination of the source, sample queues should always be randomised. Sample randomisation eliminates bias by ensuring that every experimental condition or sample type is affected equally by technical variability. For small sets, randomisation is relatively simple and can often be done within the vendor software that generates the sample queue. For larger sample sets, a randomised block design should be considered [48]. For a detailed discussion on statistics in experimental design see [49].

5.3.3 *m/z Measurement and Data Quality Control*

5.3.3.1 The Mass Spectrum

Ions derived from column eluents (incl. column bleed) at a particular time point of a sample run are scanned through the quadrupole and are displayed as a *mass spectrum*. The mass spectrum is a plot of m/z *vs.* relative ion abundance. An example of a mass spectrum is shown in Fig. 5.5. Reflecting the resolution capacity of the quadrupole mass analyser, m/z values are usually binned into 1 m/z intervals, which is why the mass spectrum is not a continuous trace but rather a needle graph. In our standard

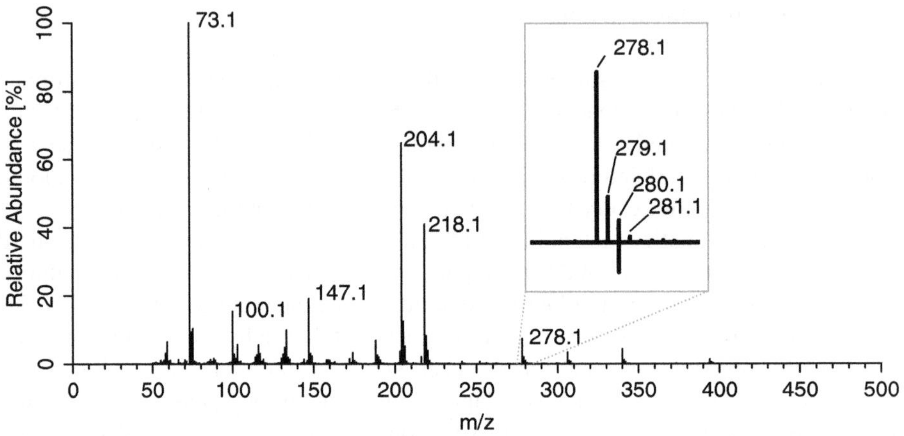

Fig. 5.5 Example of a mass spectrum. The most intense peak in the spectrum, known as the *base* peak (*m*/*z* 73), is set to 100 %. *m*/*z* 73 and 147 are contaminating ions from the TMS derivatisation agent. *m*/*z* 204 and 218 correspond to fragments of the eluting compound (in this case: serine)

method, *m*/*z* scanning is from *m*/*z* 50 to 565 with the lower mass range limit set to *m*/*z* 50 to avoid detection of traces of water (*m*/*z* 18), nitrogen (*m*/*z* 34) and oxygen (*m*/*z* 36) on the spectra.

5.3.3.2 The Total Ion Current Chromatogram (TIC)

An overview of each sample run can be obtained by plotting the *total ion current chromatogram* (often referred to simply as *TIC*). The TIC is generated by summing up all ion intensities of the same scan and plotting the total ion intensity against retention time. The TIC is very informative about the overall quality of the run. Example of typical TICs of a hexane blank and of a polar metabolite extract from MCF7 cells are shown in Fig. 5.4a and 5.4b, respectively. The start of the TIC trace at 6 min reflects a delay in ionisation and *m*/*z* scanning (solvent delay), which is scheduled in our standard method to avoid the solvent front in the TIC and to protect the ionisation filament. The TIC of blank runs is a useful indicator of column performance (discussed in Sect. 5.3.4.1). In the sample TIC, the large peak around 9 min typically corresponds to excess derivatisation agent and phosphate contamination (*m*/*z* 299) from PBS washes. From the TIC, using the analysis software, selected ion chromatograms (SIC) for a single *m*/*z* value can be extracted. Alternatively, SICs can be generated directly by running the GC/MS in fixed-mass SIM mode (see Sect. 5.3.1.3). If an ion is specific for a single compound (and not shared by classes of compounds, like *m*/*z* 205, 217 and 319 for TMS-derivatised hexoses, and *m*/*z* 218 for TMS-derivatised amino acids) the SIC can represent the chromatogram for this compound.

5.3.4 Instrument Maintenance, Quality Control and Troubleshooting

5.3.4.1 Column Performance

Given the importance of retention time and instrument sensitivity for reproducible identification and quantitation of metabolites, it is important to monitor regularly indicators of column quality deterioration. Towards this end, TICs of blank sample runs are very useful. A typical column bleed profile obtained from a blank run is shown in Fig. 5.4a and should have the following features:

- Flat baseline at lower temperatures
- Sharp rise at 30–40 °C below the upper temperature limit of the column
- Continued signal rise until upper temperature is reached
- Flat baseline when holding upper temperature

Major deviations from this profile (i.e. visible peaks) are likely due to contaminants, either originating from previously run samples or instrument parts, such as the septum. The levels of column bleed will inevitably increase during a column's lifetime but a rapid increase is usually caused by damage (e.g. prolonged heating to temperature limit, oxygen exposure via a leak or injection of damaging chemical compounds).

The accumulation of non-volatile contaminants at the inlet end of the column leads to peak shape distortions. Therefore, as part of the regular maintenance, short pieces of the column need to be removed (a.k.a. *column trimming*), using a ceramic wafer, to restore its performance. Since the column flow rate needs to be adjusted to the column length, the actual column length needs to be recorded in the GC–MS operating software.

Permanent background that is not caused by column bleed is usually independent of GC oven temperature and usually comes from the MS. If the background signal can still be detected at 50 °C, the ion source and the quadrupole should be cleaned [47]. A list of typical contaminants can be found in [47].

5.3.4.2 Column Capacity and Overloaded Peaks

The capacity of a column corresponds to the amount of analyte that can be introduced without significant peak distortion. Column capacity for a specific compound depends on the properties of the solid phase as well as the compound's retention time. The column generally has a lower capacity for analytes that elute later compared to earlier, so column capacity for each metabolite must be determined individually (i.e. some analytes might be overloaded even if others with the same concentration are not). Ideal chromatographic peaks are symmetric while overloaded peaks are asymmetric with a leading edge ('shark fin' shaped). Overloading does not damage the column but can lead to difficulty with quantification.

However, peak fronting can also be caused by reduced column capacity due to the loss of stationary phase at the head of the column, as can be the case in old or highly damaged columns.

5.3.4.3 Detector Saturation

Physical detector saturation occurs when there is no linear relationship between the increase in amount of analyte and the increase in detector signal. If the detector is physically saturated the top of the peak will be distorted or noisy. In addition, detector electronics can be saturated which results in a 'clamped' signal or peaks with a flat top.

Detector saturation inevitably leads to underestimation of metabolite abundance (and overestimation of ^{13}C labelling, since in most cases only the $M+0$ peak will be saturated, see Sect. 5.4.2.3). In addition, the detector may become contaminated. Detector saturation can be avoided by either injecting a smaller sample volume, splitting the introduced sample or diluting the sample before injection. In addition, detector parameters can be adjusted to accommodate the higher sample load.

5.4 Data Analysis and Reporting

Specific data analysis workflows depend on the scope of the experiment. Ions can be quantified without any knowledge of the metabolites they correspond to in order to select those ions that exhibit different abundances between samples. Subsequent analyses can then focus on identifying the metabolites these particular ions are derived from. However, given that sample extraction, derivatisation and chromatography methods are selected to enrich for specific classes of molecules, it is common practice to use GC–MS as a targeted method to quantify specific known metabolites. Therefore, data analysis involves the identification of metabolites that correspond to detected ion signals and quantification thereof.

5.4.1 Metabolite Identification

Similar to other chromatography methods, retention time, i.e. the time between injection and elution of a target compound peak, is one of the parameters used to identify a metabolite. However, many factors, such as the type of column, column dimensions, column degradation, derivatisation, presence of contaminants, etc. influence analyte retention time, which is why retention times are not readily comparable between GC–MS systems. In addition, retention times change over time in any GC system due to column degradation and trimming. Only the relative retention

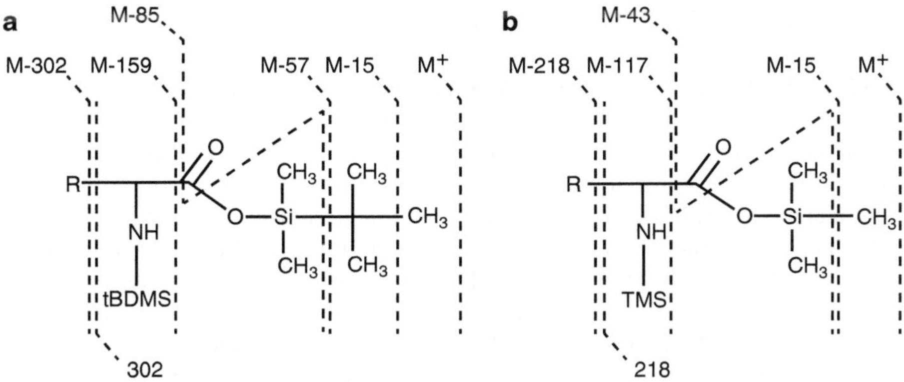

Fig. 5.6 Major ion fragments of amino acids with commonly used derivatisation agents. (**a**) Chemical structure of TBDMS-derivatised amino acids. Typical fragments resulting from breakage of indicated bonds (*dotted lines*) are (where "M" indicates the mass of the molecular ion): M-15 (loss of $-CH_3$), M-57 [loss of $-C(CH_3)_3$], M-302 (loss of the side chain), M-85 [concomitant loss of –C=O and $-C(CH_3)_3$], M-159 (loss of $-CO_2$-TBDMS) and for some amino acids also M-302 (side chain only) [63]. (**b**) Chemical structure of TMS-derivatised amino acids. Frequently observed ion fragments are: M-15 (loss of $-CH_3$), M-43 (loss of $-CO-CH_3$), M-117 (loss of $-CO_2$-TMS), M-R (i.e. *m*/*z* 218), and, for some, M-218 (side chain only) [51]

time between metabolite standards and unknowns analysed in close succession can therefore be used to assist with identification, because the influence of operational parameters will be comparable between these runs.

The most reliable features used for identification are the characteristic fragment ions and their specific *relative* intensities. It is best practice to compare these to metabolite standards analysed at the same time as the biological samples. Fragment ion *m*/*z* values can be used to deduce the atomic composition of the corresponding fragment species aided by the fact that many compound classes exhibit characteristic fragment ion patterns. The typical fragmentation patterns of amino acids are shown in Fig. 5.6. Typical fragments of TMS-derivatised sugars can be found in [52] and of TBDMS-derivatised carboxylic acids in [50].

Unknown ion fragment identities can be putatively assigned by interrogating reference mass spectral libraries. Library searching is done by probability matching comparison of the recorded and library spectra and will often return a hit list containing multiple identifications and display the best-matching spectrum. Publicly available databases include Human Metabolome Database (HMB, (http://www.hmdb.ca) [53]) and Metlin (https://metlin.scripps.edu/index.php [54]). Authentic standard(s) for one or more putatively identified compounds should be obtained or chemically synthesised, and analysed on the same instrument to determine their retention time and mass spectra. When the retention time, fragment ion *m*/*z* and relative intensities are closely similar between the authentic standard and unknown metabolite, a positive match is likely [47].

5.4.2 Metabolite Quantification

5.4.2.1 Peak Selection and Target Ion Analysis (Pre-processing)

Accurate quantification of a metabolite of interest from a GC–MS experiment relies on careful selection of an ion fragment, known as the *target ion*, which distinguishes this metabolite from other compounds co-eluting from the column with similar retention times. The SIC for the target ion within a given time window (usually 0.2-1 min) that matches the expected elution time for the corresponding metabolite is used to integrate the area under the peak (AUP). This can be done manually using the Agilent ChemStation software. This method of quantification is, however, very time-consuming and only recommended when few samples and metabolites need to be analysed.

Peak selection and target compound quantification can be performed semi-automatically using the Agilent MassHunter software. This software offers the possibility for the user to build a list of characteristic mass fragments that correspond to different metabolites associated with a retention time window. This list can then be applied to entire sample batches to identify metabolite-specific peaks and integrate their AUPs as above. Peak selection and accuracy of integration can be inspected and manually corrected by the user before exporting the data for further analysis. By adding isotopically labelled fragment masses, this programme also allows quantification of stable isotope labelling. The raw MassHunter export, in the form of comma-separated files, can then be further processed by MS Excel or using custom scripts in other software (e.g. in statistical programming packages such as R).

5.4.2.2 Relative and Semi-quantitative Analysis

The size (AUP) of a metabolite fragment peak ideally is proportional to the amount of analyte that reaches the detector if this amount lies within the linear range of the detector. Relative metabolite amounts can be compared between samples by normalising the corresponding peak area to the peak area of the internal standard thereby correcting for volume loss during phase separation (see Sect. 5.2.3.2). For semi-quantitative analysis, the *relative molar response factor* has to be calculated for every analyte by injecting a known quantity of the compound (in a standard mix or alone) and measuring the peak area. Metabolite amounts in a sample can then be estimated by comparing the normalised AUP from the experimental sample to the normalised AUP of a known amount of the metabolite in the standard sample.

Absolute quantification of a metabolite is possible by adding into every sample a known amount of this metabolite labelled with one or more stable isotopes. This needs to be done individually for every metabolite and is usually not practically feasible given the cost and limited availability of labelled standards.

5.4.2.3 Quantification of Stable Isotope-Labelled Compounds

For each fragment ion, the major peak in the mass spectrum that is used to identify that ion is accompanied by additional peaks with increasing *m/z* (increments of approx. +1 for singly charged ions) (Fig. 5.5, inset). These are called *isotopic peaks* and arise due to the presence of heavier, stable isotopes, such as ^{13}C and ^{15}N, which occur naturally in defined proportions. As a result of the specific abundance of heavier isotopes in nature compared to their light counterparts (e.g. 98.93 % for ^{12}C *vs.* 1.07 % for ^{13}C), isotopic peaks have characteristic intensities relative to each other that depend on the atomic composition of the ion.

Ion fragments derived from compounds with incorporated stable isotopes such as ^{13}C and ^{15}N can be identified by changes in the characteristic distribution pattern of isotopic peaks. If M represents the mass of a particular ion containing no heavy isotope atoms, peaks containing n number of heavy atoms are denoted as $M+n$. Isotopic labelling patterns for specific metabolite fragments can be obtained by quantifying the $M+0$ as well as each of the $M+n$ peaks for the respective fragments, as described above. A useful, non-targeted tool to find highly labelled molecular fragments derived from a stable isotope labelling experiment is non-targeted tracer fate detection (NTFD [55]). Before interpretation, the labelling pattern needs to be corrected for the natural abundance of isotopes in the fragment as well as the derivatisation agent. The discussion of the experimental design and data analysis steps necessary to qualitatively and quantitatively interpret isotope labelling patterns is beyond the scope of this chapter. A comprehensive discussion on how to interpret ^{13}C labelling patterns can be found in [28].

5.4.3 *Data Visualisation and Statistical Analysis*

Abundances of individual metabolites in different conditions can be illustrated using box plots, ideally overlaying individual data points. An often-useful representation involves the calculation of relative metabolite abundance changes between conditions. In many cases, given the significantly different pool sizes between metabolites, associated abundance changes can span over one or more orders of magnitude. Log_2 transformation is therefore commonly employed to scale metabolomics data. Log_2-transformed fold-changes over the corresponding control average for each of the individual replicates, can be plotted as a heatmap, which is an effective way to summarise global metabolite changes, identify metabolites that show similar behaviours (e.g. by clustering algorithms) but also provides a visual overview of the technical variability within the experiment. Another way to look at the magnitude of change *vs.* variability is a Z score plot, which uses both the mean and variance of the measurements.

To identify true metabolite abundance changes in a background of biological variability as well as technical fluctuations, robust statistical analysis is necessary. Univariate analysis can be used to test if an individual metabolite changes significantly between sample groups. The most commonly used tests are ANOVA (analysis of variance) and the *t*-test. It is important to keep in mind that these parametric tests assume normal distribution of the data, which is usually not possible to determine with small numbers of samples. In addition, studies with small sample sizes can often be underpowered, meaning that small differences cannot be measured with confidence [56].

If more than one metabolite is tested for significant changes between sample groups, uncorrected multiple hypothesis testing will inevitably lead to a high false discovery rate. *P* values therefore have to be adjusted for multiple tests using a suitable correction method. Although several easy-to-implement ways to correct for multiple comparisons exist, they tend to be very conservative/stringent. High stringency usually means that those methods are good at excluding false positives but increase the chances of false negatives. The choice of correction should therefore be based on the potential cost (e.g. in follow-up experiments) of false negatives *vs.* false positives. A commonly used, rather conservative, method is the Bonferroni correction, which decreases the *p* value in proportion to the number of executed tests. Guidelines on which statistical parameters should be reported for metabolomics experiments can be found in [57]. Volcano plots can then be used to illustrate $\log_2$ fold-change *vs.* *p* values, which gives a compact summary of magnitude changes as a function of their significance.

Since large numbers of metabolites are measured per sample, metabolomics data are by definition multivariate rather than univariate. An example for an unsupervised method that aims to reduce data dimensionality is principle component analysis (PCA). PCA is a good exploratory analysis tool to get a first overview over data quality and identify potential outliers, but its interpretation can be difficult [58]. However, PCA can help to get an impression of within-class variability *vs.* the difference between sample groups. If within-class variability is unusually high or there are obvious outliers, it usually points towards a technical problem (batch effects or failed injections).

PCA can be performed using open source tools such as R or commercial software (e.g. SIMCA). Importantly, the data need to be pre-processed by auto-scaling to set the mean of each metabolite to zero prior to analysis otherwise PCA will focus on the most intense signals (explained in detail in [59]). In addition, missing peaks should not be automatically filled with an arbitrary number (such as 0, sometimes automatically done by analysis software), as this creates artificial structure in the data set.

A comprehensive summary of more advanced multivariate statistical tools can be found in [56].

5.4.4 Data Curation

Metabolomics is becoming increasingly used in labs around the world. Given the inherent heterogeneity of the target molecules and analysed samples, and similarly to other -omics technologies, robust experimental methods and data reporting principles are desirable to promote experimental reproducibility longitudinally and across laboratories, but also facilitate proper data management. The Metabolomics

Standards Initiative (MSI) is driving the standardised reporting of metabolomics data and aims to define minimal reporting requirements [60, 61]. In addition, it is increasingly becoming standard practice to deposit metabolomics data in an open-source repository, such as MetaboLights [62].

5.5 Materials

5.5.1 Consumables

- Cell culture plates
- Cell culture media (w/o metabolite to be used as isotopic tracer, when applicable)
- Dialysed FCS
- Cell scrapers
- PBS
- 2 ml tubes (e.g. Eppendorf, must be solvent-resistant), 5 ml glass tubes can be used for larger extraction volumes
- GC–MS vials (e.g. Agilent, 5182-0715)
- GC–MS vial inserts (e.g. Agilent, 5183-2085)
- Screw caps for GC–MS vials (e.g. Agilent, 5185-5820)

5.5.2 Reagents

- Water, HPLC-grade (e.g. Acros Organics, 390760025)
- Methanol, HPLC-grade (e.g. Fisher Chemicals, A456-212)
- Chloroform, HPLC-grade (e.g. Fisher Chemicals, W/0106/PB17)
- Hexane, HPLC-grade (e.g. Fisher, H/0406/PB17)
- Pyridine (e.g. Sigma, 270970)
- Methoxyamine (Sigma, 226904)
- BSTFA+1 % TMCS (Sigma, 33148)
- *Scyllo*-inositol (Sigma, I8132)
- 1-^{13}C-Lauric acid (Cambridge Isotope Laboratories, CLM-1586)
- Meth-Prep™ II (Grace Discovery Sciences, 18007)

5.5.3 Equipment

- Agilent 5975C TAD Series GC/MSD System (G3440A)
- Agilent 7890A Network Gas Chromatograph (GC)
- Agilent 5975C inert XL MSD (G3122A)
- Agilent 7693 autosampler
- Merlin microseal septum (Agilent 5181-8833)
- Agilent ultra-inert injection port liner (5190-2293)

- Agilent DB-5ms column (30 m, 0.25 mm, 0.25 μm, DuraGuard, 10 m, 122-5532G)
- Aspirator
- Cooled table-top centrifuge
- Centrifugal evaporator
- Positive-displacement pipettes

Acknowledgments We would like to thank James MacRae (The Francis Crick Institute) for technical advice and comments on the content of this chapter, and the Francis Crick Institute Photographics team for help with figure preparation. Work in the Anastasiou lab is supported by MRC grant MC_UP_1202/1.

References

1. Voet D, Voet JG. Biochemistry. 4th ed. New York: Wiley Global Education; 2010.
2. Kaelin WG, Thompson CB. Q&A: cancer: clues from cell metabolism. Nature. 2010;465:562–64. doi:10.1038/465562a.
3. Schulze A, Harris AL. How cancer metabolism is tuned for proliferation and vulnerable to disruption. Nature. 2012;491:364–73. doi:10.1038/nature11706.
4. Hanahan D, Weinberg RA. Hallmarks of cancer: the next generation. Cell. 2011;144:646–74. doi:10.1016/j.cell.2011.02.013.
5. Koppenol WH, Bounds PL, Dang CV. Otto Warburg's contributions to current concepts of cancer metabolism. Nat Rev Cancer. 2011;11:325–37. doi:10.1038/nrc3038.
6. Vander Heiden MG, Cantley LC, Thompson CB. Understanding the Warburg effect: the metabolic requirements of cell proliferation. Science (New York, NY). 2009;324:1029–33. doi:10.1126/science.1160809.
7. Anastasiou D, Poulogiannis G, Asara JM, et al. Inhibition of pyruvate kinase M2 by reactive oxygen species contributes to cellular antioxidant responses. Science (New York, NY). 2011;334:1278–83. doi:10.1126/science.1211485.
8. Cairns RA, Harris IS, Mak TW. Regulation of cancer cell metabolism. Nat Rev Cancer. 2011;11(2):85–95.
9. Denko NC. Hypoxia, HIF1 and glucose metabolism in the solid tumour. Nat Rev Cancer. 2008;8:705–13. doi:10.1038/nrc2468.
10. Favaro E, Bensaad K, Chong MG, et al. Glucose utilization via glycogen phosphorylase sustains proliferation and prevents premature senescence in cancer cells. Cell Metab. 2012;16:751–64. doi:10.1016/j.cmet.2012.10.017.
11. Nieman KM, Kenny HA, Penicka CV, et al. Adipocytes promote ovarian cancer metastasis and provide energy for rapid tumor growth. Nat Med. 2011;17:1498–503. doi:10.1038/nm.2492.
12. Semenza GL. Regulation of cancer cell metabolism by hypoxia-inducible factor 1. Semin Cancer Biol. 2009;19:12–6. doi:10.1016/j.semcancer.2008.11.009.
13. Anastasiou D, Yu Y, Israelsen WJ, et al. Pyruvate kinase M2 activators promote tetramer formation and suppress tumorigenesis. Nat Chem Biol. 2012;8:839–47. doi:10.1038/nchembio.1060.
14. Galluzzi L, Kepp O, Vander Heiden MG. Metabolic targets for cancer therapy. Nat Rev Drug Discov. 2013;12:829–46. doi:10.1038/nrd4145.
15. Griffin JL, Atherton H, Shockcor J, Atzori L. Metabolomics as a tool for cardiac research. Nat Rev Cardiol. 2011;8:630–43. doi:10.1038/nrcardio.2011.138.
16. Griffin JL, Shockcor JP. Metabolic profiles of cancer cells. Nat Rev Cancer. 2004;4:551–61. doi:10.1038/nrc1390.
17. Lu W, Bennett BD, Rabinowitz JD. Analytical strategies for LC-MS-based targeted metabolomics. J Chromatogr B. 2008;871:236–42. doi:10.1016/j.jchromb.2008.04.031.

18. Patti GJ, Yanes O, Siuzdak G. Innovation: metabolomics: the apogee of the omics trilogy. Nat Rev Mol Cell Biol. 2012;13:263–9. doi:10.1038/nrm3314.
19. Souza AL, Gerszten RE, Clish CB. Targeted metabolomics. Curr Protoc Mol Biol. 2012. doi:10.1002/0471142727.mb3002s98.
20. Fiehn O. Combining genomics, metabolome analysis, and biochemical modelling to understand metabolic networks. Comp Funct Genomics. 2001. doi:10.1002/cfg.82.
21. Jerby-Arnon L, Pfetzer N, Waldman YY, et al. Predicting cancer-specific vulnerability via data-driven detection of synthetic lethality. Cell. 2014;158:1199–209. doi:10.1016/j.cell.2014.07.027.
22. Weckwerth W, Morgenthal K. Metabolomics: from pattern recognition to biological interpretation. Drug Discov Today. 2005;10:1551–8. doi:10.1016/S1359-6446(05)03609-3.
23. Büscher JM, Czernik D, Ewald JC, et al. Cross-platform comparison of methods for quantitative metabolomics of primary metabolism. Anal Chem. 2009;81:2135–43. doi:10.1021/ac8022857.
24. Lu W, Clasquin MF, Melamud E, et al. Metabolomic analysis via reversed-phase ion-pairing liquid chromatography coupled to a stand alone orbitrap mass spectrometer. Anal Chem. 2010;82:3212–21. doi:10.1021/ac902837x.
25. Jonsson P, Johansson AI, Gullberg J, et al. High-throughput data analysis for detecting and identifying differences between samples in GC/MS-based metabolomic analyses. Anal Chem. 2005;77:5635–42. doi:10.1021/ac050601e.
26. Weckwerth W. Metabolomics in systems biology. Annu Rev Plant Biol. 2003;54:669–89. doi:10.1146/annurev.arplant.54.031902.135014.
27. Sauer U. Metabolic networks in motion: 13C-based flux analysis. Mol Syst Biol. 2006. doi:10.1038/msb4100109.
28. Buescher JM, Antoniewicz MR, Boros LG, et al. A roadmap for interpreting 13C metabolite labeling patterns from cells. Curr Opin Biotechnol. 2015;34:189–201. doi:10.1016/j.copbio.2015.02.003.
29. Metallo CM, Walther JL, Stephanopoulos G. Evaluation of 13C isotopic tracers for metabolic flux analysis in mammalian cells. J Biotechnol. 2009;144:167–74. doi:10.1016/j.jbiotec.2009.07.010.
30. Zamboni N. C metabolic flux analysis in complex systems. Curr Opin Biotechnol. 2011;22:103–8. doi:10.1016/j.copbio.2010.08.009.
31. Van Winden WA, Wittmann C. Correcting mass isotopomer distributions for naturally occurring isotopes. Biotechnol Bioeng. 2002. doi:10.1002/bit.10393.
32. Jain M, Nilsson R, Sharma S, et al. Metabolite profiling identifies a key role for glycine in rapid cancer cell proliferation. Science. 2012;336:1040–4. doi:10.1126/science.1218595.
33. Munger J, Bajad SU, Coller HA, et al. Dynamics of the cellular metabolome during human cytomegalovirus infection. PLoS Pathog. 2006;2:e132. doi:10.1371/journal.ppat.0020132.st002.
34. Teng Q, Huang W, Collette TW, et al. A direct cell quenching method for cell-culture based metabolomics. Metabolomics. 2008;5:199–208. doi:10.1007/s11306-008-0137-z.
35. Lorenz MA, Burant CF, Kennedy RT. Reducing time and increasing sensitivity in sample preparation for adherent mammalian cell metabolomics. Anal Chem. 2011;83:3406–14. doi:10.1021/ac103313x.
36. Yanes O, Tautenhahn R, Patti GJ, Siuzdak G. Expanding coverage of the metabolome for global metabolite profiling. Anal Chem. 2011;83:2152–61. doi:10.1021/ac102981k.
37. Bi H, Krausz KW, Manna SK, et al. Optimization of harvesting, extraction, and analytical protocols for UPLC-ESI-MS-based metabolomic analysis of adherent mammalian cancer cells. Anal Bioanal Chem. 2013;405:5279–89. doi:10.1007/s00216-013-6927-9.
38. Rae CD. A guide to the metabolic pathways and function of metabolites observed in human brain 1H magnetic resonance spectra. Neurochem Res. 2013;39:1–36. doi:10.1007/s11064-013-1199-5.
39. Wu L, Mashego MR, van Dam JC, et al. Quantitative analysis of the microbial metabolome by isotope dilution mass spectrometry using uniformly 13C-labeled cell extracts as internal standards. Anal Biochem. 2005;336:164–71. doi:10.1016/j.ab.2004.09.001.

40. Biermann CJ, McGinnis GD. Analysis of carbohydrates by GLC and MS. Boca Raton, FL: CRC Press; 1988.
41. Zaikin V, Halket JM. A handbook of derivatives for mass spectrometry. Chichester, UK: IM Publications; 2009.
42. Kim H-Y, Salem Jr N. Separation of lipid classes by solid phase extraction. J Lipid Res. 1990;31:2285–9.
43. Snow NH. Inlet systems for gas chromatography. In: Grob RL, Barry EF, editors. Modern practice of gas chromatography. 4th ed. Hoboken, NJ: Wiley; 2004. p. 1–29.
44. Grob K. Split and splitless injection for quantitative gas chromatography. 4th ed. New York: Wiley; 2015. p. 1–477.
45. Barry EF. Columns: packed and capillary; column selection in gas chromatography. In: Grob RL, Barry EF, editors. Modern practice of gas chromatography. 4th ed. Hoboken, NJ: Wiley; 2004. p. 1–127.
46. Colon LA, Baird LJ. Detectors in modern gas chromatography. In: Grob RL, Barry EF, editors. Modern practice of gas chromatography. 4th ed. Hoboken, NJ: Wiley; 2004. p. 1–62.
47. McMaster MC. GC/MS: a practical user's guide. 2nd ed. Hoboken, NJ: Wiley; 2008. p. 1–153.
48. Baker JM, Hawkins ND, Ward JL, et al. A metabolomic study of substantial equivalence of field-grown genetically modified wheat. Plant Biotechnol J. 2006;4:381–92. doi:10.1111/j.1467-7652.2006.00197.x.
49. Oberg AL, Vitek O. Statistical design of quantitative mass spectrometry-based proteomic experiments. J Proteome Res. 2009;8:2144–56. doi:10.1021/pr8010099.
50. Mawhinney TP, Robinett RS, Atalay A, Madson MA. Gas-liquid chromatography and mass spectral analysis of mono-, di- and tricarboxylates as their tert.-butyldimethylsilyl derivatives. J Chromatogr. 1986;361:117–30.
51. Leimer KR, Rice RH, Gehrke CW. Complete mass spectra of the per-trimethylsilylated amino acids. J Chromatogr. 1977;141:355–75.
52. DeJongh DC, Radford T, Hribar JD, et al. Analysis of trimethylsilyl derivatives of carbohydrates by gas chromatography and mass spectrometry. J Am Chem Soc. 1969;91:1728–40.
53. Wishart DS, Tzur D, Knox C, et al. HMDB: the human metabolome database. Nucleic Acids Res. 2007;35:D521–6. doi:10.1093/nar/gkl923.
54. Smith CA, OMaille G, Want EJ, et al. A metabolite mass spectral database. In: Proceedings of the 9th International Congress of Therapeutic Drug Monitoring & Clinical Toxicology. Louisville, Kentucky; 2005. pp. 1–5.
55. Hiller K, Wegner A, Weindl D, et al. NTFD—a stand-alone application for the non-targeted detection of stable isotope-labeled compounds in GC/MS data. Bioinformatics. 2013;29:1226–8. doi:10.1093/bioinformatics/btt119.
56. Broadhurst DI, Kell DB. Statistical strategies for avoiding false discoveries in metabolomics and related experiments. Metabolomics. 2006;2:171–96. doi:10.1007/s11306-006-0037-z.
57. Goodacre R, Broadhurst D, Smilde AK, et al. Proposed minimum reporting standards for data analysis in metabolomics. Metabolomics. 2007;3:231–41. doi:10.1007/s11306-007-0081-3.
58. Jolliffe IT. Principal component analysis. 2nd ed. New York: Springer; 2002. p. 1–519.
59. Worley B, Powers R. Multivariate analysis in metabolomics. Curr Metabolomics. 2013;1:1–16.
60. Fiehn O, Robertson D, Griffin J, et al. The metabolomics standards initiative (MSI). Metabolomics. 2007;3:175–8. doi:10.1007/s11306-007-0070-6.
61. Goodacre R, Vaidyanathan S, Dunn WB. Metabolomics by numbers: acquiring and understanding global metabolite data. Trends Biotechnol. 2004;22:245–52. doi:10.1016/j.tibtech.2004.03.007.
62. Haug K, Salek RM, Conesa P, et al. MetaboLights—an open-access general-purpose repository for metabolomics studies and associated meta-data. Nucleic Acids Res. 2012;41:D781–6. doi:10.1093/nar/gks1004.
63. Mawhinney TP, Robinett RS, Atalay A, Madson MA. Analysis of amino acids as their tert.-butyldimethylsilyl derivatives by gas-liquid chromatography and mass spectrometry. J Chromatogr. 1986;358:231–42.

Chapter 6
Probing Cancer Cell Metabolism Using NMR Spectroscopy

Kate E.R. Hollinshead, Debbie S. Williams, Daniel A. Tennant, and Christian Ludwig

Abstract Altered cellular metabolism is now accepted to be at the core of many diseases including cancer. Over the past 20 years, NMR has become a core technology to study these metabolic perturbations in detail. This chapter reviews current NMR-based methods for steady-state metabolism and, in particular, the use of non-radioactive stable isotope-enriched tracers. Opportunities and challenges for each method, such as 1D ^{1}H NMR spectroscopy and ^{13}C carbon-based NMR spectroscopic methods, are discussed. Ultimately, the combination of NMR and mass spectra as orthogonal technologies are required to compensate for the drawbacks of each technique when used singly are discussed.

Keywords NMR • Cancer • Metabolism • ^{13}C • ^{1}H • Metabolomics • Tracer analysis • Stable isotopes • HSQC • MS

6.1 Introduction to Metabolism

Altered cellular metabolism contributes to many diseases including metabolic syndromes, neurodegenerative disorders and, of significant interest in this review, cancer. Dating back to 1924, Otto Warburg observed that malignant tissues appeared to have undergone metabolic transformation in that they produced more lactate in aerobic conditions than normal tissues—a phenomenon now known as aerobic glycolysis [1]. This feature has since been incorporated into Hanahan and Weinberg's posited hallmarks of cancer [2], whereby cancer cells undergo metabolic reprogramming to meet the increased demands of proliferation in terms of anabolism (including the production of carbohydrates, nucleotides, lipids, proteins and nucleic

K.E.R. Hollinshead • D.S. Williams • D.A. Tennant • C. Ludwig (✉)
Institute of Metabolism and Systems Research, University of Birmingham, IBR, Edgbaston, Birmingham B15 2TT, UK
e-mail: kxh879@bham.ac.uk; d.s.williams@bham.ac.uk; tennantd@bham.ac.uk; C.Ludwig@bham.ac.uk

C. Koumenis et al. (eds.), *Tumor Microenvironment*, Advances in Experimental Medicine and Biology 899, DOI 10.1007/978-3-319-26666-4_6

acids) and energy [3, 4]. The nature of these metabolic alterations has subsequently been shown to be context dependent [5–11]. As targeting tumour metabolism presents an attractive therapeutic approach [12], analytical approaches are being increasingly developed and employed to provide a better understanding of the effects of transformed metabolism in cancer.

Nuclear magnetic resonance spectroscopy (NMR) and mass spectrometry (MS) are two such suitable analytical platforms. Although MS technology developments are more advanced than NMR-based approaches and have been more widely and successfully implicated in the research of cancer metabolism, NMR is a particularly powerful tool for the elucidation of structures at the atomic level. This review provides an overview of the developments in NMR spectroscopy, with specific emphasis on the somewhat overlooked benefits of employing NMR-based technology for stable isotope-resolved metabolism, a technique that can provide valuable information generally beyond most MS methods.

6.2 Basic Principles of NMR Spectroscopy

As the name suggests, NMR spectroscopy uses the characteristics of nuclei to identify atoms within molecules. Accordingly, the number of protons and neutrons, both of which possess an intrinsic property termed spin (taking the value of plus or minus half) determine whether or not a particular atom is visible using NMR spectroscopic methods. Depending on the number of protons and neutrons inside a given nucleus, the net spin can be zero, half-integer or integer. Nuclei with a non-zero net spin behave like a magnet and it is this magnetic property that NMR spectroscopy exploits. One of the most widely used nuclei for NMR is the hydrogen nucleus (i.e. ^{1}H or proton), although other non-zero spin nuclei used include ^{13}C, ^{15}N and ^{31}P. It becomes apparent that this variety of NMR-visible nuclei could provide the opportunity to study almost any molecule in a biological system using single or multinuclear approaches. However, there are two reasons why this is frequently not possible: (1) the relative abundance of isotopes and (2) the sensitivity of the approach. In contrast to ^{1}H and ^{31}P, which are high abundance isotopes (approaching 100 %), the two other nuclei common in biological systems, ^{13}C and ^{15}N, demonstrate low natural abundance (~1 %). This means that investigating a low abundance nucleus in a biological molecule requires either long measurement times or molecules need to be artificially enriched with the NMR-visible isotope. In some cases, the molecule is of such low concentration within the cell that even with artificial enrichment, it is still not visible.

To identify different molecules within cells or tissues, NMR methods take advantage of the fact that the molecular environment subtly but measurably alters the spin of a nucleus. Therefore the protons within a CH_2 group can be differentiated depending on the group(s) in their vicinity. A good example of this is when differentiating between carbon 3 and 4 of glutamine, glutamate and alpha-ketoglutarate, which is possible due to the differences in their atomic environment (Fig. 6.1). One significant advantage of NMR over other analytical methods is that

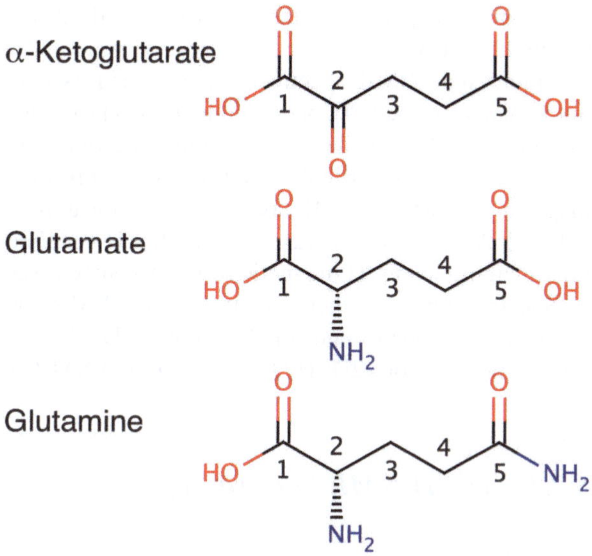

Fig. 6.1 Chemical structures of α-ketoglutarate, glutamate and glutamine. NMR spectroscopy is able to differentiate α-ketoglutarate, glutamate and glutamine based on ^{13}C and ^{1}H signals originating from C(3) and C(4)

the signal intensity in a 1D NMR spectrum is directly proportional to the number of nuclear spins contributing to that signal. This feature facilitates highly accurate metabolite quantification and, unlike other methods, does not suffer from batch effects, allowing for inter-experimental comparisons without the need for internal standards.

In addition to being one of the most widely used nuclei in NMR, 1D proton spectra constitute the most commonly used NMR experiments. However, due to the vast number of metabolites within a system (with over 40,000 identified [13]) there is a large degree of overlap in ^{1}H peaks within a proton spectrum. To reduce this overlap and allow more rigorous metabolite identification, multi-dimensional NMR spectra can be acquired where extra dimensions are added to create 2D, 3D or even 4D NMR spectra. These complex spectra utilise the long-lived property of NMR magnetisation, which permits the transfer of magnetisation across multiple nuclei. Hence, one can start from one end of a molecule and, by distributing the magnetisation across the entire molecule, obtain information on the nuclei of atoms separated by multiple chemical bonds. Although complex, this powerful approach can be used to build an unbiased picture of large numbers of known and unknown molecules within a biological system.

6.3 Measurements of Steady-State Metabolism Using NMR Spectroscopy

The term metabolomics refers to the complete study of metabolites within a biological sample and is particularly useful in determining differences in metabolic states, e.g. diseased vs non-diseased. It can also be used to reveal disease biomarkers in leading to diagnosis, prognosis and treatment outcome. NMR-based metabolomics can inform on pathway activities by providing absolute intra- or extra-cellular metabolite levels.

Liquid-state NMR spectroscopy has been used in a diverse number of bodily fluids such as urine [14], breath condensates [15], blood plasma or serum [16], liver extracts [17, 18], bile acid from human intestinal biopsy samples [19], and kidney perfusates [20]. A particularly attractive feature of liquid-state or high-resolution magic angle spinning NMR spectroscopy is the ability to reuse tissue or cell extracts [21, 22]. As it is a non-invasive method, it is beneficial for in vivo analysis or real-time imaging using ^{1}H magnetic resonance spectroscopy (MRS) [23, 24].

Spectroscopically, there are two major NMR methods used to determine the metabolome—one-dimensional proton (1D ^{1}H) NMR spectroscopy and two-dimensional proton (2D ^{1}H) J-resolved (Jres) NMR spectroscopy.

6.3.1 1D ^{1}H NMR Spectroscopy

1D ^{1}H NMR spectroscopy is the most commonly used approach in NMR-based studies of steady-state metabolism, because it provides reproducible spectra suitable for high-throughput sample analysis [25]. Dried extracts are re-suspended in an aqueous solution containing a known concentration of an internal reference standard in water and/or heavy water. A 1D ^{1}H NMR experiment, also known as a pulse sequence, contains an element to suppress the (residual) water signal [26], which is followed by an excitation pulse to generate observable magnetisation prior to the acquisition of the NMR signal. An entire NMR experiment typically takes less than 20 min per sample.

1D ^{1}H NMR is the simplest and most sensitive NMR method, where the area under each signal (or the intensity of signal) in a spectrum is directly proportional to the number of ^{1}H nuclei contributing to this signal. As such, it can accurately quantify metabolite concentrations without the need for prior assumption of metabolite composition [27], exemplified in Fig. 6.2a. Indeed, reliable and reproducible detection of metabolite concentrations from 40 to 50 μM are achievable with a sufficient magnetic field strength and an appropriate (e.g. cryogenically cooled) probe. 1D ^{1}H NMR spectroscopy therefore provides an untargeted and sensitive method for steady-state metabolite analysis in complex biological mixtures.

Since biological samples for metabolomic studies, such as body fluids, tissue and cell extracts, are themselves complex mixtures with hundreds of dissolved metabolites, the resulting NMR spectra become difficult to interpret. This is a result of each proton within a metabolite resonating at a specific frequency that depends on its chemical environment. Different protons therefore have NMR peaks with different spectral positions, where multiple ^{1}H peaks exist per metabolite. Multivariate statistical methods such as principle component analysis (PCA) are common approaches used to reduce spectral complexity and uncover those changes in metabolite concentrations that vary significantly between different sample groups [28]. PCA is an unsupervised method that compresses data sets to investigate biological

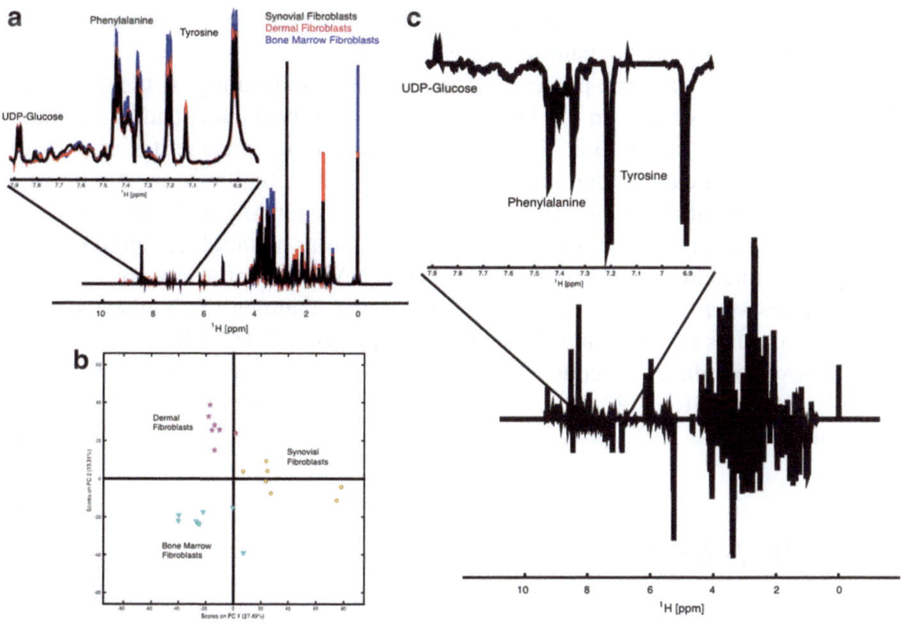

Fig. 6.2 Statistical analysis of 1D ^{1}H NMR spectra. Cultured fibroblasts from the synovium, skin and bone marrow of arthritic patients. (**a**) The mean 1D ^{1}H NMR spectra for each sample group. (**b**) Principle component analysis illustrating statistically significant separation between the fibroblast groups. (**c**) Loading plot back calculated from principle component 1 (PC1). The assigned aromatic amino acids are an example of the metabolic differences between fibroblasts originating from the synovium and fibroblasts originating from the skin or bone marrow

significance and naturally separates data based on biological variance, as shown in Fig. 6.2b. This method determines variations in metabolite concentrations across sample groups to identify significant differences. Whilst PCA is an unbiased analysis, additional supervised analytical methods are available to narrow the selection criteria to distinguish between different sample groups. As with many other statistical tests, PCA is most effective if the probability of the sample data follows a Gaussian distribution.

A series of data pre-processing steps are necessary prior to statistical analysis, without which the quality of analysis is compromised [29, 30]. Typical pre-processing operations include global alignment, baseline correction, exclusion regions, segmental alignment, global scaling, bucketing and non-linear scaling. Collectively, these necessary steps improve PCA separation between sample classes. For example, exclusion regions avoid unwanted parts of the NMR spectra such as the solvent peak or spectral edges. Segmental alignment corrects for pH differences and sample inconsistencies, and global scaling is used predominately for body fluids where the total amount of metabolites is assumed to be consistent across samples. Additionally, non-linear scaling, such as the generalised log-transform, is used to stabilise variance between small and large signals in the NMR spectrum. A large variance originates on account of the large dynamic range of metabolite concentrations quantified by NMR [14].

With optimum data pre-processing, the signals contributing to the separation between different classes in the PCA analysis can be back calculated as loadings plots, exemplified in Fig. 6.2c. From these loading plots, metabolites responsible for the separation can be identified. Mapping these metabolites to metabolic pathways can be an initial step towards a molecular understanding of the disease.

Whilst this approach is effective for analysing polar metabolites, including carbohydrates, nucleotides and amino acids, 1D ^{1}H NMR cannot resolve other metabolite classes such as lipids or polyamines, as the chemical shift dispersion for these metabolites is very small. An additional issue of 1D ^{1}H NMR is that metabolites in low abundance or concentration cannot be detected owing to the limited sensitivity of NMR itself. Therefore adequate sample amounts, be it tissue or cells, are required.

6.3.2 2D J-Resolved NMR Spectroscopy

The problem of overcrowded spectra raised above is further exacerbated through J coupling, also known as spin–spin coupling, which splits each signal into several components based on the number of protons attached to the adjacent carbon. Collectively, this compromises unambiguous peak identification and accurate metabolite quantification. To offset this issue, an independent second dimension is introduced.

An example is 2D J-resolved NMR spectroscopy (2D-Jres), which was first introduced by Richard Ernst and co-workers in the 1970s [31]. A typical 2D-Jres spectrum can be acquired in less than 30 min, facilitating rapid sample throughput [32]. The reduction in overlap is achieved by separating the chemical shift from the signal splitting through J coupling, as shown in Fig. 6.3. The projection of such a 2D spectrum onto the chemical shift axis, known as pJres, removes the multiple peaks observed through J coupling, thereby reducing overcrowding in the 1D spectrum.

In addition to the reduction in peak overlap, another significant advantage of 2D-Jres, or pJres, spectra is the ability to directly compare spectra acquired at different magnetic field strengths. NMR spectra become more or less field independent as a result of separating the chemical shift axis and the effects of J coupling into two orthogonal dimensions. This is not possible using a 1D ^{1}H NMR spectroscopic approach. Metabolites in 2D-Jres spectra can still be quantified using spectral databases [33].

Despite minimising signal overlap, ^{1}H–^{1}H 2D NMR spectra are still affected by the large number of signals present within an NMR spectrum. Employing other nuclei with greater chemical shift dispersion, such as ^{13}C, may be attractive to avoid this. However, the lower natural abundance of these NMR active isotopes decreases the sensitivity: 1.07 % ^{13}C natural abundance compared to ~100 % ^{1}H natural abundance. This approach has decreased sensitivity compared to ^{1}H. As a result, the most sensitive nuclei (e.g. ^{1}H) tend to be employed for metabolomic studies.

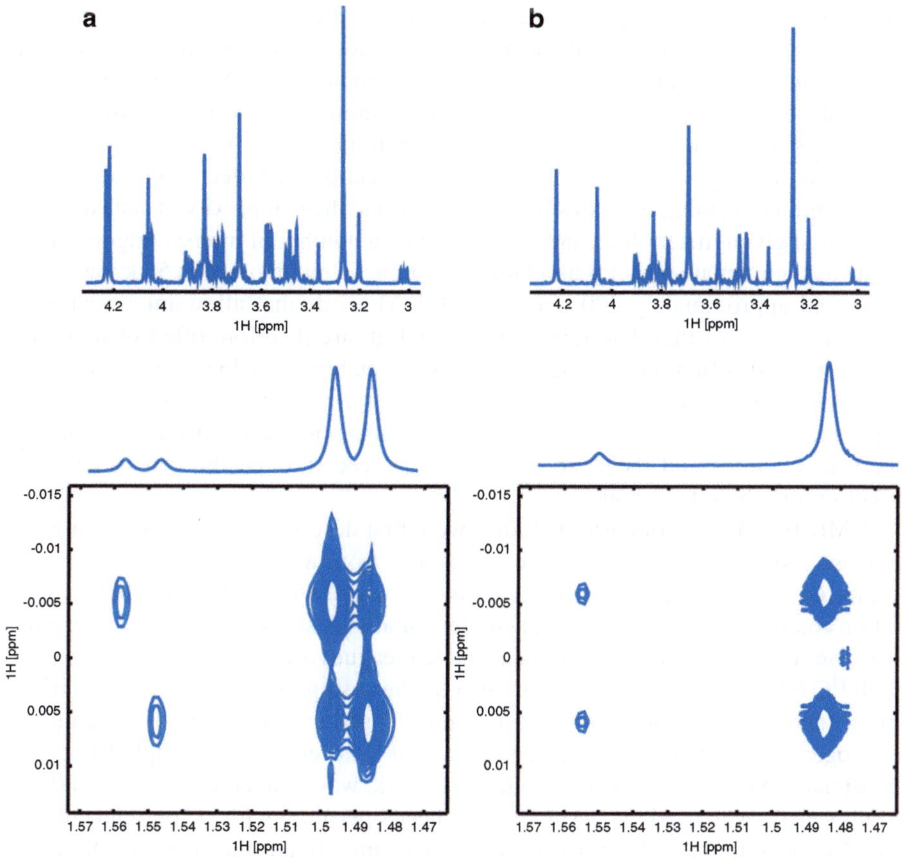

Fig. 6.3 2D J-resolved NMR spectra and 1D projections. (**a**) 2D Fourier transformed spectra and projection onto the horizontal axis (pJres). (**b**) Data tilted by 45° and symmetrised after Fourier transform. These pJres spectra no longer contain ^{1}H–^{1}H splitting and therefore have reduced peak overlap

These untargeted ^{1}H NMR spectroscopic approaches require no prior assumptions about metabolite composition or concentrations and are therefore a useful tool in metabolic fingerprinting. The speed of acquisition in these spectral types enables high-throughput sample analysis. Several spectral databases and software tools facilitate automatic metabolite quantification. At this stage, these NMR approaches are beneficial for metabolic profiling.

6.4 Tracer-Based Metabolism

Whilst being an untargeted tool, and therefore useful for gaining an overview of a system, the metabolomic approach offers limited mechanistic information. Concentration changes of intracellular metabolites indicate altered activity of connected consuming or producing reactions—be it enzymatic, non-enzymatic or transporters. However, such concentration changes do not readily allow conclusions on metabolic rates or flux, nor do they provide information on changes in nutrient source [34]. They also give no indication of the directionality of flux changes, since an increase in metabolite concentration could be indicative of either increased activity of metabolite-producing reactions or decreased activity of metabolite-consuming reactions [34]. In addition to the complexity of such dynamic systems, a given metabolite can be produced by a number of intersecting metabolic pathways: glutamate presents as an ideal example being involved in 55 known pathways and approximately 200 reactions [35]. Methods that allow interrogation of pathway usage, or that determine flux through it, are therefore often of more use. These methods often rely on the use of novel metabolite analogues (such as ^{18}F-2-deoxyglucose) or naturally occurring metabolites enriched in a relatively rare isotope, such as $^{13}C_{1-5}$ glutamine. If these isotopes also possess a non-integer spin, then these metabolites and their products can be traced through the cell using NMR spectroscopy-based methods.

NMR-based metabolic tracer studies were first described in the 1970s using $^{13}C_1$ glucose [36]. ^{13}C NMR spectra were acquired from a suspension of *E. coli* cells subjected to aerobic and anaerobic conditions, where within 15 min, label incorporation could be traced into lactate, alanine, glutamate, succinate, acetate, valine and fructose 1,3 bisphosphate. Shulman and colleagues made further developments with ^{13}C NMR spectra in subsequent liver studies using rat hepatocytes and purified mitochondria. They used $^{13}C_{1,3}$ glycerol and $^{13}C_2$ glycerol tracers to investigate gluconeogenesis and to calculate the percentage of hexoses cycled through the pentose phosphate cycle [37]. Further pioneering work was conducted in the 1980s by Malloy et al., who used ^{13}C NMR from rat hearts perfused with ^{13}C enrichment such as $^{13}C_{1,2}$ acetate and $^{13}C_3$ pyruvate in vivo to investigate the relative activity of anaplerotic and oxidative reactions in the TCA cycle [38].

Unlike metabolic steady-state analysis, which addresses the state of metabolism, the introduction of a stable isotope metabolic tracer can be used to highlight the use of specific nutrients and infer activity of specific metabolic pathways. Two of the most common atoms in biological systems are carbon and nitrogen but their NMR active isotopes, ^{13}C and ^{15}N, have low natural abundances (1.07 % and 0.364 %, respectively). However, these can be enriched in metabolic tracers (e.g. 98 atom % $^{13}C_{1-6}$ glucose), thereby enabling investigations to probe intracellular metabolism as a dynamic system. With the correct samples and analytical techniques, this can provide valuable qualitative and quantitative information on metabolic pathway fluxes.

The most often used isotope for the analysis of metabolism by NMR spectroscopy is ^{13}C. Experimentally, cells are exposed to ~100 % ^{13}C-enriched metabolic tracer: common examples include ^{13}C-labelled glucose or glutamine. Metabolism of the tracer results in increasingly ^{13}C-enriched downstream metabolites until a steady state is reached. This metabolism can take minutes, as is the case for glycolysis, to hours, and is highly dependent on the system being studied. The capability of NMR spectroscopy to resolve ^{13}C incorporation at an atomic level enables the determination of labelling patterns in intracellular metabolites to provide crucial information on pathway activity, be it the analysis of isotopomers (metabolites with the same number of ^{13}C nuclei present, but differing in position) or isotopologues (metabolites containing different quantities of ^{13}C nuclei).

Different metabolic tracers, which can be the metabolite itself or its isotopic labelling position can be used to provide information on differential pathway activity. Therefore, the choice of metabolic tracer should be dictated by the biological hypothesis. For example, compared to other isotopic-labelled glucose tracers, $^{13}C_{1,2}$-glucose yields the most precise information on glycolysis and the pentose phosphate pathway (PPP) [39]. Furthermore, the use of labelled tracers in combination can provide specific pathway information, e.g. using $^{13}C_{1,6}$ glucose and $^{13}C_3$ glutamine to investigate the contribution of glutaminolysis and glycolysis for fatty acid synthesis [40]. Ultimately, the combination of multiple complementary tracers can resolve metabolism to a greater extent than single tracer approaches.

NMR-based metabolic tracer studies can be used to quantify fluxes when samples from multiple time points are analysed in parallel and combined with metabolite levels from 1D ^{1}H NMR spectra resulting in metabolite amount converted/cell/time. However, NMR is limited by sensitivity, and data analysis tends to focus only on those metabolites whose concentrations are sufficient to be NMR-visible. In typical mammalian cell culture flux experiments and with current instrumentation, NMR spectroscopy cannot detect most intermediates of glycolysis and the TCA cycle. Instead, label incorporation into metabolites such as lactate, glutamate and aspartate can be considered metabolic readouts of pathway activity.

Figure 6.4a highlights the use of $^{13}C_{1,2}$ glucose to provide information on the differential pathway contribution of glycolysis and the PPP to the lactate and alanine pools. Both lactate and alanine are produced directly from pyruvate—the end-product of glycolysis. Labelling in lactate could be used as a readout of pathway activity: $^{13}C_{2,3}$ lactate is formed from pyruvate produced from carbons coming directly from glycolysis, whereas $^{13}C_3$ lactate is the product from pyruvate that was formed from those molecules of glucose-6-phosphate that diverted through the oxidative PPP before continuing through the rest of glycolysis. The analysis of each of these isotopomers from either tissue or cell extracts, in addition to the microenvironment, allows the relative contributions of each pathway to be assessed. As the oxidative PPP is a major source of cellular antioxidants in the form of NADPH, the information gained from this type of analysis can provide important knowledge about more diverse aspects of cellular metabolism and the tumour microenvironment than just glycolysis. A further example using the same tracer ($^{13}C_{1,2}$ glucose), is the ability to investigate mitochondrial activity using the enrichment of ^{13}C into glutamate and aspartate. Pyruvate that enters the mitochondrion can be oxidised by pyruvate dehydrogenase to form acetyl CoA, which then condenses with oxaloacetate to form citrate, entering the TCA cycle, as shown in Fig. 6.4b. This set of reactions eventually results in the enrichment of the glutamate pool with $^{13}C_{4,5}$ glutamate, and the aspartate pool with two isotopomers of

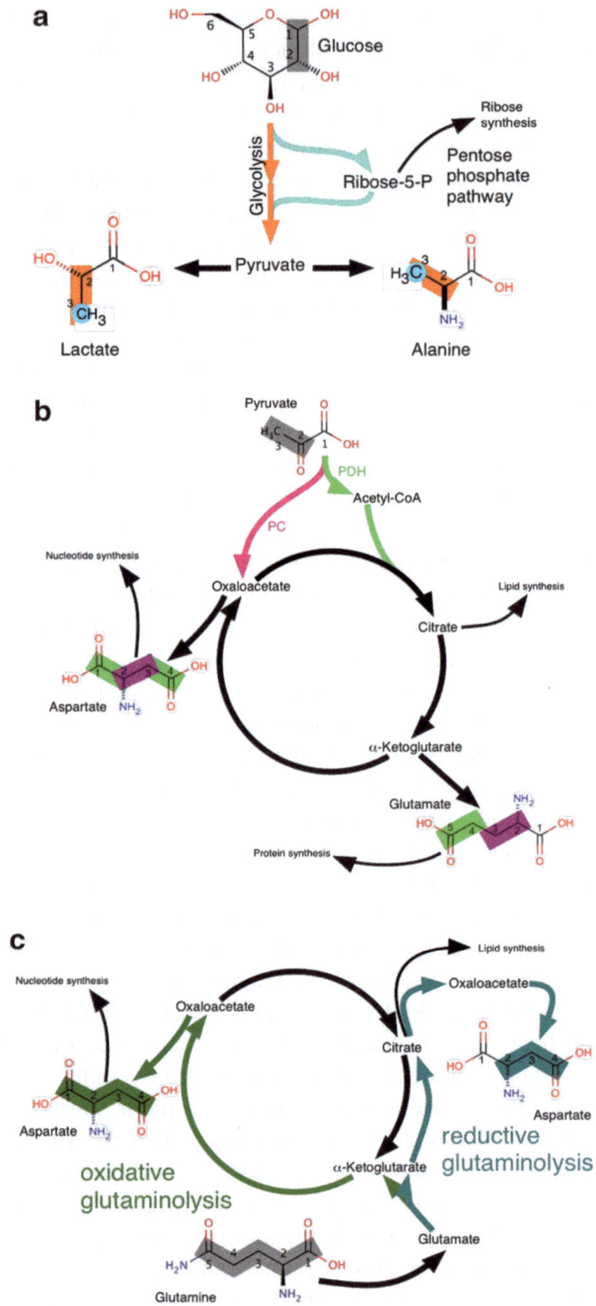

Fig. 6.4 Metabolic pathway tracking using $^{13}C_{1,2}$ glucose and $^{13}C_{1\text{–}5}$ glutamine tracers by NMR spectroscopy. Lactate, glutamate and aspartate are NMR-visible metabolites that can be considered metabolic readouts of pathway activity using $^{13}C_{1,2}$ glucose and $^{13}C_{1\text{–}5}$ glutamine as metabolic tracers. (**a**) $^{13}C_{2,3}$ lactate is formed from glycolytic pyruvate whereas $^{13}C_{3}$ lactate is made from pentose phosphate pathway derived pyruvate. (**b**) In the TCA cycle, $^{13}C_{2,3}$ pyruvate is oxidised by pyruvate dehydrogenase to form $^{13}C_{4,5}$ glutamate and $^{13}C_{1,2}$ or $^{13}C_{3,4}$ aspartate. $^{13}C_{2,3}$ pyruvate can also be carboxylated by pyruvate carboxylase to form $^{13}C_{2,3}$ glutamate and $^{13}C_{2,3}$ aspartate. (**c**) $^{13}C_{1\text{–}5}$ glutamine can either be converted oxidatively into $^{13}C_{1\text{–}4}$ aspartate or reductively into $^{13}C_{2,3,4}$ aspartate

aspartate: the $^{13}C_{1,2}$ and $^{13}C_{3,4}$ forms. However, in certain conditions and in some organs, pyruvate can be carboxylated to form oxaloacetate. This anaplerotic pathway, which relies on the activity of pyruvate carboxylase (PC), can be identified by virtue of the evolution of alternative isotopomers of aspartate and glutamate: $^{13}C_{2,3}$ aspartate and $^{13}C_{2,3}$ glutamate. Additionally, reductive glutamine metabolism is a metabolic perturbation recently described in cancer cells. In conditions where oxidative TCA metabolism is compromised, the relative use of reductive carboxylation of glutamine-derived α-ketoglutarate to produce sufficient citrate required for lipid synthesis may increase [5, 6, 8]. Using a $^{13}C_{1-5}$ glutamine tracer, label incorporation into aspartate can provide an insight into the activities of these two pathways: $^{13}C_{1-4}$ aspartate is produced as a consequence of oxidative TCA metabolism whereas $^{13}C_{2,3,4}$ aspartate is initially formed from reductive glutamine metabolism, as shown in Fig. 6.4c.

Complete isotope distribution analysis into these key NMR-visible metabolites allows us to determine differential pathway activities, which is often vital in determining how alterations in genetics, environment or organ function impinge upon the metabolic network. Importantly, a number of NMR spectroscopy methods can be exploited for this type of analysis, including 2D ^1H–^1H TOCSY, quantitatively isotope filtered 1D ^1H, 1D ^{13}C and 2D ^1H–^{13}C HSQC.

6.4.1 2D ^1H–^1H TOCSY NMR Spectroscopy

The majority of biological molecules under consideration in metabolic analysis consist of protons bound to ^{12}C atoms. ^{12}C atoms are not visible by NMR, as ^{12}C nuclei have a zero spin (see above). As a consequence, signals originating from ^1H attached to ^{12}C appear at the normal chemical shift, unlike ^1H with ^{13}C attached, which show as two signals symmetrical about the ^{12}C bound ^1H signal. These ^{13}C satellite signals, usually minor components (0.5 %) of the main NMR signal, become visible when ^{13}C is enriched. This consequently enables study of metabolism using nutrients enriched with ^{13}C. Further information about the chemical environment of the nucleus bound to the ^1H can also be obtained, as this influences the degree of splitting of the ^{13}C satellite signals (known as the $1J_{CH}$-coupling constant). However, this method significantly increases the complexity of the NMR spectrum and exacerbates the previously highlighted issue of signal overlap. Hence, the introduction of a second dimension to increase resolution of the spectrum is paramount, as illustrated in Fig. 6.5.

2D ^1H–^1H TOCSY NMR spectra are used to determine relative pathway information in tracer studies by assessing isotopic enrichment (such as ^{13}C) into downstream detectable metabolites. In this method, signal overlap is overcome by the use of cross peaks, where signals from different ^1H nuclei bound to different carbon

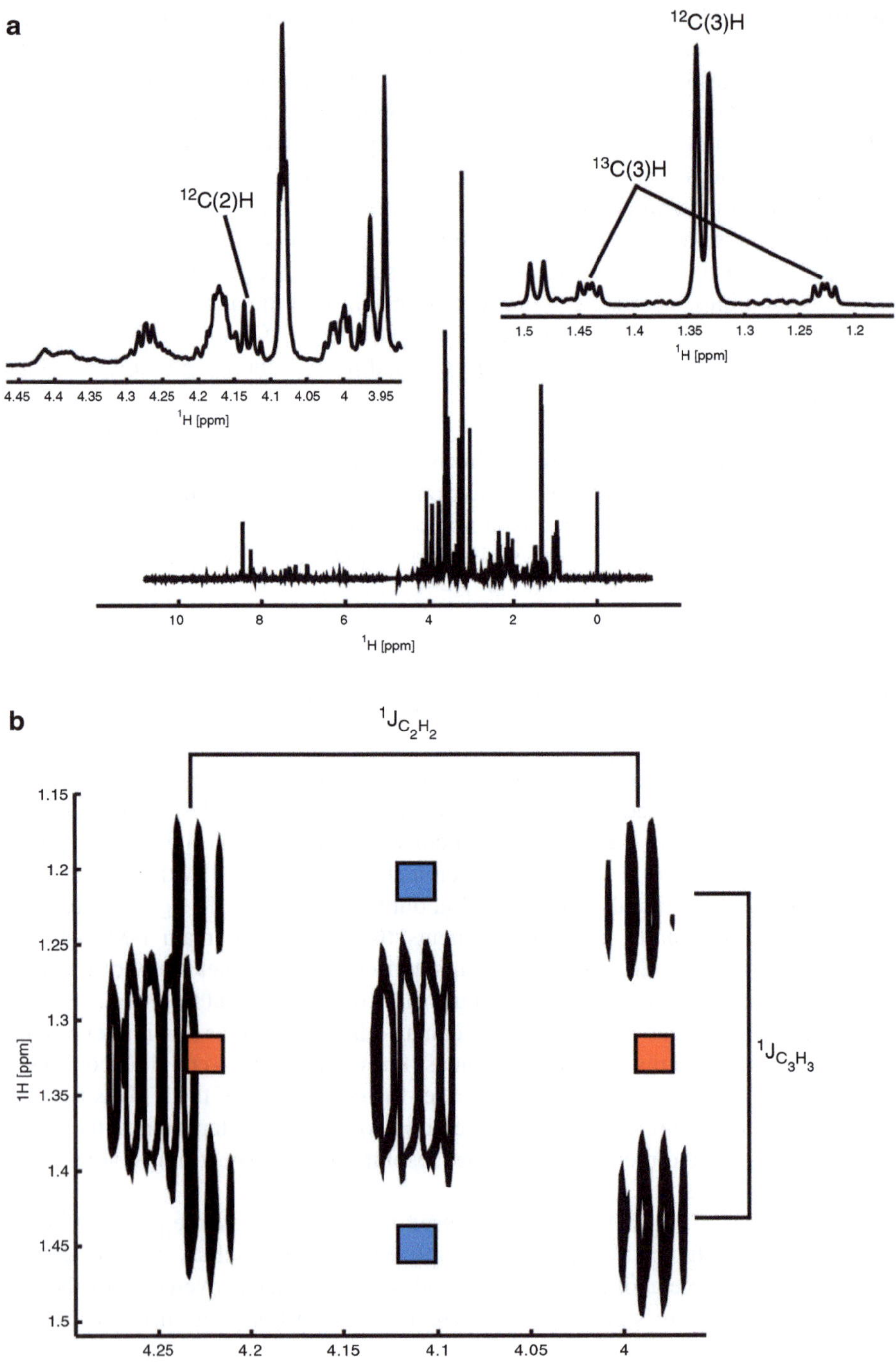

Fig. 6.5 ^{13}C tracer incorporation using 2D ^{1}H–^{1}H TOCSY spectra. (**a**) A 1D ^{1}H NMR spectrum acquired from a OE33 cell extract exposed to $^{13}C_{1,2}$ glucose for 6 h. As an example, the two protonFig. 6.5 (continued) signals (C(2) and C(3)) of lactate are highlighted. C(3) of lactate is

atoms are split across two axes. In the 2D spectrum, a cross peak occurs if two protons belong to the same spin system, which consists of nuclei connected through J coupling. Most protons within a metabolite belong to the same spin system, with the exception of quaternary carbon atoms (those with no bound protons), which separate these proton spin systems.

Each cross peak in 2D ^{1}H–^{1}H TOCSY consists of several components. If both protons contributing to the cross peak are bound to ^{12}C, a single peak appears in the 2D spectrum at the frequency of each proton in the direct and indirect dimension. If one or both of them are bound to a ^{13}C nucleus, the signal is split either in the direct dimension, indirect dimension, or both, depending on which carbon nuclei are ^{13}C. This splitting information can be used to determine the percentage of ^{13}C incorporation per carbon and, to a limited extent, to obtain information on simultaneous ^{13}C incorporation into two carbon nuclei within the same molecule. This can be particularly important when attempting to resolve the use of different pathways by a nutrient, such as in the example above of lactate production from glycolysis. However, to obtain detailed pathway information, a model simulation of the entire pathway is usually required [41].

6.4.2 *Quantitatively Isotope Filtered 1D ^{1}H NMR Spectroscopy*

An alternative to the use of 2D ^{1}H–^{1}H TOCSY spectra is the isotope filtered 1D ^{1}H NMR spectrum. In this approach, two ^{13}C decoupled 1D NMR spectra are acquired per sample. ^{13}C decoupling removes the signal splitting of ^{1}H signals. The first spectrum is simply a relaxation compensated 1D spectrum, where every proton attached to either a ^{12}C or ^{13}C nucleus contributes to the signal intensity in the 1D spectrum. A second spectrum is then acquired where the proton signals arising from ^{12}C bound ^{1}H nuclei are filtered. An alternative to the second spectrum would be to acquire a spectrum where the magnetisation is edited through ^{13}C-bound protons. However, if the latter approach is used, the intensities of the two spectra need to be calibrated with respect to one other, which is usually carried out on the assumption that the majority of protons are only bound to ^{12}C neighbours [42]. If quantitative filters are used, no assumptions about ^{13}C incorporation are necessary.

Fig. 6.5 (continued) well resolved and ^{13}C incorporation can be easily derived from a 1D ^{1}H NMR spectrum. C(2) of lactate resonates in a region with considerable signal overlap from other metabolites. (**b**) 2D ^{1}H–^{1}H TOCSY cross peak between proton signals attached to C(2) and C(3) of lactate. The cross peak between C(2) and C(3) is well resolved. The middle signals arise from protons attached to ^{12}C, whereas the surrounding signals originate from protons attached to $^{13}C_{2,3}$ lactate. The *coloured squares* indicate where signals would appear if $^{13}C_2$ lactate (*orange*) or $^{13}C_3$ lactate (*blue*) were present

Owing to the speed with which these 1D spectra can be acquired, this approach lends itself to real-time metabolic flux analysis. Live tissue or cells can be monitored in real-time, enabling a kinetic analysis of cell metabolism without the need for metabolite extraction [43], which is typically performed for most biological samples. Extraction of metabolites from cultured tissue or cells allows NMR spectra to be acquired at higher resolution, thus obtaining a more comprehensive overview of the metabolism. The typical aqueous extraction procedure, however, introduce an unavoidable bias into the analysis towards polar metabolites.

Whilst compared to conventional 1D ^{1}H NMR spectra, where the split ^{13}C bound proton signals are observed, all carbon bound proton signals in a filtered 1D ^{1}H NMR appear at the same chemical shift. This leads to metabolite peak overlap in the spectrum, complicating the analysis.

6.4.3 1D ^{13}C NMR Spectroscopy

1D ^{13}C NMR spectra can provide high-resolution data and localised information on simultaneous ^{13}C incorporation into the same molecule by virtue of signal multiplets. An example of how this splitting information is used to differentiate $^{13}C_{1,2}$ glutamate from $^{13}C_{2,3}$ glutamate is illustrated in Fig. 6.6. In this method, a single ^{13}C nucleus produces a single peak. If a neighbouring carbon is also ^{13}C, then the signal is split into two peaks, known as a doublet. The degree of splitting depends on the chemical environment of the neighbouring carbon, providing important information about the nature of the molecule. If two carbon atoms surround the carbon nucleus, and all three carbon nuclei are ^{13}C, the signal splits into either three peaks, known as a pseudo triplet (providing the J-coupling constant is the same for both coupling partners) or four peaks, known as a doublet of doublets (if the J-coupling constants for adjacent carbon nuclei are different). The ability of NMR to distinguish not only isotopologues but also isotopomers is crucial to differentiate relative pathway activity accurately.

It cannot be ignored that the lengthy acquisition time inherent in this approach is not compatible with most biological projects. This arises because ^{13}C-based NMR studies are significantly less sensitive than 1D ^{1}H spectra (approximately 16× less, based solely on gyromagnetic ratios). However, the overlap of ^{13}C-based NMR studies is significantly improved due to the fourfold chemical shift dispersion of 1D ^{13}C NMR spectra compared to 1D ^{1}H NMR spectra. Where 1D ^{1}H spectra are dominated by ^{1}H signals attached to ^{12}C, ^{1}H-decoupled 1D ^{13}C NMR spectra cannot see ^{12}C nuclei and as a result have reduced background. This means that low-moderate label incorporation is more reliably detected in a 1D ^{13}C NMR compared to proton-based equivalents, and is further explained in the HSQC section. This approach may therefore be useful for precise detection of multiple isotopomers in a metabolite from single samples only, unlike some other methods where ambiguity may exist.

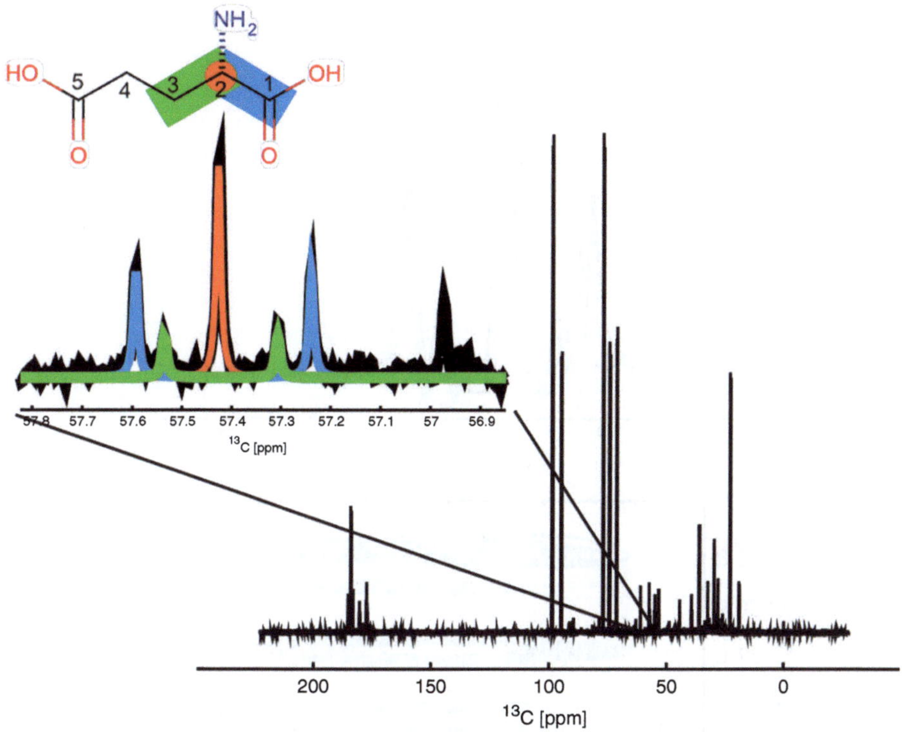

Fig. 6.6 1D ^{13}C NMR on OE33 cell extracts. Signals from C(2) of glutamate are highlighted. The multiplet components are fitted to the experimental spectrum. The *orange* signal appears if only C(2) is ^{13}C and C(1) and C(3) are ^{12}C. The *blue* doublet represents simultaneous ^{13}C incorporation into C(1) and C(2) ($^{13}C_{1,2}$ glutamate). A similar doublet can be observed if there is simultaneous ^{13}C incorporation into C(2) and C(3) ($^{13}C_{2,3}$ glutamate, *green curve*). The different chemical nature of C(1) and C(3) result in different J-coupling constants and hence can be resolved spectroscopically

6.4.4 2D ^{1}H–^{13}C HSQC NMR Spectroscopy

2D ^{1}H–^{13}C HSQC spectroscopy is an attractive alternative to conventional 1D ^{13}C spectra and ^{1}H–^{1}H TOCSY spectra having improved sensitivity over the former and decreased spectral overlap, relative to the latter. This spectroscopy type correlates the resonance frequencies of ^{1}H and ^{13}C that are directly bound, where each ^{1}H–^{13}C pair gives rise to a signal at the proton chemical shift in the horizontal (direct) and the ^{13}C chemical shift in the vertical (indirect) dimension. The ^{13}C–^{13}C multiplets as seen in the 1D ^{13}C NMR spectrum can therefore be observed in the indirect dimension, as highlighted in Fig. 6.7a.

To retain multiplicity information, HSQC spectra need to be acquired at high resolution, such as 16,384 increments (Fig. 6.7b). This results in long acquisition times (up to 16 h per sample) to observe the ^{13}C–^{13}C scalar couplings, which may be

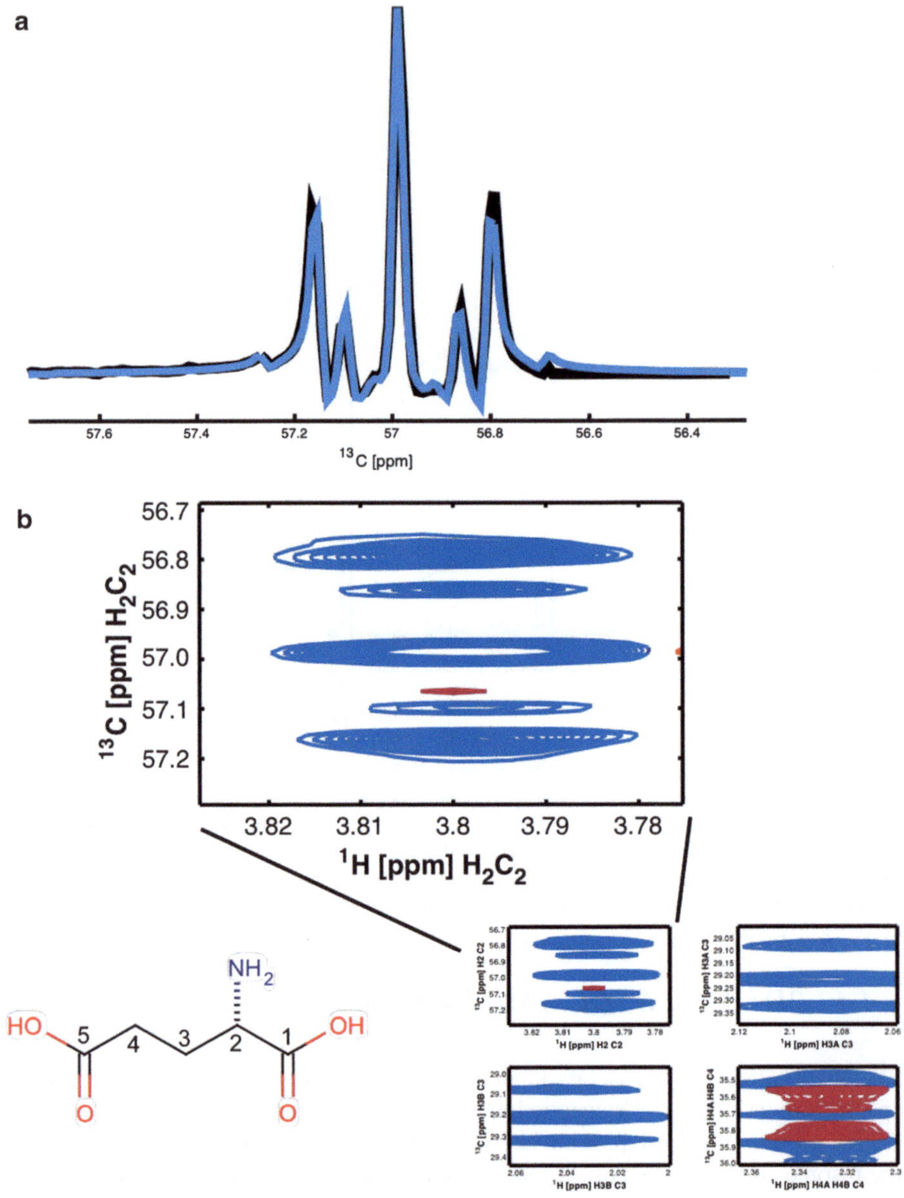

Fig. 6.7 HSQC analysis of glutamate. (**a**) Multiplet analysis of glutamate where all major and minor components comprising this multiplet are fitted to a theoretical model. (**b**) Four signals are visible in an HSQC spectrum. Only proton bearing carbon nuclei ($C_{2,3,4}$) are observed. As both protons attached to C(3) of glutamate are not equivalent, they resonate at different chemical shifts. Signals split into multiplets in the indirect (*vertical*) dimension owing to simultaneous ^{13}C incorporation into adjacent carbon atoms. As an example C(2) of glutamate is highlighted

impractical or too costly for some studies. A pragmatic alternative to reduce acquisition time by up to 70 % and increase sample throughput for HSQC spectra is to acquire them using a technique termed non-uniform sampling, where only a subset of increments is sampled. The 2D spectrum is then reconstructed using an algorithm, examples of which include compressed sensing, maximum entropy or discrete Fourier transform compressed sensing [44–46]. These reconstruction methods can require substantial computational capability, such as access to high-performance computing clusters.

Sufficient relaxation delays between transients are required for accurate metabolite quantification. 2D ^{1}H–^{13}C HSQC NMR spectra therefore have the additional benefit of quicker acquisition times compared to 1D ^{13}C NMR due to the differences between ^{13}C and ^{1}H relaxation times themselves. Unlike 1D ^{13}C NMR, which relies on ^{13}C relaxation rates, 2D ^{1}H–^{13}C HSQC NMR relies on ^{1}H relaxation rates and, as ^{13}C requires a longer relaxation time than ^{1}H, the resulting delay time between scans for HSQCs is shorter.

Similar to 1D ^{13}C NMR, ^{12}C bound protons are not visible in a 2D ^{1}H–^{13}C HSQC NMR spectra, which facilitates the detection of low percentage ^{13}C-labelled metabolites with increased confidence, as demonstrated in Fig. 6.8. This feature is unlike 2D ^{1}H–^{1}H TOCSY, where low to moderate percentage ^{13}C label incorporation into metabolites is obscured by ^{12}C bound ^{1}H signals. Both 2D TOCSY and 2D HSQC spectra are blind to quarternary carbons. However, in HSQC spectra indirect information can be obtained by splittings if there is simultaneous label incorporation into adjacent non-quarternary carbon nuclei. However, a combination of NMR and MS data can be used to derive information about NMR invisible carbons, as explained in the next section.

6.5 Isopologue/Isotopomer Analysis

Whilst quantitative multiplet analysis provides localised information only, overlapping two and three carbon fragments originating from neighbouring carbon atoms within a metabolite can be used to derive more accurate isotopologue or isotopomer distributions. In some circumstances, this information can be used directly to decipher alternative pathway usage, such as aspartate labelling from $^{13}C_{1,2}$ glucose (see beginning of Sect. 6.4). A detailed knowledge of all isotopomers and isotopologues is required to perform a comprehensive analysis on cellular metabolic processes.

Another important consideration is that in specific metabolites some ^{1}J-coupling constants are too similar (if not the same) and therefore contribute to the same signal. This can be illustrated in glutamate where the J-coupling constants in $^{13}C_{2,3}$ and $^{13}C_{3,4}$ glutamate cannot be resolved spectroscopically. It is unknown whether the doublet component of C(3) glutamate multiplet is caused by $^{13}C_{2,3}$ or $^{13}C_{3,4}$ glutamate: information that would shed light on the synthetic route for oxaloacetate. This information is encoded in the multiplets of C(2) and C(4) of glutamate; therefore

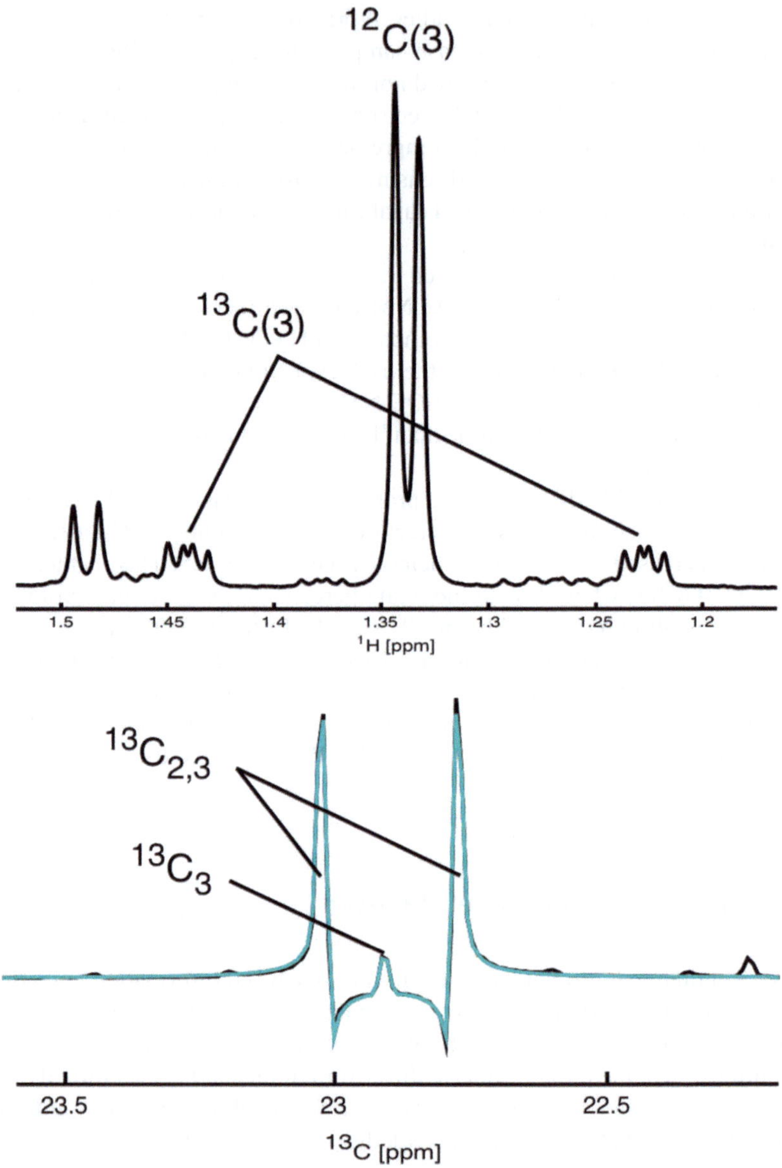

Fig. 6.8 1D ^{1}H tracer vs 2D HSQC analysis of lactate. (**a**) 1D ^{1}H NMR signals of protons attached to C(3) of lactate. In this example, ~25 % of all C(3) nuclei in lactate are labelled with ^{13}C. Despite a significant proportion of carbon nuclei being enriched with ^{13}C, the 1D signals (and therefore the 2D ^{1}H–^{1}H TOCSY cross peaks) only show a minor signal component in the spectrum. Hence, it can be difficult to estimate lower contributions to the NMR multiplet. 2D ^{1}H–^{13}C HSQC spectra on the other hand enhance the ^{13}C contribution and therefore are more sensitive to minor ^{13}C-multiplet contributions. As only protons bound to ^{13}C nuclei give rise to a signal in HSQC spectra, $^{13}C_{2,3}$ and $^{13}C_{3}$ isotopomers lead to different splittings as shown in the lower panel

simultaneous analysis of all glutamate multiplets is required to resolve this ambiguity. Similar ambiguity can exist for other metabolites, typically those with long aliphatic chains such as proline.

Additionally, HSQC multiplets alone cannot determine if the middle signal originates from ^{13}C natural abundance only, or if there is an additional single label incorporated into that carbon nucleus. This issue can be clarified by providing an absolute amount of ^{13}C incorporation into the carbon of interest, independent of ^{13}C incorporation into adjacent nuclei. There are several methods used to ascertain relative concentrations of labelled metabolites. The first acquires spectra from two samples produced in parallel, where one sample is unlabelled material and the other is enriched with ^{13}C metabolic precursors. However, in this approach, inconsistent concentrations between the two samples may lead to misguided results and incorrect biological interpretation. Other methods to determine absolute ^{13}C incorporation can use a single sample only. However, certain analytical assumptions have to be made, such as the middle peak of the multiplet consisting only of natural abundance ^{13}C contributions. Alternatively, either 2D TOCSY spectra or filtered 1D spectra can be used, but are limited by overlap and consequently can be problematic for even simple metabolites such as lactate.

Combining NMR multiplets with MS data provides all the relevant information to determine the correct ^{13}C incorporation percentage in addition to long-range isotopomers or isotopologues. For example, using NMR data only, a glutamate molecule labelled in carbon positions 1,2, 4 and 5 would be impossible to distinguish from two independently labelled glutamate molecules labelled with either carbon 1 and 2, or carbon 4 and 5. Using MS data only, it would also be impossible to distinguish all possible isotopomers that contain four ^{13}C nuclei without fragmentation-based approaches. Metabolic flux data are typically analysed using an appropriate metabolic model for MS and/or 2D TOCSY data. Combining information derived from HSQC multiplets and MS permits the analysis of an unbiased model-free pathway, whereby no prior knowledge of metabolic pathway activities is required to derive the whole isotopomer or isotopologue distribution. Figure 6.9 illustrates how well NMR and MS data can be fitted simultaneously. Isotopomers or isotopologues derived in this way can then be used as an input to a metabolic pathway simulation, rather than being derived from it.

6.6 Discussion and Future Outlook

Targeting tumour-specific metabolic alterations presents as an attractive therapeutic approach in anti-cancer therapy [12]. Analytical platforms, such as NMR spectroscopy, are being increasingly developed and employed to aid our understanding of the perturbed metabolism identified in cancer cells. NMR is a particularly powerful tool for the elucidation of structures at the atomic level, resulting in highly reproducible and quantitative data. As a non-invasive technique, it has the versatility of being used in vivo, ex vivo and in vitro, making it a highly powerful method,

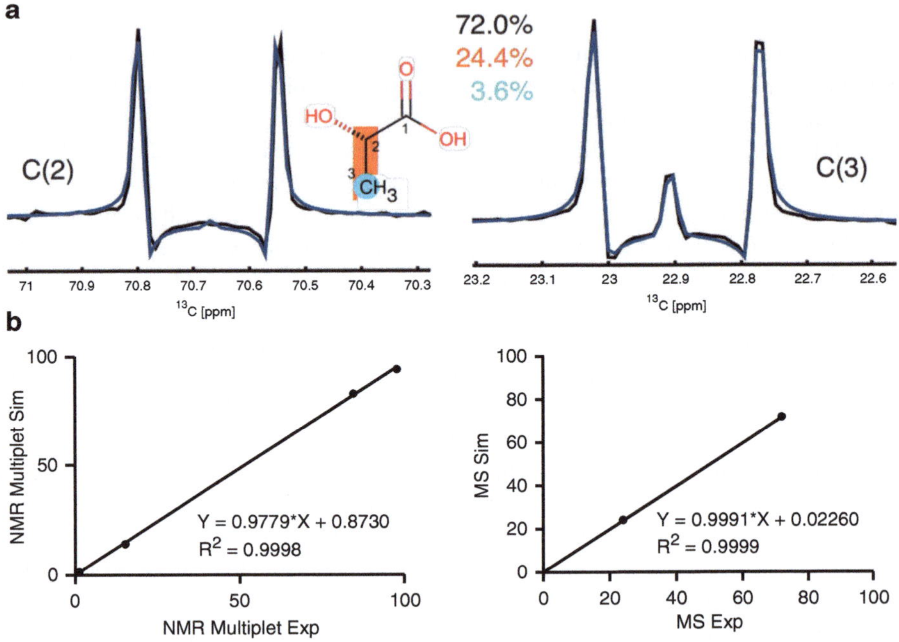

Fig. 6.9 Combination of NMR and MS data. (**a**) Experimental (*black*) and fitted (*blue*) ^{13}C multiplets for C(2) and C(3) of lactate. (**b**) Fitted and experimental percentages for NMR multiplet composition and MS data. Incorporating the resulting NMR multiplet with the MS isotopologue distribution simulates the fitted data. This is based on the proposed isotopologue distribution of 72 % unlabelled, 24.4 % $^{13}C_{2,3}$ lactate and 3.6 % $^{13}C_3$ lactate

suitable for a variety of biological applications that have potential to translate into a clinical setting [20]. However, it is limited by lower sensitivity than other approaches, such as MS, and the ability to detect and distinguish reliably only between some limited classes of molecules.

Steady-state metabolism analysis provides relative or absolute information on intra- or extra-cellular metabolite levels, which can be used to distinguish metabolic differences and so can provide an initial insight into disease biochemistry. Owing to the untargeted nature of metabolomics, analysis of steady-state metabolites presents as a suitable method for discovery studies. This is further enhanced by the speed of experimental acquisition and sensitivity of ^1H nuclei. However, metabolomics provides no information on flux changes, directionality of flux changes or changes in nutrient source/metabolite usage. The use of metabolic tracers artificially enriched with low abundance NMR active isotopes compensates for some of these limitations. Therefore, steady-state metabolism analysis is frequently used as an initial platform to distinguish whether metabolic differences exist, after which a more targeted analysis is made using isotopic-labelled metabolic tracers to examine why. For example, glutamate concentration changes may only be indicative of changes in net production or consumption fluxes, whereas labelling distributions in glutamate with the use of $^{13}C_{1,2}$ glucose tracer reveal potentially differential pyruvate pathway activity on entry into the TCA cycle ($^{13}C_{4,5}$ glutamate is indicative of pyruvate oxidation and $^{13}C_{2,3}$ glutamate by pyruvate carboxylation).

Differential metabolic pathway activity can be obtained by NMR spectroscopy due to its capability to resolve ^{13}C incorporation at an atomic level, which can be quantified when combined with total metabolite concentrations. As NMR is limited by sensitivity, data analysis tends to focus on those metabolites whose concentrations are sufficient to be NMR-visible. The use of complementary tracers and analysis of labelling patterns in multiple downstream metabolites increases understanding of and confidence in biological conclusions. Labelled glucose can reveal information on oxidative TCA cycle metabolism; labelled glutamine can provide complementary information such as reductive glutaminolysis.

Tracer-based metabolism studies tend to be analysed on whole cell extracts, which can complicate data analysis and interpretation. In particular, cell compartmentalisation, where the dynamic exchange of metabolites between the mitochondria and the cytosol can obscure findings. An example is the production of lactate and alanine from cytosolic and/or mitochondrial pyruvate pools, respectively. Additionally, metabolites formed from multiple intersecting pathways, such as glutamate, can result in ambiguous results and incorrect conclusions being drawn from resulting data. The incorporation of NMR and MS, along with the use of multiple complementary tracers, has the potential to resolve these issues.

A major drawback in the development of NMR-based approaches for metabolic tracer studies has been the lack of available software tools required to support data analysis and interpretation. Whilst numerous software tools exist for metabolomics spectra [33, 47–49], the information content of NMR multiplets in tracer studies is far more complex, and existing basic software requires further development to extract the necessary information [29, 50]. This type of software also needs to be readily available and amenable to non-NMR specialists. With the ongoing developments in novel labelling strategies, data software tools must continue to develop in parallel, an area that is currently poorly represented in the field. The combination of NMR and MS data resolves metabolic ambiguity better than if each were used alone thereby providing a greater insight into the metabolic network. Further developments are required to use these model-free labelling distributions as an input for dynamic metabolism simulations to result in an unbiased, more representative overview of metabolism.

Acknowledgements The authors thank BBSRC and AstraZeneca for supporting Kate Hollinshead with a CASE studentship, the Wellcome Trust for supporting the HWB-NMR facility in Birmingham and lastly Sylvia C Miller and Jay Nath for critical reading of the manuscript.

References

1. Warburg O, Posener K, Negelein E. On the metabolism of carcinoma cells. Biochem Z. 1924;152:309–44.
2. Hanahan D, Weinberg RA. Hallmarks of cancer: the next generation. Cell. 2011;144(5):646–74.
3. Dang CV, Semenza GL. Oncogenic alterations of metabolism. Trends Biochem Sci. 1999;24(2):68–72.

4. Vander Heiden MG, Cantley LC, Thompson CB. Understanding the Warburg effect: the metabolic requirements of cell proliferation. Science. 2009;324(5930):1029–33.
5. Metallo CM, et al. Reductive glutamine metabolism by IDH1 mediates lipogenesis under hypoxia. Nature. 2012;481(7381):380–4.
6. Wise DR, et al. Hypoxia promotes isocitrate dehydrogenase-dependent carboxylation of alpha-ketoglutarate to citrate to support cell growth and viability. Proc Natl Acad Sci U S A. 2011;108(49):19611–6.
7. Frezza C, et al. Haem oxygenase is synthetically lethal with the tumour suppressor fumarate hydratase. Nature. 2011;477(7363):225–8.
8. Mullen AR, et al. Reductive carboxylation supports growth in tumour cells with defective mitochondria. Nature. 2012;481(7381):385–8.
9. Possemato R, et al. Functional genomics reveal that the serine synthesis pathway is essential in breast cancer. Nature. 2011;476(7360):346–50.
10. Le A, et al. Glucose-independent glutamine metabolism via TCA cycling for proliferation and survival in B cells. Cell Metab. 2012;15(1):110–21.
11. Yuneva MO, et al. The metabolic profile of tumors depends on both the responsible genetic lesion and tissue type. Cell Metab. 2012;15(2):157–70.
12. Tennant DA, Duran RV, Gottlieb E. Targeting metabolic transformation for cancer therapy. Nat Rev Cancer. 2010;10(4):267–77.
13. Wishart DS, et al. HMDB 3.0-the human metabolome database in 2013. Nucleic Acids Res. 2013;41(D1):D801–7.
14. Parsons HM, et al. Improved classification accuracy in 1- and 2-dimensional NMR metabolomics data using the variance stabilising generalised logarithm transformation. BMC Bioinformatics. 2007;8:234.
15. Marek EM, et al. Measurements of lactate in exhaled breath condensate at rest and after maximal exercise in young and healthy subjects. J Breath Res. 2010;4(1):017105.
16. Sinclair AJ, et al. NMR-based metabolomic analysis of cerebrospinal fluid and serum in neurological diseases—a diagnostic tool? NMR Biomed. 2010;23(2):123–32.
17. Viant MR, et al. International NMR-based environmental metabolomics intercomparison exercise. Environ Sci Technol. 2009;43(1):219–25.
18. Sands CJ, et al. Data-driven approach for metabolite relationship recovery in biological 1H NMR data sets using iterative statistical total correlation spectroscopy. Anal Chem. 2011;83(6):2075–82.
19. Swann JR, et al. Systemic gut microbial modulation of bile acid metabolism in host tissue compartments. Proc Natl Acad Sci U S A. 2011;108 Suppl 1:4523–30.
20. Guy AJ, et al. Metabolomic analysis of perfusate during hypothermic machine perfusion of human cadaveric kidneys. Transplantation. 2015;99(4):754–9.
21. Wilson M, et al. A constrained least-squares approach to the automated quantitation of in vivo H-1 magnetic resonance spectroscopy data. Magn Reson Med. 2011;65(1):1–12.
22. Chung YL, Griffiths JR. Using metabolomics to monitor anticancer drugs. Ernst Schering Found Symp Proc. 2007;4:55–78.
23. Davies NP, et al. Non-invasive detection of glycine as a biomarker of malignancy in childhood brain tumours using in-vivo 1H MRS at 1.5 tesla confirmed by ex-vivo high-resolution magic-angle spinning NMR. NMR Biomed. 2010;23(1):80–7.
24. Mirbahai L, et al. 1H magnetic resonance spectroscopy metabolites as biomarkers for cell cycle arrest and cell death in rat glioma cells. Int J Biochem Cell Biol. 2011;43(7):990–1001.
25. Dona AC, et al. Precision high-throughput proton NMR spectroscopy of human urine, serum, and plasma for large-scale metabolic phenotyping. Anal Chem. 2014;86(19):9887–94.
26. Gueron M, Plateau P, Decorps M. Solvent signal suppression in NMR. Prog Nucl Magn Reson Spectrosc. 1991;23:135–209.
27. Levitt M. Spin dynamics. 2nd ed. Chichester: Wiley; 2008.
28. Ramadan Z, et al. Metabolic profiling using principal component analysis, discriminant partial least squares, and genetic algorithms. Talanta. 2006;68(5):1683–91.

29. Ludwig C, Gunther UL. MetaboLab—advanced NMR data processing and analysis for metabolomics. BMC Bioinformatics. 2011;12:366.
30. Viant MR. Improved methods for the acquisition and interpretation of NMR metabolomic data. Biochem Biophys Res Commun. 2003;310(3):943–8.
31. Aue WP, Karhan J, Ernst RR. Homonuclear broad-band decoupling and 2-dimensional J-resolved NMR-spectroscopy. J Chem Phys. 1976;64(10):4226–7.
32. Ludwig C, Viant MR. Two-dimensional J-resolved NMR spectroscopy: review of a key methodology in the metabolomics toolbox. Phytochem Anal. 2010;21(1):22–32.
33. Ludwig C, et al. Birmingham Metabolite Library: a publicly accessible database of 1-D H-1 and 2-D H-1 J-resolved NMR spectra of authentic metabolite standards (BML-NMR). Metabolomics. 2012;8(1):8–18.
34. Buescher JM, et al. A roadmap for interpreting C metabolite labeling patterns from cells. Curr Opin Biotechnol. 2015;34:189–201.
35. Fan TW, et al. Stable isotope-resolved metabolomics and applications for drug development. Pharmacol Ther. 2012;133(3):366–91.
36. Ugurbil K, et al. High-resolution 13C nuclear magnetic resonance studies of glucose metabolism in Escherichia coli. Proc Natl Acad Sci U S A. 1978;75(8):3742–6.
37. Shulman RG, et al. Cellular applications of 31P and 13C nuclear magnetic resonance. Science. 1979;205(4402):160–6.
38. Malloy CR, Sherry AD, Jeffrey FM. Evaluation of carbon flux and substrate selection through alternate pathways involving the citric acid cycle of the heart by 13C NMR spectroscopy. J Biol Chem. 1988;263(15):6964–71.
39. Metallo CM, Walther JL, Stephanopoulos G. Evaluation of 13C isotopic tracers for metabolic flux analysis in mammalian cells. J Biotechnol. 2009;144(3):167–74.
40. DeBerardinis RJ, et al. Beyond aerobic glycolysis: transformed cells can engage in glutamine metabolism that exceeds the requirement for protein and nucleotide synthesis. Proc Natl Acad Sci U S A. 2007;104(49):19345–50.
41. Lane AN, et al. Stable isotope-resolved metabolomics (SIRM) in cancer research with clinical application to nonsmall cell lung cancer. OMICS. 2011;15(3):173–82.
42. Howe PW, et al. Combined use of filtered and edited 1 H NMR spectroscopy to detect 13 C-enriched compounds in complex mixtures. NMR Biomed. 2012;25(11):1217–23.
43. Xin LJ, et al. Assessment of metabolic fluxes in the mouse brain in vivo using H-1-[C-13] NMR spectroscopy at 14.1 Tesla. J Cereb Blood Flow Metab. 2015;35(5):759–65.
44. Kazimierczuk K, Orekhov VY. Accelerated NMR spectroscopy by using compressed sensing. Angew Chem Int Ed Engl. 2011;50(24):5556–9.
45. Hyberts SG, et al. Ultrahigh-resolution (1)H-(13)C HSQC spectra of metabolite mixtures using nonlinear sampling and forward maximum entropy reconstruction. J Am Chem Soc. 2007;129(16):5108–16.
46. Stanek J, Kozminski W. Iterative algorithm of discrete Fourier transform for processing randomly sampled NMR data sets. J Biomol NMR. 2010;47(1):65–77.
47. Ravanbakhsh S, et al. Accurate, fully-automated NMR spectral profiling for metabolomics. PLoS One. 2015;10(5):e0124219.
48. Xia J, et al. MetaboAnalyst 3.0-making metabolomics more meaningful. Nucleic Acids Res. 2015;43(W1):W251–7.
49. Fitzpatrick MA, McGrath CM, Young SP. Pathomx: an interactive workflow-based tool for the analysis of metabolomic data. BMC Bioinformatics. 2014;15(1):396.
50. Lewis IA, Schommer SC, Markley JL. rNMR: open source software for identifying and quantifying metabolites in NMR spectra. Magn Reson Chem. 2009;47:S123–6.

Chapter 7
Measuring the Impact of Microenvironmental Conditions on Mitochondrial Dehydrogenase Activity in Cultured Cells

Ramon C. Sun, Albert Koong, Amato Giaccia, and Nicholas C. Denko

Keywords Enzymatic activity • Colorimetric detection • Hypoxia • Hypoglycemia • Dehydrogenase

7.1 Introduction

Mitochondria are powerhouses of a cell, producing much of the cellular ATP. However, mitochondrial enzymes also participate in many cellular biosynthetic processes. They are responsible for helping to maintain NAD(P)/H and redox balance, supplying metabolic intermediates for cell growth, and regulating several types of programed cell death. Several mitochondrial enzymes have even been shown to participate in the oncogenic process such as isocitrate dehydrogenase, succinate dehydrogenase, and fumarate hydratase. Recent advances have identified significant metabolic changes in the mitochondria that are regulated by malignant transformation and environmental stimuli. Understanding the biological activity and regulation of mitochondrial enzymes can provide insight into how they

R.C. Sun
Center for Environmental and Systems Biochemistry, Mackey Cancer Center, University of KentucKY Lexington, KY 40536, USA

Department of Radiation Oncology, Ohio State University Wexner School of Medicine and Comprehensive Cancer Center, Ohio Sate University, Columbus, OH 43210, USA
e-mail: ramon.sun@uky.edu

A. Koong • A. Giaccia
Department of Radiation Oncology, Stanford University School of Medicine, Stanford, CA 94305, USA
e-mail: albert.koong@stanford.edu; amato.giaccia@stanford.edu

N.C. Denko (✉)
Department of Radiation Oncology, Ohio State University Wexner School of Medicine and Comprehensive Cancer Center, Ohio Sate University, Columbus, OH 43210, USA
e-mail: Nicholas.denko@osumc.edu

C. Koumenis et al. (eds.), *Tumor Microenvironment*, Advances in Experimental Medicine and Biology 899, DOI 10.1007/978-3-319-26666-4_7

participate in the process of oncogenic transformation and work to sustain malignant growth. This chapter describes a technique to measure mitochondrial dehydrogenase activities that is faster and more cost effective which can also be scaled up for high throughput.

7.2 General Method

Conventional methods of measuring dehydrogenase activity involve biochemical isolation of whole enzyme complexes. Crude preparations can be made by subcellular fractionation and disruption of intracellular compartments with weak ionic detergent. Isolated enzyme complexes can either be further purified via size or affinity-based fractionation methods for more accurate measurement of specific activity or used as a crude complex mixture containing other enzymes. Depending on the extent of purification, the results can be more qualitative rather than quantitative. Recently, antibodies have been employed for even more specific immune capture and purification of enzymes. For example, the PDH assay sold by Mitoscience purifies the entire core PDH complex, but does not retain regulatory kinases and phosphatases.

Conventional methods have been used for the past century as a cornerstone of many reports that built our understanding of fundamental biochemical processes. However, significant limitations to the approach exist. Due to their low abundance and low recovery, it often takes large amounts of starting material (in some cases kilograms of tissue). Biochemical purification also requires technical skill and time for high activity preparations. Procedures can take days with multiple steps of centrifugation and dialysis. On a more theoretical note, it is hard to guarantee the integrity of the enzymatic complex. Critical components of the active complex could be lost in purification, or regulatory elements that are specific to the growth conditions (i.e., modification of critical regulatory residues, or associated regulatory kinases or phosphatases).

Here, we describe a method-of measuring mitochondrial dehydrogenase activities that overcomes many of these limitations. First, the method requires only a few thousand adherent cells. Second, it keeps the enzyme complex in its native environment with only minimal disruption of the cell by permeabilization of the membranes to facilitate substrate entry. Finally, and perhaps most important is that it can be performed in a 96-well format to allow real time, replicate comparison of multiple treatment conditions. This technique is based on P. Kugler's microscopic histochemistry method to detect dehydrogenase activity in brain tissue slices [1]. This method uses a two-step biochemical reaction that produces a colorimetric detection of dehydrogenase activity which is much more sensitive than the traditional absorbance-based assays. In the first reaction the dehydrogenase carries out its dehydrogenation with the concurrent conversion of NAD/NADP to NADH/NADPH. In the second reaction NAD(P)H is oxidized via phenazine methosulfate which in turn donates the electron to nitroblue tetrazolium to produce a blue-stained

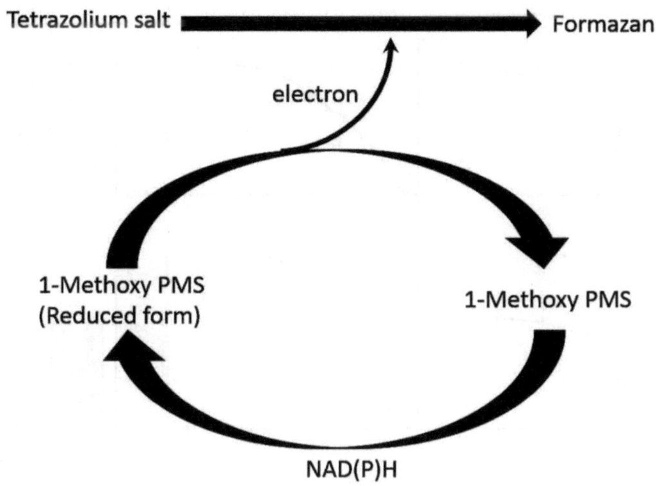

Fig. 7.1 Generation of the blue formazan precipitate through the transfer of electrons from NAD(P)H to the nitroblue tetrazolium to form the purple-blue precipitate

water-insoluble formazan (Fig. 7.1) [2–4]. The dark formazan is then solubilized with 10 % SDS in 0.01 N HCl overnight in a CO_2 incubator and the optical density measured at 540 nm in a plate reader. The optical density is a measure of NAD(P)H produced, which is a function of the amount of enzyme activity because substrates are in excess.

7.2.1 *List of Stock Reagents*

HBSS—See below for recipe, once made stable for up to 3 months at 4 °C.

Assay buffer-50 mM Tris-Cl, 0.05 mM EDTA, pH 7.8, stable for up to 3 months at room temperature.

1 M αKG made up in MilliQ water and stored at −20 °C for up to 1 month.

1 M $MgCl_2$ made up in MilliQ water and stored at −20 °C for up to 1 month.

1 M $CaCl_2$ made up in MilliQ water and stored at −20 °C for up to 1 month.

1 M Na pyruvate made up in MilliQ water and stored at −20 °C for up to 1 month.

1 M Glucose made up in MilliQ water and stored at −20 °C for up to 1 month.

100 mM Isocitrate made up in MilliQ water and stored at −20 °C for up to 1 month.

200 mM ThDP made up in MilliQ water and stored at −20 °C for up to 1 month.

300 mM NAD made up in MilliQ water and stored at −20 °C for up to 1 week.

100 mM CoA made up in MilliQ water and stored at −20 °C for up to 1 week.

10 mg/ml Nitroblue tetrazolium made up in MilliQ water and stored at −20 °C for up to 1 month.

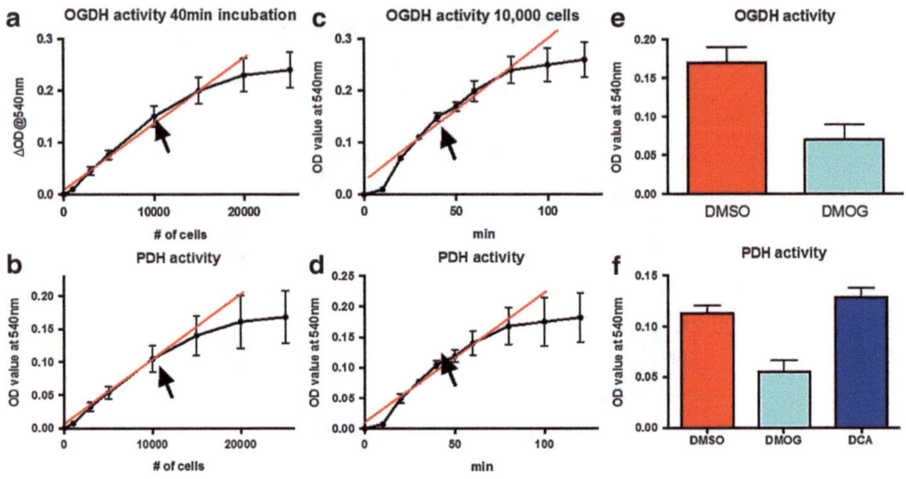

Fig. 7.2 (**a**–**d**) Determination of reaction parameters for adherent RKO colorectal cancer cells for both αKGDH and PDH assays. Note that cell number (**a**, **b**) and time of reaction (**c**, **d**) are both chosen to be in the linear portion of the curve. (**e**, **f**) determination of the effect of HIF1 stabilization by DMOG on aKGDH and PDH activities, and determination of the effect of the pyruvate dehydrogenase kinase inhibitor dichloroacetate on PDH activity

31.25 mg/ml Phenazine methosulfate made up in MilliQ water and stored at −20 °C for up to 1 month.

0.5 mg/ml Rotenone made up in DMSO or ethanol and stored at −20 °C.

7.2.2 *Method for Selected Enzymes*

The following steps for αKGDH, PDH, and IDH are optimized for RKO human colorectal cancer cells (Fig. 7.2). Cell density, time of incubation, and substrate concentrations may need to be adjusted for cell lines of different origins.

1. Seed cells in a 96-well plate at a seeding density of 1×10^4/well overnight in 200 μl of growth medium. Plates can be treated with hypoxia or other experimental conditions such as treatment with DMOG to induce HIF-1 activity.

   Low-glucose DMEM with 10 % FBS should be used to grow cells overnight since glucose has been shown to suppress mitochondrial oxygen consumption and enzyme activities. The even seeding of adherent cells can be achieved by allowing cells to attach on a 360° orbital (i.e., "belly dancer") plate shaker at 37 °C if possible.
2. On the day of the measurement, the medium is aspirated, and the cells are washed once with balanced salt solution (BBS) [140 mM NaCl, 5 mM KCl, 2.5 mM $CaCl_2$, 1 mM $MgCl_2$, 5 mM glucose, and 10 mM HEPES (pH 7.4)]. To test the activity of enzymatic inhibitors in vivo, treat cells with the desired inhibitor in BSS for up to 2 h.

PBS can be used in place of BSS. BSS is crucial to maintain normal cellular homeostasis for slow-acting inhibitors.

3. At the end of the treatment, or if there is no treatment, wash the cells with 200 μl of Hanks' balanced salt solution (HBSS) containing 0.1 % (v/v) Triton X-100.

   Due to its activity as a weak detergent, Triton X-100 produces permeabilization of the cells and entry of small molecules without compromising cell or enzyme complex integrity.

4. Incubate with 200 μl of either complete assay mixture or the assay mixture without substrate as the blank for background dehydrogenase activity, and incubate for 40 min at 37 °C.

   (a) The reaction mixture for alpha-ketoglutarate dehydrogenase (αKGDH) also known as 2-oxoglutarate dehydrogenase (2oxGDH) contains 50 mM Tris–HCl (pH 7.6), 1 mM $MgCl_2$, 0.1 mM $CaCl_2$, 0.05 mM EDTA, 0.3 mM ThDP, 0.5 μg/ml rotenone, 0.2 % Triton X-100, 3 mM KG, 3 mM NAD+, 1 mM CoA, 0.75 mM nitroblue tetrazolium, and 0.05 mM phenazine methosulfate [5–12].

   Nitroblue tetrazolium and phenazine methosulfate should be added immediately before the reaction. Control buffer should not contain αKG or CoA. NADH ubiquinone reductase (mitochondrial complex 1) is a main enzyme consuming NADH; therefore suppressing its activity with rotenone is important. Correct pH is also crucial at this step for optimal enzyme activity. Different cell lines have different amounts of αKGDH activity; therefore longer or shorter incubation may be required for optimal detection.

   (b) Reaction buffer for pyruvate dehydrogenase (PDH) activity consists of 1 mM $MgCl_2$, 0.05 mM EDTA, 0.2 % Triton X-100, 0.3 mM ThDP, 10 μM rotenone, 10 mM pyruvate, 3 mM NAD, 1 mM Co-A, 2 mM bromopyruvate, 0.75 mM nitroblue tetrazolium, and 0.05 mM phenazine methosulfate in 50 mM Tris–HCl pH 7.8 [13–17].

   Nitroblue tetrazolium and phenazine methosulfate were added immediately before the reaction. Control buffer should not contain pyruvate and CoA. In the case of PDH activity, both rotenone (complex 1 inhibitor) and bromopyruvate (glyceraldehyde phosphate dehydrogenase inhibitor) are needed to minimize background reading due to high levels of NADH and pyruvate produced from glycolysis.

   (c) Reaction buffer for NAD/NADP isocitrate dehydrogenase (IDH) activities consists of 8 mM $MgCl_2$, 1 mM $MnCl_2$, 0.05 mM EDTA, 0.2 % Triton X-100, 10 μM rotenone, 2 mM NAD/0.5 mM NADP, 1.5 mM isocitrate, 10 mM citrate, 2 mM ADP, 0.75 mM nitroblue tetrazolium, and 0.05 mM phenazine methosulfate in 50 mM Tris–HCl pH 7.5 [18–21].

   (d) Reaction buffer for glutamate dehydrogenase (GDH) activity consists of 1 mM $MgCl_2$, 0.1 mM $CaCl_2$, 0.05 mM EDTA, 0.2 % Triton X-100, 10 μM rotenone, 2 mM ADP, 3 mM glutamate, 3 mM NAD, 0.75 mM nitroblue tetrazolium, and 0.05 mM phenazine methosulfate in 50 mM Tris–HCl pH 7.6 [22, 23].

5. After incubation, aspirate the treatment medium, and gently wash cells with Ca^{2+}- and Mg^{2+}-free HBSS. Add 200 μl of 10 % (w/v) SDS in 0.01 N HCl to solubilize the dark blue formazan overnight at 37 °C in a CO_2 incubator.

   Red formazan should be fairly visible to the naked eye after wash. Plates need to be sealed with parafilm to prevent uneven evaporation of buffer. Alternatively, plates can be placed carefully in a water bath sonicator for up to 1 h for reading on the same day.
6. Measure absorbance (OD) at 540 nm on any compatible plate reader.
7. Activity is calculated by subtraction of the absorbance of the well containing the blank control (without substrate) from the absorbance of the well containing the reaction with the specific substrate.

7.3 Results and Discussion

Here we used RKO colorectal cells as a model to measure the effect of HIF1α stabilization on both αKGDH and PDH activities. Both cell density and incubation time were chosen for optimal absorbance while still being in the linear range of the reaction. For the best result, it is important to find the linear range or both parameters, shown in red in Fig. 7.2. Arrows indicate optimal cell density and incubation time for RKO cells specifically for the 96-well plate reaction, which is at 10,000 cells and 40 min, respectively. Both parameters should be determined empirically for other cell lines of interest.

In order to validate the method, we treated RKO cells overnight with 500 nM DMOG in order to stabilize HIF1α. Previous reports have shown that HIF1 activation suppresses both αKGDH and PDH activities [24, 25]. This experiment)shows approximately 50–70 % inhibition of these regulatory dehydrogenases in response to HIF1 activation, consistent with reported values [24, 25]. The mechanisms of inhibition of PDH and αKGDH by hypoxia are very different, but both serve to decrease mitochondrial oxygen consumption and still provide the necessary macromolecules for growth of the tumor cells. An additional series of RKO cells were also treated with dichloroacetate (DCA), a pyruvate mimetic that also activates PDH through the inhibition of the inhibitory pyruvate dehydrogenase kinases. Treatment of normoxic cells with DCA showed a modest 10–20 % increase in activity. Normoxic PDH activity is near maximal, so this increase is in agreement with the literature.

7.4 Final Remarks

The method described above is faster, requires less starting material, has higher throughput, and most important of all measures enzyme activity while they are in their native cellular compartment. Different assay conditions and buffers should be tested for enzymes not described here. The limitations include the following: only adherent cell lines that grow as monolayers can be used for this assay, the formazan can be hard to dissolve, and background activities can be high depending on the substrate used. Appropriate inhibitors should be used in this assay to eliminate confounding activities, such as NADH dehydrogenase.

References

1. Kugler P. Quantitative enzyme histochemistry in the brain. Histochemistry. 1988;90(2):99–107.
2. Feinstein RN, Lindahl R. Detection of oxidases on polyacrylamide gels. Anal Biochem. 1973;56(2):353–60.
3. Fried R. Enzymatic and non-enzymatic assay of superoxide dismutase. Biochimie. 1975;57(5): 657–60.
4. Rajagopalan KV, Handler P. Oxidation of phenazine methosulfate by hepatic aldehyde oxidase. Biochem Biophys Res Commun. 1962;8(1-2):43–7.
5. Bunik VI, et al. Phosphonate analogues of alpha-ketoglutarate inhibit the activity of the alpha-ketoglutarate dehydrogenase complex isolated from brain and in cultured cells. Biochemistry. 2005;44(31):10552–61.
6. Mizuno Y, et al. An immunohistochemical study on α-ketoglutarate dehydrogenase complex in Parkinson's disease. Ann Neurol. 1994;35(2):204–10.
7. Mastrogiacomo F, Bergeron C, Kish SJ. Brain α-ketoglutarate dehydrogenase complex activity in Alzheimer's disease. J Neurochem. 1993;61(6):2007–14.
8. Lai JCK, Cooper AJL. Brain α-ketoglutarate dehydrogenase complex: kinetic properties, regional distribution, and effects of inhibitors. J Neurochem. 1986;47(5):1376–86.
9. Patel MS. Inhibition by the branched chain 2 oxo acids of the 2 oxoglutarate dehydrogenase complex in developing rat and human brain. Biochem J. 1974;144(1):91–7.
10. Linn TC. Studies on the apparent instability of bovine kidney α-ketoglutarate dehydrogenase complex. Arch Biochem Biophys. 1974;161(2):505–14.
11. Imai K, Tomita Y. Interaction of the α ketoglutarate dehydrogenase complex with basic polypeptides. J Biochem. 1974;75(4):699–705.
12. Bowden JA, McArthur Iii CL, Fried M. Metabolic diseases and mental retardation. I. The chick embryo as a model system in branched-chain ketoaciduria; the effect of α-ketoisocaproic acid. Int J Biochem. 1974;5(4):391–6.
13. Humphries KM, Szweda LI. Selective inactivation of α-ketoglutarate dehydrogenase and pyruvate dehydrogenase: reaction of lipoic acid with 4-hydroxy-2-nonenal. Biochemistry. 1998;37(45):15835–41.
14. Bowker-Kinley MM, et al. Evidence for existence of tissue-specific regulation of the mammalian pyruvate dehydrogenase complex. Biochem J. 1998;329(1):191–6.
15. Stanley CJ, Perham RN. Purification of 2-oxo acid dehydrogenase multienzyme complexes from ox heart by a new method. Biochem J. 1980;191(1):147–54.
16. Stansbie D, et al. Acute effects in vivo of anti insulin serum on rates of fatty acid synthesis and activities of acetyl coenzyme A carboxylase and pyruvate dehydrogenase in liver and epididymal adipose tissue of fed rats. Biochem J. 1976;160(2):413–6.
17. Kerbey AL, et al. Regulation of pyruvate dehydrogenase in rat heart. Mechanism of regulation of proportions of dephosphorylated and phosphorylated enzyme by oxidation of fatty acids and ketone bodies and of effects of diabetes: role of coenzyme A, acetyl-coenzyme A and reduced and oxidized nicotinamide-adenine dinucleotide. Biochem J. 1976;154(2):327–48.
18. Hurley JH. Catalytic mechanism of NADP+-dependent isocitrate dehydrogenase: implications from the structures of magnesium-isocitrate and NADP+ complexes. Biochemistry. 1991;30(35):8671–8.

19. Thorsness PE, Koshland Jr DE. Inactivation of isocitrate dehydrogenase by phosphorylation is mediated by the negative charge of the phosphate. J Biol Chem. 1987;262(22):10422–5.
20. Lai JCK, et al. Synaptic and non synaptic mitochondria from rat brain: isolation and characterization. J Neurochem. 1977;28(3):625–31.
21. Alp PR, Newsholme EA, Zammit VA. Activities of citrate synthase and NAD+ linked and NADP+ linked isocitrate dehydrogenase in muscle from vertebrates and invertebrates. Biochem J. 1976;154(3):689–700.
22. Gouia H, Habib Ghorbal M, Meyer C. Effects of cadmium on activity of nitrate reductase and on other enzymes of the nitrate assimilation pathway in bean. Plant Physiol Biochem. 2000;38(7-8):629–38.
23. Benzi G, Moretti A. Age- and peroxidative stress-related modifications of the cerebral enzymatic activities linked to mitochondria and the glutathione system. Free Radic Biol Med. 1995;19(1):77–101.
24. Papandreou I, et al. HIF-1 mediates adaptation to hypoxia by actively downregulating mitochondrial oxygen consumption. Cell Metab. 2006;3(3):187–97.
25. Sun RC, Denko NC. Hypoxic regulation of glutamine metabolism through HIF1 and SIAH2 supports lipid synthesis that is necessary for tumor growth. Cell Metab. 2014;19(2):285–92.

Chapter 8
Measuring Autophagy in the Context of Cancer

Michael J. Morgan and Andrew Thorburn

Abstract Autophagy plays multiple roles in the formation and progression of cancer, including both suppressive and promotive roles. It not only impacts cancer cell growth and viability directly but also has a significant role through its effects on the tumor microenvironment. Measurement of autophagy can be confusing and sometimes misleading due to the inherent difficulty of measuring both the formation and turnover of molecules involved in the autophagic process. The LC3 proteins serve as autophagosomal markers and are the basis for most of the assays used for measuring autophagy. Since each of the current assays for autophagy has significant limitations, the use of multiple assays for the analysis of autophagy in most contexts is highly advised. Here we outline three assays that are commonly used to evaluate autophagic flux in cells. These assays include the determination of LC3II formation and LC3II and p62 turnover by use of Western Blotting, quantification of LC3 puncta, and the measurement of autophagic flux using tandem labeled mCherry-GFP-LC3.

Keywords Autophagy • Autophagic flux • Cancer • Tumor progression • Cancer therapy

8.1 Introduction

8.1.1 The Process of Autophagy

Macroautophagy (hereafter autophagy) is a highly conserved cellular process in all eukaryotic cells by which the cell targets defective organelles, protein aggregates, long-lived proteins, as well as bulk cytoplasm for degradation by the lysosome.

M.J. Morgan, Ph.D. (✉)
Department of Pharmacology, University of Colorado School of Medicine, 12801 East 17th Avenue, Rm. L18-6110, MS 8303, Aurora, CO 80045, USA
e-mail: Michael.Morgan@ucdenver.edu

A. Thorburn
Department of Pharmacology, University of Colorado School of Medicine, 12801 East 17th Avenue, Rm. L18-6105, MS 8303, Aurora, CO 80045, USA
e-mail: Andrew.Thorburn@ucdenver.edu

C. Koumenis et al. (eds.), *Tumor Microenvironment*, Advances in Experimental Medicine and Biology 899, DOI 10.1007/978-3-319-26666-4_8

Autophagy allows the reuse of components to maintain and sustain the metabolic and catabolic activities of the cell [1]. Greater than 30 autophagy-related (ATG) genes direct this process, which includes the formation of a double membrane vacuole called the autophagosome that contains the organelles, proteins, and cytoplasm to be recycled [2]. Autophagosomes then fuse with lysosomes to form autolysosomes, where these contents are broken down by the lysosomal hydrolases. Not surprisingly, the process of autophagy is activated in response to cell stressors and promotes cell survival during nutrient deprivation by providing a source of material and energy for cellular functions [3, 4]. A basal amount of autophagy also exists in most cells even in the presence of nutrients. Both basal and induced autophagy maintain cellular homeostasis and help to prevent and to remedy oxidative damage. Autophagy is also important in different contexts for development, cellular differentiation or maintenance of pluripotence, intracellular elimination of pathogens, the presentation of antigens, and in protein trafficking and secretion.

Autophagy also has a complex relationship with cell death pathways, with which it often acts antagonistically as a survival pathway. For instance, autophagy suppresses cell death induced by matrix detachment (anoikis) [5]. Thus, inhibition of autophagy can often sensitize a cell to death induced through many stimuli [6, 7]. On the other hand, autophagy can promote cell death in other specific contexts [6, 8, 9]. We recently reported in several cases that differences in basal autophagy determine future fate of a cell in response to death stimuli [9, 10], implying that basal autophagy can be key regulatory factor in cell death/survival decisions. The relationship between autophagy and cell death and survival is currently being studied in the hopes that the modulation of autophagy may provide a pharmacologic target in the treatment of cancer and other diseases [7]. In the next section we shall briefly summarize some of what is known about the relationship between autophagy and cancer. For further information on role of autophagy with regard to different aspects of cancer and its progression or suppression, the reader is referred to a recent review representing a consensus of investigators in the fields of cancer and autophagy [11].

8.1.2 Autophagy and Cancer

Tumor suppressive effects of autophagy are evident in systems where genes that control or regulate autophagy are inactivated or deleted. For example, increased spontaneous malignancies are observed upon heterozygous deletion of Beclin-1 in mice [12, 13], and heterozygous deletions are observed in multiple human tumors. In addition, several interactors/regulators of the Beclin-1 complex have similar phenotypes: Bif-1 (SH3GLB1) knockout mice [14] and AMBRA1 haploinsufficient mice [15] develop spontaneous tumors, and UVRAG suppresses the growth of human cancers in mouse tumor models [16]. Deficiencies in all three of these molecules are found in varying human tumors.

Moreover, chimeric Atg5 mice or liver-specific knockout mice of Atg7 develop spontaneous liver tumors [17] and Atg4c mice are sensitive to the development of fibrosarcomas induced by chemical carcinogens [18]. The development of oncogene-driven lung carcinomas induced by $BRAF^{V600E}$ and $KRAS^{G12D}$ expression is promoted by lung-specific deletion of Atg5 or Atg7 [19, 20]. Premalignant pancreatic tumors driven by $KRAS^{G12D}$ are also promoted by pancreas-specific knockout of Atg5 or Atg7 [21, 22].

However, despite such evidence for a tumor suppressive function of autophagy, it is also clear that autophagy is required for the progression of many cancers. For instance, conditional Atg3 deletion in hematopoietic cells precludes the development of BCR-Abl-mediated leukemia [23]. In the case of the aforementioned spontaneous liver tumors occurring in the liver-specific absence of Atg7 or Atg5, the tumors remained benign [17]. In the case of the $KRAS^{G12D}$- and $BRAF^{V600E}$-driven lung tumors where Atg7 is deleted, benign oncocytomas predominate rather than adenocarcinomas [19, 24], and other studies have also shown that Atg5-deficient $KRAS^{G12D}$-driven lung tumors do not progress [20]. Similarly, in models of $KRAS^{G12D}$-driven pancreatic carcinogenesis, the tissue-specific deletion of Atg7 or Atg5 blocks the progression to later stage disease [21, 22]. Acute autophagy oblation (whole body Atg7 knockout) in mice with preexisting $KRAS^{G12D}$-driven Tp53 deficient lung cancers promotes tumor cell death and inhibits tumor growth [25]. In addition, Atg7 deficiency prevents melanoma progression induced by $Braf^{V600E}$ and allelic Pten loss [26].

Thus there is abundant evidence that autophagy acts in tumor supportive roles. The current consensus is that while autophagy may suppress tumor development, its tumor supportive role in fully formed cancers may therefore make such tumors sensitive to autophagy inhibitors, making autophagy inhibition a potentially useful pharmacological strategy in cancer. However, we have previously reported that some tumor cells are more dependent on autophagy than others [27–30], and there is a wide range of responses of cancer cells to autophagy inhibition. Breast cancer cell lines illustrate this variability. For example, the murine breast cell line 67NR is highly dependent on efficient basal autophagy to maximize its growth even under nutrient replete conditions [27]. In human breast cancer cell lines, MCF7 cells are minimally affected by autophagy inhibition, with a small amount of growth inhibition. MDA-MB-231 cells, on the other hand, are largely growth inhibited and some cells die in response to inhibition; while MDA-MB-468 cells mostly undergo cell death in response to autophagy inhibition [28]. Several phase I trials with chloroquine or hydroxychloroquine have recently concluded with positive, but mixed results [31–36], making it increasingly important to be able to measure autophagy in tumor cells, tumor tissue, and in the tumor microenvironment so as to be able to identify cases where autophagy is relevant to patient treatment.

8.1.3 General Considerations of Using LC3 and p62 as Markers for Autophagy

Observation of the double membrane autophagosome by transmission electron microscopy is often considered a gold standard in the detection of autophagy (please see Chap. 9). However, this method requires access to expensive equipment and trained personnel with significant experience. Sample preparation for this methodology is a highly time- and labor-intensive process and is limited to observations of fixed cells, which limits the kinds and amounts of samples that can be analyzed. Additionally, by its nature, electron microscopy must be done in fixed cells/tissue and therefore cannot follow dynamic changes in autophagy over time. Therefore, most current studies focus on assessing autophagy by following markers of the process and it is these methods that we will discuss below.

The microtubule-associated protein 1 light chain 3 proteins, MAP1LC3A, MAP1LC3B, and MAP1LC3C (herein these proteins are referred to nonspecifically as a group in the singular as LC3) are human homologs of the yeast protein Atg8, an autophagy-related protein involved in the elongation of the isolation membrane in autophagosome biogenesis. Since LC3 is one of very few proteins associated with the autophagosome from its initial formation through its fusion with the lysosome, LC3 serves as an autophagosomal marker and is the basis for most of the assays used for measuring autophagy. The 22 C-terminal residues of LC3 are constitutively removed by the proteolytic activity of ATG4 and is designated LC3-I. LC3-I is subsequently conjugated with phosphatidylethanolamine (PE) in a series of ubiquitination-like reactions that involves ATG7 (an E1-like enzyme), ATG3 (an E2-like enzyme), and an Atg5-Atg12:Atg16L complex (with E3-like activity). The PE conjugate of LC3 is designated as LC3-II, which, due to its lipidation, associates with both outer and inner membranes of the autophagosome and, if visualized, is seen in a punctate pattern as opposed to the largely diffuse localization pattern seen with LC3-I. PE-conjugated LC3-II also has a higher mobility than LC3-I when running an SDS-PAGE gel. After autophagosome-lysosomal fusion is completed, LC3 on the outer membrane is recycled by the ATG4-catalyzed reversal of the lipidation reaction, while the LC3 that was associated with the inner autophagosomal membrane is degraded by lysosomal proteases. One common confusion in the literature is that while increases in LC3II are often interpreted as a sign of increased autophagy, the fact that LC3II is also degraded in the lysosome means that this may not always be the case. For example, under conditions of high flux the steady state amounts of LCII may actually decrease due to its degradation. And secondly, inhibition of the autophagic process at late stages, such as when autophagosomal-lysosomal fusion is prevented, or when lysosomal function is disturbed, may lead to increased amounts of LC3-II and autophagosomes even though autophagic flux has been prevented. Additionally genetic inhibition of autophagy at some early stages may prevent autophagosome formation without preventing the generation of LC3-II. For instance loss of the autophagy-specific PI3-kinase complex proteins Beclin-1 or VSP34 expression prevents the formation of autophagosomes, but since these proteins participate in a parallel pathway, loss of these proteins does not directly prevent LC3-II formation itself, though it obviously does prevent LC3-II from interacting with autophagosomal membranes. Thus experiments that simply measure the overall level of LC3-II and that detect changes in LC3-II levels (either up or down) as a result of a stimulus are unable to discriminate between that stimulus serving to increase or decrease autophagy. Similarly an experiment that measures LC3-II before and after a stimulus and detects no apparent difference cannot exclude the possibility that there was in fact a change in autophagy caused by the stimulus. To resolve this problem, autophagic flux must be inhibited at or immediately preceding the lysosomal degradation step, then changes in the levels of LC3-II with and without inhibition of lysosomal degradation must be assessed. This is often done with inhibitors of lysosomal proteases, as well as interfering with lysosomal pH using bafilomycin A_1 (Baf A) or chloroquine (CQ), both of which also prevent autophagosomal-lysosomal fusion events.

Changes in the amounts of the cargo adapter protein SQSTM1 (commonly known as p62) can also be used as a marker for autophagy. The p62 protein binds to autophagosomes through its association with LC3-II and also direct interactions with the autophagosomal membrane, and, like LC3-II, is degraded after autophagosomal-lysosomal fusion occurs. Therefore, whereas amounts of LC3-II are often correlated with increased autophagy, p62 levels are generally inversely correlated with autophagic flux. It should be noted, however, that p62 is also highly transcriptionally regulated and often transcriptionally induced by similar stimuli that induce autophagy, particularly after extensive time has occurred since the beginning of the autophagic stimulus. Thus, although the expression of endogenous p62 often is quite nicely inversely correlated with increased autophagy, this by itself is not especially strong evidence of altered autophagy and the ectopic expression of p62 fusion proteins is sometimes necessary to properly observe effects on autophagy using p62.

The methodologies we will present here using these two markers are the three most often used assays for measurement of autophagy: (1) western blotting for LC3-II and autophagic degradation substrates such as p62, (2) observation and quantification of autophagosomal puncta, and (3) measurement of autophagic flux using a tandem mCherry-GFP- LC3 assay. It should be emphasized that while these assays are among the best currently available, all have limitations and no single assay on its own is typically accepted by the field for evaluation of autophagic flux in and of itself. In most cases multiple assays will be required to confirm effects on autophagy, and we strongly recommend that investigators adopt complementary approaches whenever possible.

8.2 Measuring Autophagic Flux Using Western Blotting of LC3II

A frequent approach for examining autophagy in many publications has been to follow LC3-II formation by western blotting using an LC3-specific antibody. Although, in our view, this particular technique has significant disadvantages, such as a very limited dynamic range, and is semiquantitative at best, this popular assay remains the most common technique for assessment of autophagy.

8.2.1 Assay Considerations

Since western blotting is often only linear within a specific range of protein amounts and exposures, the main concern with this assay is to make sure that the signal stays within the linear range and that saturation of the signal is prevented. For quantification of Western blot bands, camera-based systems typically have a lower sensitivity than film, and additionally the images can tend to be a bit grainier. However, camera-based systems have a larger linear range than film and have better capability of integrating over multiple exposures, allowing one to find the best exposure to stay within the linear range.

As mentioned previously, autophagic flux must be blocked to be accurately measured. Importantly, in addition to saturation of signal from the enhanced chemiluminescence exposure, it is also possible in some cell lines to saturate the amount of protein trapped in autophagosomes when flux is blocked. When this happens, the signal obtained from a Western blot does not accurately reflect differing amounts of flux when comparisons are made. We believe that this is the most frequent error made in autophagy publications. Often researchers will present two different conditions that are both treated with a late stage autophagy inhibitor (i.e., a lysosomal inhibitor) for a long period of time, and it will be claimed that no difference exists in autophagic flux, when in reality the amount of LC3 in autophagosomes has reached close to maximum levels when compared to a low amount of LC3 protein synthesis. The best way to avoid this problem is to compare autophagic flux after treating for multiple time points with late stage autophagy inhibitors and compare the time courses side-by-side on the same gel and western blot membrane. If this is done multiple times at a variety of early to late timepoints, it will typically avoid a saturation problem with respect to LC3 in autophagosomes.

One other potential issue is that if the lysosomal inhibitor block in autophagic flux at the endpoint is not complete, then in situations of high flux, LC3 may still be degraded, preventing proper interpretation. It is therefore advisable that multiple concentrations of inhibitor be used to discern the concentration at which increases in inhibitor give no further increase in LC3 at the last given time point to be measured. Remember also when working with lysosomotropic drugs such as chloroquine, the actual concentration of drug in the lysosome (that raises the pH of the lysosome and therefore prevents autophagosome-lysosome fusion) is a product of both the time of treatment and the concentration placed in the media. While a small amount of chloroquine can be sufficient to completely achieve flux inhibition when used overa long period of time such as overnight, over shorter time courses it will be necessary to increase the amount of chloroquine in order to completely block flux.

8.2.2 Procedures

(a) Plate cells in a 6-well tissue culture plate or the equivalent amount of 35 mm dishes. Ideally multiple (about 4–6) wells should be compared for each condition in which autophagy is to be measured. The cell density should be approximately 40–80 % confluent at the time the assay is performed. Avoid using cell densities approaching complete confluency, as we have observed that in some cell types, autophagy in highly induced or repressed when cells become overconfluent. For nonadherent cells, make sure that the cells are in normal log-phase growth and are not grown too densely, as this can also affect basal autophagy. Although replating cells can induce autophagy, most cell types will revert to normal basal state autophagy when returned to normal tissue culture conditions overnight. Thus, for most tumor cell lines, plating cells at 18–24 h before the assay is suggested. However, there are some cell types in which very high autophagy induction occurs when cells are in suspension during the replating process (this appears to be especially true for cells that take a long time to re-attach to the culture plates). For these cell types, plating 36–48 h before the assay is recommended so that cells may recover (media may need to be replaced with fresh media 24 h before the assay if cells grow quickly and use up the media nutrients).

(b) If basal autophagy is to be measured, treat some wells with 10 nM Bafilomycin A_1 at various timepoints (1, 2, 3, 4, and 6 h, for example) before cell harvest to inhibit autophagic flux, making sure to have one or more untreated control wells. If induced autophagy is to be measured after stimuli (e.g., amino acid starvation), it is usually desirable to pretreat at least one well with Bafilomycin A_1 for an hour before adding a given stimulus. Then, all the wells in the stimulus plate are simultaneously treated with the stimulus and Bafilomycin A_1 is added at various timepoints concurrently and after stimulus treatment. Shorter timepoints of flux inhibition (0.5, 1, 1.5, 2, 4 h) are typically used while measuring strong inducers of autophagy, such as serum/amino acid starvation in EBSS (Earle's Balanced Salt Solutions) (Sigma, E2888). The main concern is to avoid exceeding the linear range of the assay by getting too much LC3-II accumulation. In the cases where cell types have very small amounts of basal autophagy or have a very small amount of autophagy induction, flux may need to be blocked for a longer amount of time to reliably see differences in LC3-II formation.

(c) When the time course is completed, remove the media and rinse cells with PBS (Cellgro, 21-040-CV) and then lyse the cells on the plate by addition of stringent RIPA buffer with protease inhibitors (typically 100–300 μl for one well of a six-well plate). Incubate the plate on ice for 2–3 min and then scrape the cells with a cell scraper and remove the cell lysate to a microfuge tube.

(d) Sonicate the samples briefly to shear the DNA and then spin tubes at 13,000 rpm in a microfuge for 5 min. Remove the supernatant to a new microfuge tube.

(e) Measure the protein concentration using Bradford (Bio Rad) or other assay. Add 5× Laemmli (SDS) sample buffer and boil at 95 °C for 5 min.

(f) Load 5–15 mg of protein in each lane (5 mg of protein is sufficient for most cell lines using the antibodies that we use) of a 12 or 15 % SDS-PAGE gel. Gel density is critical for this step. Separation of LC3-II from LC3I requires a higher percentage SDS-PAGE gel (at least 12 % and preferably 15 %). Precast 4–20 % gradient gels also work OK. In our experience, however, on a typical 7 cm 10 % gel it is impossible to distinguish LC3I from LC3-II, as they run with a similar mobility. Run sample at 100 V until good separation of low molecular weight markers is achieved. LC3-II runs at approximately 16-17 kDa (LC3-I runs just under 20 kDa), so be sure to stop running the gel before LC3 runs off the bottom!

(g) Transfer the proteins from the gel using wet or semi-dry apparatus. Using semi-dry apparatus one usually observes good transfers of LC3 on small blots for 45 min to 1 h at 15 V, while wet transfer works sufficiently at 100–120 V for 1 h or 37 V overnight at 4 °C. One must be careful not to transfer for too long at high voltage—since LC3 is small it is possible to transfer some of the protein all of the way through the membrane. The transfer buffer is the same in both cases (Towbin transfer buffer: 25 mM Tris, 192 mM glycine, pH 8.3, 20 % methanol).

(h) Probe membranes overnight with anti-LC3 or anti-p62 antibodies diluted in 5 % milk in TBST buffer (50 mM Tris, 150 mM NaCl, 1 % Tween 20, pH 7.5). For antibodies, we recommend Novus-Biologicals (NB100-2220) for anti-LC3 (Rabbit, 1:2000–5000) and Abnova (H00008878-M01) for anti-SQSTM1/p62 (Mouse, 1:5000).

(i) Incubate with HRP conjugated anti-rabbit (Cell signaling, #7074, 1:2000–5000) for LC3 or anti-mouse (Cell signaling, #7076, 1:2000–5000) for p62 diluted in 5 % milk in TBST buffer.

(j) Visualize by enhanced chemiluminescence. Immobilon Western Chemiluminescent HRP Substrate from Millipore (WBKLS0500) is recommended for stronger amplification, while ECL from Pierce (32106) is recommended if the signal is too high. If quantification is desired it is preferable to use an electronic CCD imaging system with software to detect saturated signals. If film is used, multiple exposures should be used to find the right unsaturated exposures. Density analysis is performed using Image J 1.43 m (NIH, USA), or comparable software and typically quantification of three or more independent experiments is required so that one can generate statistically useful data.

8.2.3 *Interpretation and Analysis*

In principle, the analysis of LC3 western blots is relatively straightforward. Some antibodies recognize both LC3I and LC3II, while others more strongly recognize LC3II. LC3I is typically detected at 18–19 kDa, while LC3II appears at 16–17 kDa. When doing density quantification, the quantified LC3II bands are typically normalized to Actin or other housekeeping genes. (However, there are some cases where the amounts of Actin decrease when autophagy is induced, so it is wise to be careful and make sure that Actin remains constant in your system.) One then averages these values over 3–4 experiments. Typically one analyzes two sets of comparisons (three comparisons if one is looking at effects of gene modifiers on autophagy induction by a stimulus). The first comparison is made between each sample in the presence and absence of CQ at the various timepoints. The comparison that is made between cells with the presence and absence of flux is really a measurement of amount of basal autophagy (i.e., under normal growth conditions)

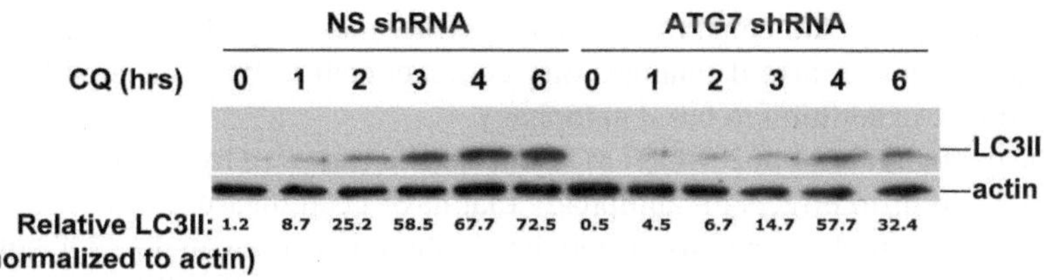

Fig. 8.1 Examination of basal flux by inhibition of LC3II turnover. A stable variant of the T24t cell line was infected with lentivirus expressing ATG7 or non-silencing shRNA. Cells were treated with 100 μM chloroquine for the indicated times and lysates were probed for LC3 and Actin by immunoblotting. Quantification of the LC3II and Actin bands was conducted using Image J software on inverted blot images. Normalization was done by dividing the LC3 band value by the associated Actin band value and multiplying by 100

in each condition. For instance, one can see in Fig. 8.1 that infection with an ATG7 shRNA in these cells has not completely inhibited basal flux (due to incomplete knockdown), since there is an increase in LC3II over time when treated with chloroquine. The second comparison is made between the amount of accumulation under one condition and the amount of accumulation under a second condition. For example, in Fig. 8.1, one can see that although basal flux was not eliminated completely by the ATG7 shRNA, there is a substantial reduction in the time-dependent LC3II accumulation in the presence of chloroquine when compared to the non-silencing control cells. Therefore we conclude that basal autophagic flux was greater in the non-silencing control cells and that (not surprisingly) ATG7 knockdown reduces basal autophagic flux.

Experimental interpretation can be slightly more complex when one is trying to determine if a modifier has an effect on induced flux. One must then make the first two comparisons as explained above, and then make a third comparison as to how this changes when autophagy is induced by a stimulus. This may be straightforward if the modifier only affects "induced" autophagy, since one will see that there is no difference under basal conditions, but will see an effect after the stimulus. However, if something affects basal autophagy, it can be difficult to distinguish between effects solely on basal autophagy versus affecting both basal and induced autophagy, since there is already a difference to be seen in LC3II. It is often useful in this situation to establish a "fold change value" that is based on the approximate rate of change in LC3II over the linear part of the blot. For example, in Fig. 8.1 the rate of change (i.e., a slope of a line with x representing the time and y the normalized intensity of the LC3II band) of the basal increase in the non-silencing control over the first 0–3 h (we exclude the 4 and 6 h time points, because the blot is approaching saturation as seen in the quantification) is calculated at 18.8 and the ATG7 samples is calculated at 4.5 over this same set of timepoints. This represents an approximate fourfold change in the rate of LCII formation between the control and modifier cells. One then compares the same rates of change when an autophagic stimulus is applied over the same time course (assuming the blots are still linear; one has to reduce the time, of course, if it is not). If the fold change remains a fourfold change or less, then one could conclude that the modifier may only affect basal autophagy; if higher than a fourfold change, one could conclude that the modifier affects induced flux in addition to basal autophagy.

The degradation of p62 (SQSTM1) can also be followed by western blotting and may help confirm effects on autophagy that have been measured by LC3II. p62 is substrate for autophagy and its protein levels should decrease under high autophagy additions. Changes in p62 are however not consistent in all cell lines due to transcriptional regulation of p62 protein levels, especially under long-term conditions where the cell senses changes in autophagy resulting in feedback inhibition. Typically under strong autophagy stimuli one will observe a decrease over the first few hours. Importantly, the decrease in p62 should be inhibited by late stage flux inhibitors such as CQ and Baf A. One sometimes may also observe an increase in p62 levels in the presence of these inhibitors in cells with very high basal autophagy. To get around the transcriptional regulation of p62, some researchers have made stable cell lines that express tagged versions of p62 expressed of a constitutive promoter. One powerful approach utilizes a HaloTag-p62 fusion protein and labeling with the fluorescent HaloTag ligand, which is not influenced by de novo protein synthesis [37].

8.3 Measurement of Autophagy Using LC3 Puncta Formation

When autophagy is not induced, LC3-positive puncta are typically few in most cells, although this can vary with cell type. Therefore, increases in the amount of GFP-LC3 positive puncta in a cell can indicate the induction of autophagy. Although this assay can be time-consuming to properly analyze, it is very useful for quantification of differences in autophagy. One especial advantage to this assay is that autophagy may be followed in the same individual cells pre- and post-treatment by the use of time-lapse video microscopy.

8.3.1 Assay Considerations

One main consideration in this assay is that high overexpression of GFP-LC3 can sometimes result in GFP-LC3 aggregates independent of the induction of autophagy. It is therefore recommended that stable cell lines be produced that express GFP-LC3 at more moderate levels. (This makes the analysis of some cell types, such as primary cells, more challenging.) If transient introduction of GFP-LC3 is necessary, the use of a conjugation-incompetent mutant form of GFP-LC3 as a negative control is often essential [38]. When genetic manipulations are to be made for comparison, it is also recommended that parental GFP-LC3 expressing cells be made first before the genetic manipulation (i.e., gene overexpression, shRNA knockdown, etc.) is done, rather than attempting to make differing cell lines that possess equivalent GFP-LC3 levels. Flow cytometry can be used to sort GFP-LC3 expressing cells and remove those cells that have excessively high or low expression.

As discussed in Sect. 8.1.3, a static picture of a cell with GFP-LC3 puncta gives little information about autophagic flux, since this does not distinguish between induction of early-stage autophagy and a block in late stage autophagy that prevents turnover of the autophagosome puncta. Therefore comparisons should be made between any two conditions in both the presence and the absence of late stage autophagy inhibitors that block flux. Like western blotting, analysis of multiple time points following treatment of such inhibitors is recommended to determine the best time for such treatment. As an example of the importance of this consideration, let us consider the situation where one wishes to examine the effect of a genetic negative modifier of autophagy on a strong autophagy stimulus, such as amino acid starvation. Since a negative modifier's effect most likely will not result in complete inhibition, if one were to follow GFP-LC3 puncta formation after long a stimulus with a strong inducer of autophagy, eventually all cells would have numerous GFP puncta, which when quantified would underestimate the effect of the negative regulator examined. In addition, if one looked at GFP-LC3 puncta before puncta had properly formed in the positive control, one might conclude that there is no effect for the opposite reason. If however, one looked at GFP-LC3 puncta at the optimal timepoint, where puncta formation was evident in the positive control, but before a substantial amount of puncta formation was evident in the modifier cells, it would be evident that the modifier had an inhibitory effect on the induction of autophagy.

8.3.2 Procedures

(a) Create appropriate GFP-LC3 stable adherent cell line by infecting cells with GFP-LC3 retrovirus or by transfection, followed by selection with a selectable marker. Stable moderate fluorescent GFP-expressing cells should be selected by flow cytometry. We do not recommend using cells with transient transfection as most transfection protocols/agents induce autophagy. In addition high transient expression of GFP-LC3 can lead to nonautophagosomal aggregates that can interfere with the quantification of puncta. If transient transfection must be used, the concentration of GFP-LC3 plasmid should be reduced to eliminate high expression and very bright cells ignored in subsequent analysis.

(b) Wash glass coverslips overnight in a 2:1 mixture of nitric and hydrochloric acids. Rinse coverslips well with water and then place in 95–100 % ethanol until coverslips are needed. When ready for the experiment remove coverslips from ethanol and place coverslips in sterile plastic tissue culture plates and allow coverslips to dry. If necessary, coverslips may be coated by incubating in

0.1 mg/ml collagen I or IV (in 0.1 M acetic acid) OR 1 mg/ml polylysine (in 0.15 M borate buffer, pH 8.3) OR 1 mg/ml laminin (in PBS) OR 1 mg/ml fibronectin (in PBS). Coverslips are then washed with PBS. Alternatively, for time-lapse imaging using an epifluorescent (thin cells work better for this) or confocal (a spinning disk system is preferable) microscope, one can plate on 35 mm No. 1.5 coverslip bottom dishes (MatTek).

(c) Approximately 24–48 h before the beginning of the experiment, plate cells onto coverslips such that cells are about 50–75 % confluent at the time of the experiment. [This confluency is recommended for short experiments (3–10 h); if an experiment is expected to last overnight or longer, it may be necessary to reduce confluency somewhat.] Also plate additional cells for controls where flux is inhibited with CQ or Bafilomycin for each condition to be measured, as well as for treatment with flux inhibitors alone.

(d) Pretreat control cells with sufficient Bafilomycin or CQ for 1 h to block flux. Then treat cells with autophagy stimuli (for instance, 4 h with EBSS ± Bafilomycin). For certain treatment conditions (e.g., EBSS or trehalose), it may be necessary to wash cells, including the flux inhibitor control cells before the addition of treatment media. In this case replace the flux inhibitors as soon as possible after treatment so as to prevent the stimuli from degrading the autophagosomes. In certain long-term stimuli, the long-term combination of flux inhibitors and autophagy stimulation may be toxic to cells. In this case, it may be necessary to reduce the length of flux inhibition to the last 4–6 h before the end of the experiment (in this case, it is necessary to have a matching untreated control for flux inhibitor treatment at this late stage for comparison). Although there may be some turnover in these cases, one can still usually get informative data on the comparative amount of autophagosome formation by using flux inhibitors at this late stage so long as flux inhibitor treatments are consistent between experimental samples and controls. If basal autophagy is to be measured, it may be necessary to treat with flux inhibitors for more extensive time to observe differences in autophagosome formation, since basal flux is often low in many cell types. This is not always the case, however, since cell types that have high amount of basal autophagy can usually be observed after 2–4 h treatments with Bafilomycin or CQ.

(e) After the treatment has been completed, wash cells on coverslips in PBS and then fix in 3.7 % formaldehyde for 10 min at room temperature. Wash with PBS again and mount on slides using ProLong Gold antifade (Life Technologies) or other equivalent mountant. Allow slides to dry for 24 h. If live cells are to be observed, then immediate visualization is required.

(f) Visualize green fluorescence on a microscope at 60× or 100× magnification. Analysis is easier if pictures are taken (this is especially true of living cells) of multiple fields of cells (preferably more than 20 fields representing a total cell population > 100 cells) and then the number of puncta for each cell is counted either manually (blinded counting is better) or by using computerized software image analysis programs, such as Image J.

8.3.3 Interpretation and Analysis

There are two different ways that are typically used to present data from the puncta formation assay. One can present the average number of GFP-LC3 puncta per cell in each sample, or one can report the number of cells having at least a given amount of puncta. It is generally uninformative to simply report the total number of cells with puncta, as during basal autophagy most cells will have at least a few puncta. Thus, it is useful to establish a cutoff value that represents the difference in the number of puncta per cell during conditions of "low" and "high" autophagy. This number may be different between different cell lines and must be empirically determined by treating a cell type with known autophagy stimuli (preferably both strong and weak inducers) to be compared with basal conditions. It is often useful to then use these values to define "normal," "high," or "low" autophagy for a particular cell line.

It is usually informative, in addition to presenting data classifying cells as having increased autophagy (i.e., cells with puncta over the cutoff value), to divide the amount of increase into two or more groups. For instance, when one looks at a data set as presented in the left figure of Fig. 8.2b, one can tell that TRAIL likely causes increased autophagy in the cells; however, upon CQ treatment it is not completely evident that TRAIL causes further increase in puncta, although the data trends in this direction. One could conclude that the assay might be close to saturated in the presence of chloroquine and that a shorter CQ treatment is necessary (this may be somewhat true), or one might falsely conclude that instead of increasing autophagy, TRAIL was actually inhibiting autophagy here at a late stage since there are no statistically significant differences in the CQ-treated samples in the presence and absence of TRAIL. However, by looking at "low," "medium," and "high" populations, as presented in Fig. 8.2b on the right side, it is clear that TRAIL induced further accumulation of autophagosomes in the presence of CQ, since there is a shift between "low" and "medium" cells to those with "high" amount of puncta. Therefore the graph on the right represents a more informative way of presenting the data.

8.4 Measurement of Autophagic Flux Using Flow Cytometric Analysis of Tandem Labeled mCherry-EGFP-LC3

The principle behind this assay is that GFP fluorescence is quenched in the acidic environment of the autolysosome, while the red fluorophore (we prefer the use of mCherry) remains fluorescent at low pH until it is degraded. The main advantage of the tandem tagged-LC3 assay is that it more directly measures the step of autophagy associated with the delivery of LC3 to the lysosome (and hence actual flux) as opposed to autophagosome formation. One can follow puncta formation using time-lapse microscopy. However, the tandem label makes it amenable to measure

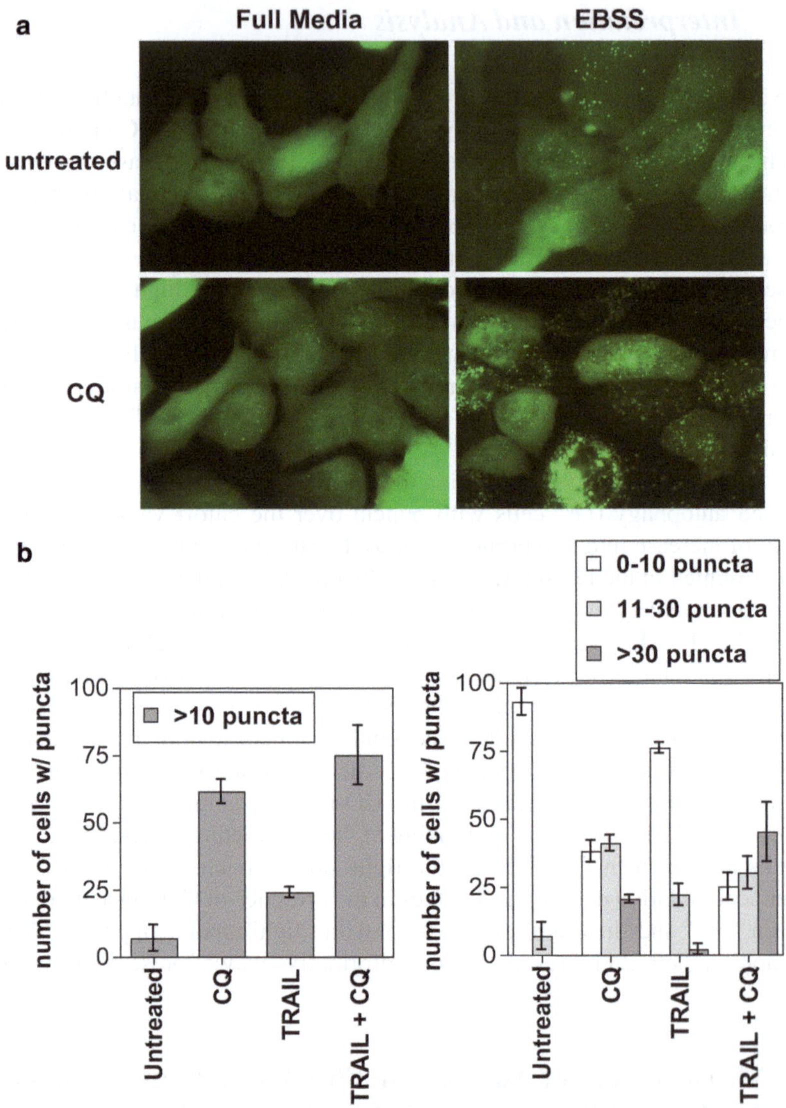

Fig. 8.2 Measurement of GFP-LC3 puncta formation. Stable cell lines were generated from MCF10A cells infected with a pBabe retrovirus that encoded GFP-LC3 followed by antibiotic selection. Cells were sorted for fluorescence uniformity by flow cytometry, and used for experiments in A and B. (**a**) Cells were washed and treated with EBSS or 100 ng/ml TRAIL in the presence or absence of CQ for 5 h. Pictures were taken of live cells on a fluorescence microscope. (**b**) Graphs show two different presentation of quantification of GFP-LC3 puncta in pictures of ten fields (each treatment) of cells from the experiment as indicated in (**a**)

autophagy using flow cytometry, which has substantial advantages in terms of the ease of quantification and reduction of subjective and unconscious operator biases that can arise when choosing fields to image by microscopy.

8.4.1 Assay Considerations

This assay, unlike others, more directly measures flux, meaning that it may not always be necessary to block flux with late stage autophagy inhibitors to get a measurement of flux. However, since there is a background amount of red fluorescence that is left over from autophagosome delivery to lysosomes during previous time periods when basal autophagy was occurring, in practice it is quite useful to block flux with late stage autophagy inhibitors and determine the amount of background signal that is not related to the flux presently being measured.

It is possible to analyze the tandem assay by microscopy, in which case, one would simply use the procedures in Sect. 8.3 using mCherry-EGFP-LC3 instead of EGFP-LC3, and then would visualize both red and green signal instead of just green signal. In this case one quantifies and compares the amount of red-only puncta to the total amount of red-only plus yellow (both red and green fluorescent) puncta. If live cell imaging is not done, the conditions of fixation may need to be modified to keep the pH of the total cell from going down (thus quenching the GFP in the whole cell) and the pH of the lysosome unperturbed (such that the GFP signal does not return).

As with the other assays, the confluency of the cells has important effects on the amount of autophagic flux a cell undergoes, and may mask the effects of stimuli that are being examined. We have found that the high sensitivity of this assay makes it more likely that confluency-specific effects will be measured in some cell lines, even when such differences in flux are not detectable by western blotting. Of course, it is often important to examine flux under more physiological conditions, such as when cells are grown in 3D cultures, or in a primary tumor mass. One advantage of the tandem-LC3 assay is that it is possible to measure flux in such cells by dissociating them and analyzing them using flow cytometry.

A major consideration in the use of flow cytometry in adherent cells is the amount of time that is necessary to detach them from the culture dish until the time in which the cells are analyzed. Since cell detachment can induce autophagy, one must keep this in mind when designing large experiments. We have observed that some tumor cells are especially sensitive to detachment-induced autophagy. Ideally, the time between detachment and analysis should be as short and in every case, it is critical to be as consistent as possible (i.e., controls and experimental treatments should be detached for the same amount of time before analysis) to ensure reliable measurements.

8.4.2 Procedures

(a) Create appropriate mCherry-EGFP-LC3 stable cell line by infecting cells with mCherry-EGFP-LC3 retrovirus, followed by selection with a selectable marker. For best results we recommend selection for uniform fluorescence by using flow cytometry to sort fluorescent cells and removing those cells with very low or very high fluorescence. We typically sort on a Moflo XDP 100 machine (Beckman Coulter) using 488 and 561 nM lasers for red and green fluorophore excitation, respectively.

(b) About 24 h before the beginning of the experiment, plate cells onto 60 mm culture plates. Plate adherent cells such that cells are at about 50–80 % confluency at the time of the experiment.

(c) Pretreat (typically treat overnight, where possible) separate sets of cells for each condition to be measured with chloroquine or bafilomycin A_1 or other flux inhibitors. This is needed as a control to show that the mCherry/GFP fluorescence ratio properly decreases in the absence of autophagic flux during the stimuli. IMPORTANT: In addition to acting as a control this step allows one to determine the amount of "red-only" background in the cells and to properly set flow cytometry gates that define where the "high autophagy" cells are found in a population. Some tumor cell types lose viability in response to long-term CQ or Bafilomycin treatment. It is best to treat these cells for as long as possible without losing viability. The long-term treatment with these drugs allows the cells to degrade the remaining amount of mCherry-EGFP-LC3 left over from autophagosome delivery during previous time periods without further replenishing it.

(d) Treat cell with appropriate stimuli (e.g., amino acid deprivation, serum starvation, glucose deprivation) for which one wishes to measure autophagic response. This may be done on the day after controls are treated with flux inhibitors in the previous step, or a few hours after the inhibitors were added on the previous day if a long-term treatment is necessary (trehalose, for instance often requires overnight treatment to observe flux). Remember to re-add flux inhibitors to any control samples in which it was removed during the treatment. The length of treatment varies depending on the stimulus. With strong inducers, such as EBSS, it may not be necessary to treat more than a few hours.

(e) After completion of the treatment. Detach adherent cells by trypsinization, followed by neutralization of the trypsin with medium with 10 % serum.

(f) Pellet cells by centrifugation, remove media and wash with PBS.

(g) Pellet cells by centrifugation and then remove PBS. Resuspend in a small amount (typically 0.3–0.4 mL) flow cytometry buffer (1× PBS (Ca/Mg2+ free), 1 mM EDTA, 25 mM HEPES, pH 7.0) and place in flow cytometry tubes. For cells that are especially sensitive to serum/amino acid withdrawal, it may be advantageous to add a small amount of serum or amino acid mixture to the buffer. We have had good success measuring autophagy induction by other stimuli in such cell lines by resuspending in ~25 % DMEM (without phenol red) in PBS containing 1 % FBS. However, as calcium chloride in some media formulations may crystallize with phosphate component of the instrument sheath buffer in the cytometer, it is best to use as little media as possible. The inclusion of EDTA keeps the cells from clumping together, and the HEPES helps to maintain pH.

(h) Flow Cytometry in our hands is performed with a Moflo XDP 100 machine (Beckman Coulter) or a Gallios 561 (Beckman Coulter) or equivalent apparatus using 488 and 561 nM lasers for red and green fluorophore excitation, respectively.

8.4.3 *Interpretation and Analysis*

We have developed multiple, equally valid, ways of analyzing and presenting the flow data obtained by flow cytometry from this assay. We shall consider two methods and one variation of the first method. There are advantages and disadvantages to each methodology of analysis. In all methods, any nonviable cells should first be excluded from analysis by gating on the appropriate forward/side scatter profile. Dead cells should not typically be included in the analysis because the pH of both their cytoplasm and lysosomes is altered giving aberrant results. Any nonfluorescent cells should also be removed from the analysis by appropriate gating.

8.4.3.1 Method 1: Ratiometric Analysis

Most flow cytometry software allows one to determine a linear fluorescence ratio between two fluorescence channels for each cell. In some cases, the software calculates this ratio during data acquisition and this number is then saved as one of the parameters associated with a cell. In other cases the ratio is calculated when the analysis is conducted and must be defined separately. Keep in mind that this ratio is not a constant for a given cell with a certain amount of autophagosomes and will change somewhat if the voltage is altered on one of the channel detectors, making it important to run comparisons at the same time using the same parameters.

For analysis, it is useful to plot a histogram that shows the amount of cells having each ratio, as is shown in Fig. 8.3. For practical purposes, we largely define cells having substantial autophagic flux as those cells having a higher mCherry/GFP fluorescence ratio than cells treated with autophagic flux inhibitors. For different tumor cell types, as noted previously, the amount of red fluorescence background may differ depending on how much fusion protein is still within the lysosome that has not yet been degraded. In Fig. 8.3, the bafilomycin A_1-treated control cells are shown in yellow (solid filled, indicated by triangle). Since bafilomycin A_1 inhibits autophagic flux, the bottom of the gate (R3) that defines the cells having substantial autophagic flux is set at the rightward base of the bafilomycin A_1-treated cells. The cells under the bafilomycin A_1 curve should represent cells with little to no autophagic flux, and the cells to the right of this curve would have higher autophagic flux (it is important to verify that this amount of flux inhibitor completely inhibits flux over the time course of treatment). It is more difficult to decide where specifically the bottom of this gate should be set, since there is, as mentioned, a certain amount of background that trails rightward. We have found that it is typically best to set the quantification gate such that no more than 2–5 % of bafilomycin A_1-treated cells from every given condition would be included within the gate. However, there are certain cell lines that have a more significant amount of red background in the absence of flux, so it may be necessary to increase this percentage in such cells. In these cases it is usually apparent that the rightward tail of the curve is more substantial than the left tail. In the case of such high background (where we are certain

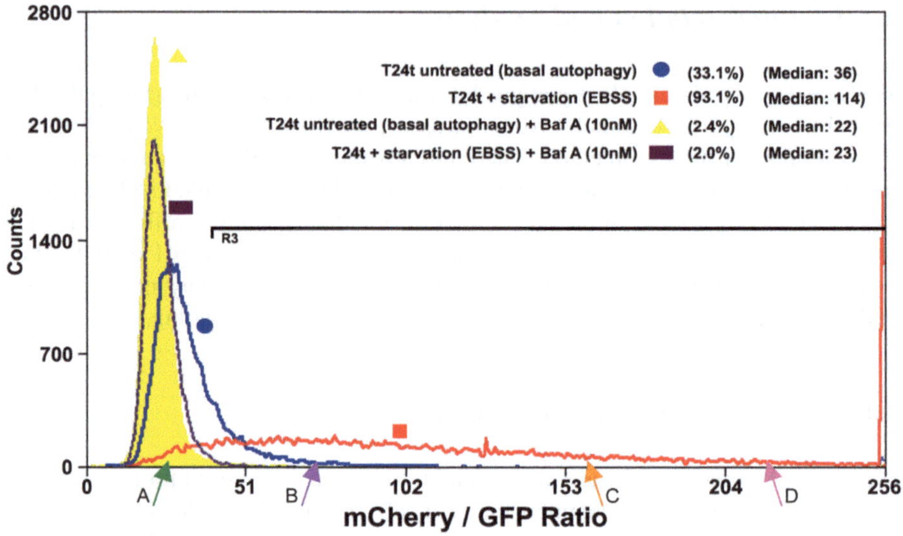

Fig. 8.3 Ratiometric analysis of mCherry-GFP-LC3 cells using flow cytometry. Stable cell lines were generated from T24t cells infected with a pBabe retrovirus that encoded mCherry-GFP-LC3 followed by antibiotic selection. Cells were sorted for fluorescence uniformity by flow cytometry. Cells were treated with or without bafilomycin A1 for 1 h and were washed and then treated overnight with EBSS and/or bafilomycin A1 and analyzed by flow cytometry

that flux has completely been blocked) we believe that it is valid to set the gate up to 15 % or more, and then subtract out the amount of bafilomycin A_1 or CQ-treated cells that are found in this gate for each individual treatment. We would, however, suggest in these cases that the gate intersect the control (Baf A treated) curve at no more than 20 % of the height of the curve. Whatever variation is introduced in setting the gate due to background, it is obviously important to be consistent in applying the same standard to all of the cells in order to have a valid measurement.

Once we have a definition of cells with substantial flux, one can measure the amount of cells within these gates as a percentage of all cells within the population. For instance in Fig. 8.3, the basal number of T24t cells having measurable autophagy in the presence of normal nutrients is around 33 % (this is indicative of quite a high rate of basal autophagy in these cells which have a HRAS mutation that is thought to drive high constitutive autophagy even in the absence of starvation), and this number increases to 93 % when the cells are starved overnight in EBSS. Once percentages are determined using the proper gates, data from these gates in multiple experiments are averaged together. These numbers are useful for comparison between samples where a gene of interest is being manipulated and comparing effects on basal autophagy, or negative effects on EBSS-induced autophagy, but it should be apparent from the figure that in the case where one wishes to examine a positive effect on EBSS-induced autophagy, the time course shown in Fig. 8.3 would be too long for this analysis, and a shorter time course would be necessary to reduce the amount of EBSS-treated cells within the gate, so as to observe an effect.

To extend the analysis one can measure the intensity of flux by gating further. For instance, it is readily apparent that cell populations with ratios indicated by the different arrows differ in the amount of autophagic flux. With cells indicated by the green arrow (arrow A), one can conclude that little flux is happening, since the ratios are similar to no-flux cells. However, our previous gate, defined such that no more than 2–5 % of bafilomycin A_1-treated cells are included, makes no distinction in differences of flux between cells indicated by the purple (arrow B), orange (arrow C), and pink (arrow D) arrows, even though it is likely that the orange arrow population has substantially more flux than that indicated by the purple arrow, and the blue arrow population likewise more than the orange arrow. At this point, one could now set arbitrary gates that define cells with low, medium, or high autophagy. This would be valid as long as the gates are applied consistently; however, significant variations can arise in these arbitrary gate populations when one tries to repeat the experiment in a different flow cytometer or when a cytometer has had some changes introduced by new maintenance, hardware, or other variables. The raw ratio for a given cell with a certain amount of autophagosomes is unfortunately not completely constant. We have not yet been able to come up with a definitive solution for setting alternative gates under such changes but separate gates can be defined based on other criteria that might more consistently control for such variations. For instance one could define a gate that includes no more than 10 % of cells under basal autophagy conditions. One can also increase the number of experimental repetitions until the variations average out, there are clear statistical differences, and it is then obvious that an arbitrary (but consistently applied) gate represents real differences.

8.4.3.2 Variation on Ratiometric Analysis

In some of our previous publications, we have presented flow cytometry ratiometric data by comparing the median mCherry/GFP ratio values in two or more populations of cells. One advantage of this method is that it is not as easily affected by experiment-to-experiment variation in the shape of the ratiometric curve. A comparison between the numbers obtained in this analysis compared to the gating method is shown in the inset for Fig. 8.3. The median for the bafilomycin control, in which there is no flux, is quantified as approximately 22, while the median for the basal autophagy and starved groups is 36 and 114, respectfully. In this case it is clear that there is a certain amount of basal autophagy in the cells and that the amount of EBSS-induced autophagy is substantially higher. The median of several different experiments is then averaged together for comparison. This can be useful both for comparing different sets of cells where a gene product has been manipulated and comparing the amount of flux induced by various stimuli.

One disadvantage of using the median is that it may not detect changes in autophagy if only a part of a cell population has changes in autophagy (for instance, if one was able to only affect certain subpopulations of tumor cells in a population). A second disadvantage is that it does not indicate the amount of cells with little or no autophagy, as does the percentage gating method in the previous section; only

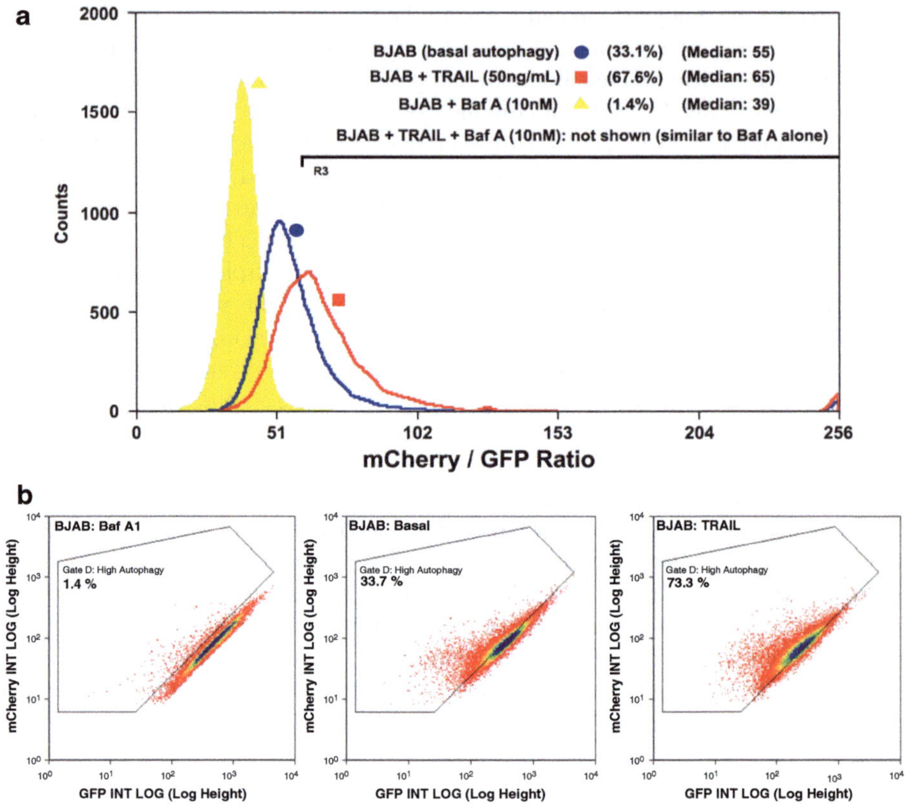

Fig. 8.4 Alternative analysis of mCherry-GFP-LC3 cells using flow cytometry. Stable cell lines were generated from BJAB cells infected with a pBabe retrovirus that encoded mCherry-GFP-LC3 followed by antibiotic selection. Cells were sorted for fluorescence uniformity by flow cytometry. Cells were treated with or without bafilomycin A1 for overnight and then washed and treated for 5 h with or without 100 ng/ml TRAIL and then analyzed by flow cytometry. The (**a**) panel shows cell analyzed by the ratiometric histogram gating method, while the (**b**) panel shows the same data as analyzed by gating a two-dimensional dot plot. The gating for both panels was set by the gate limit set by 1.5 % background in the Baf A gate

the overall effect on autophagy is indicated. These two considerations can have a profound effect when examining stimuli that are less robust than amino acid/serum starvation, and where a significant amount of cells do not respond.

A second comparison of the two ratiometric methods is shown in Fig. 8.4a. In this experiment BJAB cells were treated with the death receptor ligand TRAIL. One can see from the inset that the median of the Baf A-treated cells was 39, and the median fluorescence ratio increases to 55 in the cells under basal conditions and 65 under TRAIL-treated conditions. The percentage quantification shows about 33 % of the cells have a significant amount of basal autophagy and the amount of cells with autophagic flux increased to 68 % when the cells were treated for 5 h with TRAIL (1.5 % of Baf A-treated cells were included as background within the gate).

The percentage gating methodology may be more appropriate in this case, since it is clear from that method that there is a twofold increase in autophagy, whereas in the median reporting method one can tell that TRAIL increases autophagy, but the amount of increase is not as apparent.

8.4.3.3 Method 2: Gating a Two-Dimensional Dot Plot

Some flow cytometry software lacks the ability to quantify mCherry/GFP ratios. In this case a dot plot is created that graphs the log of the mCherry fluorescence intensities versus the log of the GFP fluorescent intensities of each cell (see Fig. 8.4b). As in the method in Sect. 8.4.3.1, the flux inhibitor controls are used to set the gate for high autophagy. The edge of the gate should run parallel to the line of cells in the flux inhibitor control, and then should be adjusted leftward to contain no more than 1–5 % of cells in this sample (Fig. 8.4b, left). When the gate is set, it is then applied to the samples with flux and the total percentage of cells in the gate compared to the total cells on the dot plot is calculated.

One can see from Fig. 8.4 that this method compares favorably with the ratio gating method. The same data is shown in Fig. 8.4a, b, but is analyzed by the two methods. In both cases background is defined at about 1.5 % of Baf A-treated cells. In both cases the amount of basal autophagy is consistent at 33 %. The amount of TRAIL-induced autophagy is quantified at 73 % in the dot plot method and 68 % in the ratiometric gating method.

The only disadvantage of this method compared to the ratio gating method is that it is not as easy to distinguish red fluorescence background. In the ratio gating method, background is apparent by comparing the amount of rightward tail to the total height profile of the bell-shaped curve. In the dot plot analysis, the proper placing of the gate should be limited to a set percentage of flux inhibitor-treated cells that should be allowed within the gate, but the gate must be determined empirically after shifting the population around with inducers and inhibitors.

8.5 Conclusions

We have presented several different assays that are commonly used to measure autophagy. There are other less commonly applied assays that may also be used [39]. Each of the three assays we have presented is widely accepted, but each also has limitations and advantages. There is currently no one ideal method to assess autophagy and changes in autophagy even in easily manipulated cancer cell lines. Moreover, when one wants to examine primary cells there may be added difficulties. Our primary recommendation is that researchers interested in establishing whether autophagy is affected in their experimental system should utilize several approaches together and only when reliable changes occur as measured by more than one assay should firm conclusions about whether one has altered autophagy be made.

References

1. Mizushima N. Autophagy: process and function. Genes Dev. 2007;21(22):2861–73.
2. Klionsky DJ. Autophagy: from phenomenology to molecular understanding in less than a decade. Nat Rev Mol Cell Biol. 2007;8(11):931–7.
3. Galluzzi L, Vicencio JM, Kepp O, et al. To die or not to die: that is the autophagic question. Curr Mol Med. 2008;8(2):78–91.
4. Yang ZJ, Chee CE, Huang S, Sinicrope FA. The role of autophagy in cancer: therapeutic implications. Mol Cancer Ther. 2011;10(9):1533–41.
5. Fung C, Lock R, Gao S, Salas E, Debnath J. Induction of autophagy during extracellular matrix detachment promotes cell survival. Mol Biol Cell. 2008;19(3):797–806.
6. Gump JM, Thorburn A. Autophagy and apoptosis: what is the connection? Trends Cell Biol. 2011;21(7):387–92.
7. Thorburn A, Thamm DH, Gustafson DL. Autophagy and cancer therapy. Mol Pharmacol. 2014;85(6):830–8.
8. Shen HM, Codogno P. Autophagic cell death: Loch Ness monster or endangered species? Autophagy. 2011;7(5):457–65.
9. Gump JM, Staskiewicz L, Morgan MJ, et al. Autophagy variation within a cell population determines cell fate through selective degradation of Fap-1. Nat Cell Biol. 2014;16(1):47–54.
10. Yonekawa T, Gamez G, Kim J, et al. RIP1 negatively regulates basal autophagic flux through TFEB to control sensitivity to apoptosis. EMBO Rep. 2015;16(6):700–8.
11. Galluzzi L, Pietrocola F, Bravo-San Pedro JM, et al. Autophagy in malignant transformation and cancer progression. EMBO J. 2015;34(7):856–80.
12. Qu X, Yu J, Bhagat G, et al. Promotion of tumorigenesis by heterozygous disruption of the beclin 1 autophagy gene. J Clin Invest. 2003;112(12):1809–20.
13. Yue Z, Jin S, Yang C, Levine AJ, Heintz N. Beclin 1, an autophagy gene essential for early embryonic development, is a haploinsufficient tumor suppressor. Proc Natl Acad Sci U S A. 2003;100(25):15077–82.
14. Takahashi Y, Coppola D, Matsushita N, et al. Bif-1 interacts with Beclin 1 through UVRAG and regulates autophagy and tumorigenesis. Nat Cell Biol. 2007;9(10):1142–51.
15. Cianfanelli V, Fuoco C, Lorente M, et al. AMBRA1 links autophagy to cell proliferation and tumorigenesis by promoting c-Myc dephosphorylation and degradation. Nat Cell Biol. 2015;17(1):20–30.
16. Liang C, Feng P, Ku B, et al. Autophagic and tumour suppressor activity of a novel Beclin1-binding protein UVRAG. Nat Cell Biol. 2006;8(7):688–98.
17. Takamura A, Komatsu M, Hara T, et al. Autophagy-deficient mice develop multiple liver tumors. Genes Dev. 2011;25(8):795–800.
18. Marino G, Salvador-Montoliu N, Fueyo A, et al. Tissue-specific autophagy alterations and increased tumorigenesis in mice deficient in Atg4C/autophagin-3. J Biol Chem. 2007;282(25):18573–83.
19. Strohecker AM, Guo JY, Karsli-Uzunbas G, et al. Autophagy sustains mitochondrial glutamine metabolism and growth of Braf(V600E)-driven lung tumors. Cancer Discov. 2013;3(11):1272–85.
20. Rao S, Tortola L, Perlot T, et al. A dual role for autophagy in a murine model of lung cancer. Nat Commun. 2014;5:3056.
21. Rosenfeldt MT, O'Prey J, Morton JP, et al. p53 status determines the role of autophagy in pancreatic tumour development. Nature. 2013;504(7479):296–300.
22. Yang A, Rajeshkumar NV, Wang XX, et al. Autophagy is critical for pancreatic tumor growth and progression in tumors with p53 alterations. Cancer Discov. 2014;4(8):905–13.
23. Altman BJ, Jacobs SR, Mason EF, et al. Autophagy is essential to suppress cell stress and to allow BCR-Abl-mediated leukemogenesis. Oncogene. 2011;30(16):1855–67.
24. Guo JY, Karsli-Uzunbas G, Mathew R, et al. Autophagy suppresses progression of K-ras-induced lung tumors to oncocytomas and maintains lipid homeostasis. Genes Dev. 2013;27(13):1447–61.

25. Karsli-Uzunbas G, Guo JY, Price S, et al. Autophagy is required for glucose homeostasis and lung tumor maintenance. Cancer Discov. 2014;4(8):914–27.
26. Xie XQ, Koh JY, Price S, White E, Mehnert JM. Atg7 overcomes senescence and promotes growth of Braf(V600E)-driven melanoma. Cancer Discov. 2015;5(4):410–23.
27. Maycotte P, Aryal S, Cummings CT, et al. Chloroquine sensitizes breast cancer cells to chemotherapy independent of autophagy. Autophagy. 2012;8(2):200–12.
28. Maycotte P, Gearheart CM, Barnard R, et al. STAT3-mediated autophagy dependence identifies subtypes of breast cancer where autophagy inhibition can be efficacious. Cancer Res. 2014;74(9):2579–90.
29. Levy JM, Thompson JC, Griesinger AM, et al. Autophagy inhibition improves chemosensitivity in BRAFV600E brain tumors. Cancer Discov. 2014;4(7):773–80.
30. Morgan MJ, Gamez G, Menke C, et al. Regulation of autophagy and chloroquine sensitivity by oncogenic RAS in vitro is context-dependent. Autophagy. 2014;10(10):1814–26.
31. Rosenfeld MR, Ye XB, Supko JG, et al. A phase I/II trial of hydroxychloroquine in conjunction with radiation therapy and concurrent and adjuvant temozolomide in patients with newly diagnosed glioblastoma multiforme. Autophagy. 2014;10(8):1359–68.
32. Mahalingam D, Mita M, Sarantopoulos J, et al. Combined autophagy and HDAC inhibition A phase I safety, tolerability, pharmacokinetic, and pharmacodynamic analysis of hydroxychloroquine in combination with the HDAC inhibitor vorinostat in patients with advanced solid tumors. Autophagy. 2014;10(8):1403–14.
33. Vogl DT, Stadtmauer EA, Tan KS, et al. Combined autophagy and proteasome inhibition A phase 1 trial of hydroxychloroquine and bortezomib in patients with relapsed/refractory myeloma. Autophagy. 2014;10(8):1380–90.
34. Rangwala R, Chang YYC, Hu J, et al. Combined MTOR and autophagy inhibition Phase I trial of hydroxychloroquine and temsirolimus in patients with advanced solid tumors and melanoma. Autophagy. 2014;10(8):1391–402.
35. Barnard RA, Wittenburg LA, Amaravadi RK, et al. Phase I clinical trial and pharmacodynamic evaluation of combination hydroxychloroquine and doxorubicin treatment in pet dogs treated for spontaneously occurring lymphoma. Autophagy. 2014;10(8):1415–25.
36. Rangwala R, Leone R, Chang YYC, et al. Phase I trial of hydroxychloroquine with dose-intense temozolomide in patients with advanced solid tumors and melanoma. Autophagy. 2014;10(8):1369–79.
37. Ben Younes A, Tajeddine N, Tailler M, et al. A fluorescence-microscopic and cytofluorometric system for monitoring the turnover of the autophagic substrate p62/SQSTM1. Autophagy. 2011;7(8):883–91.
38. Tanida I, Yamaji T, Ueno T, et al. Consideration about negative controls for LC3 and expression vectors for four colored fluorescent protein-LC3 negative controls. Autophagy. 2008;4(1):131–4.
39. Klionsky DJ, Abdalla FC, Abeliovich H, et al. Guidelines for the use and interpretation of assays for monitoring autophagy. Autophagy. 2012;8(4):445–544.

Chapter 9
Methods for Studying Autophagy Within the Tumor Microenvironment

Sengottuvelan Murugan and Ravi K. Amaravadi

Abstract Defective autophagy has been linked with many pathologies, including cancer, diabetes, infectious disease, myopathies, heart, liver, lung, and neurodegenerative disease. Autophagy has therefore become an important target in drug discovery. Recent advances have identified new ways to monitor autophagy in vitro and in vivo. Many assays rely on visualizing autophagy-related intracellular markers such as microtubule-associated protein light chain 3 (LC3) II, which have posed issues with in vivo and clinical translation of the in vitro assays. Here, we present an overview of current in vitro and in vivo methodologies to measure autophagy with a special focus on the tumor microenvironment.

Keywords Autophagy • Tumor microenvironment • Autophagy modulators • Autophagic flux • Automated quantitative analyses (AQUA) • Comparative secretome analysis • High-autophagy cells • Low-autophagy cells

9.1 Introduction

Autophagy is a dynamic and tightly regulated homeostatic process. Autophagy is characterized by sequestration of cellular organelles and proteins into autophagic vesicles and fusion of these vesicles with lysosomes. Under normal conditions, basal autophagy plays an important role in the housekeeping of the cell via disposal of waste, which includes removal of damaged subcellular organelles and protein aggregates. Under stress conditions, including starvation, intracellular pathogens,

S. Murugan, Ph.D.
Hematology/Oncology Division, Perelman School of Medicine, University of Pennsylvania, Clinical Research Building Room No: 120, Philadelphia, PA 19104, USA
e-mail: murugan@mail.med.upenn.edu

R.K. Amaravadi, M.D. (✉)
The Department of Medicine and Abramson Cancer Center, University of Pennsylvania School of Medicine, 777 South Tower 34th St and Civic Center Blvd, Philadelphia, PA 19104, USA
e-mail: ravi.amaravadi@uphs.upenn.edu

C. Koumenis et al. (eds.), *Tumor Microenvironment*, Advances in Experimental Medicine and Biology 899, DOI 10.1007/978-3-319-26666-4_9

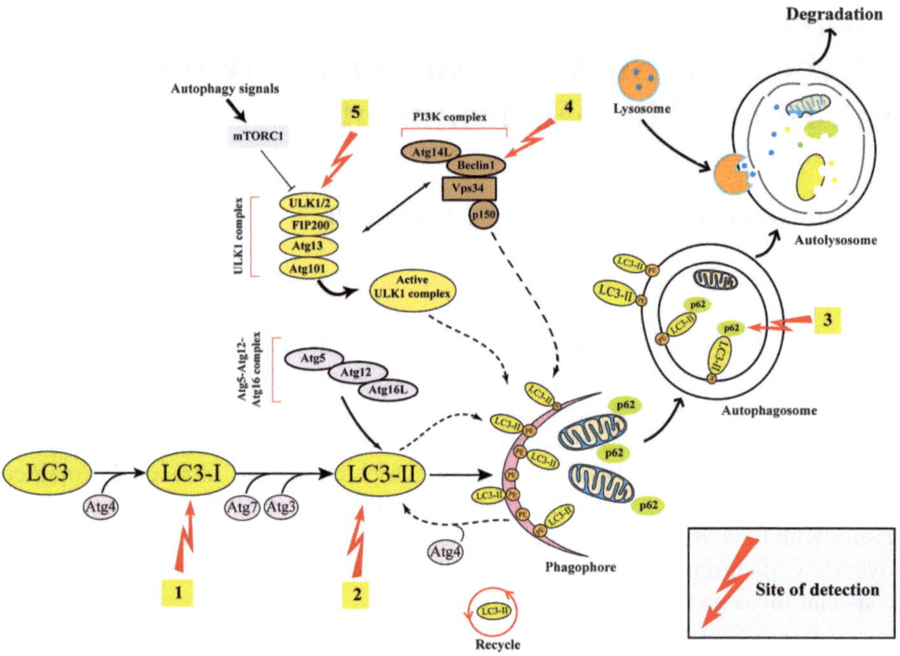

Fig. 9.1 Formation of autophagic vesicles and the site of autophagy measurement

and reactive oxygen species, autophagy supplies the cell with an internal source of nutrients (amino acids, sugars, and nucleic acids). This recycling capacity helps cells adapt and survive in the face of unfavorable conditions. The autophagy pathway occurs in many distinct stages, including autophagic vesicle initiation, nucleation, elongation, fusion, and degradation (Fig. 9.1). These stages are tightly regulated by several autophagy-related (Atg) proteins. Activation or suppression of autophagic machinery is regulated through a number of signaling networks including the mammalian target of rapamycin (mTOR) or AMPK signaling, the ER stress response, and the DNA damage response. For example a signaling kinase called unc-like kinase 1 (Ulk1)/Atg 1 complex is responsible for initiation autophagy. Phosphorylation of Ulk1 at Ser 317 and Ser 777 by the energy-sensing AMP-activated protein kinase (AMPK) activates autophagy, whereas phosphorylation of Ulk1 at ser 757 by mammalian target of rapamycin (mTOR) dissociates Ulk1 from AMPK and suppresses autophagy [1]. In addition, many posttranslational modifications including acetylation, ubiquitination, and oxidation of sulfhydryls regulate the autophagic process. After initiation and activation, the Ulk1/Atg 1 complex guides the localization of class III phosphoinositide 3-kinase (PI3K) complex for the regulation of nucleation and assembly of the phagophore membrane. In addition, a ubiquitin-like conjugation system involving ATG7 and ATG3 guides the formation of the Atg5-Atg12-Atg16L complex. This complex in turn is responsible for conjugating LC3 to phosphatidylethanolamines (PE), thereby promoting the elongation and closing of the autophagosomal membrane [1]. The sequestering of cargo substrates (protein aggregates, mitochondria, and other organelles) into the autophagosomes is mainly guided by cargo receptor proteins such as P62/SQSTM1. Finally, autophagosomes fuse with lysosomes to form autolysosomes, where the degradation of cargo is mainly achieved by acid hydrolases (for more details of molecular machinery of autophagy see [2]).

Given the well-known role of autophagy in normal physiology, recent evidence suggests that autophagy in cancer cells plays a dual role, to either suppress early carcinogenesis or support the survival and growth of advanced tumors [3]. The role of autophagy within the tumor microenvironment (TME) is being increasingly recognized as a key factor in cancer progression. Evidence indicates that autophagy promotes tumor progression [4], resistance to therapy [5, 6], a blunting of immune effector cell function [7–9], and metastasis [10]. A study shows that in a mouse model of ductal adenocarcinoma of the pancreas (PDAC), high levels of basal autophagy support malignant growth. Inhibition of autophagy by chloroquine (CQ) or silencing of Atg5 induced tumor regression [11]. In addition, recent data suggest that autophagy is involved in the cross talk between the cancer cell and tumor stroma, where Atg5 expressed in endothelial cells mediates starvation and hypoxia-induced angiogenesis by high mobility group box1 (HMGB1), a pro-autophagic factor [12]. In pancreatic cancer cells a protein called receptor for advanced glycation end products (RAGE) overexpression and interaction with HMGB1 causes resistance to apoptosis and induces autophagy as pro-survival mechanism [13]. Taken together these capacities of autophagy contribute to its role as a resistance mechanism to multiple cancer therapeutics. Despite a large volume of data that supports targeting autophagy in cancer, development of autophagy inhibitors has been slow. One reason for this is that the methods used to monitor autophagy have significant limitations. Despite these limitations some of these assays have been applied to human samples effectively to fuel translational research. Here we will provide detailed information for each assays and report on their strengths and weaknesses.

9.2 Autophagy Modulators

Even though numerous reports have validated the role of autophagy as a potential therapeutic target for diseases [14], the role of autophagy in anticancer treatment is complex and may be dependent heavily on the tumor microenvironment [15]. On the one hand unfettered autophagy induced by specific anticancer agents can promote autophagic cell death in vitro. On the other hand, there is mounting evidence that in the context of an advanced cancer, intratumoral autophagy promotes growth and resistance of cancers [16]. Although a growing number of reports on the discovery of small-molecule autophagy modulators have been published, concern is raised that some of the hits in these screens modulate autophagy through off-target or indirect effects. Many new autophagy modulators appear to be effective only in cell culture systems but little is known about their safety or efficacy in preclinical and clinical uses. Given the complexity of interpreting the autophagy process, one should consider using multiple methods to discover more selective agents that can efficiently modulate autophagy either alone or in combination. At present, many autophagy modulating agents serve as a potential anticancer therapeutics and here is the partial list of widely used autophagic modulators (Table 9.1) and site of action in the autophagy pathway.

Table 9.1 List of compounds with known mechanism of autophagy modulation

Autophagy inducers	
AMPK activators and mTORC1 inhibitors	• Rapamycin • Temsirolimus (CCI-779) • Everolimus (RAD001) • Deforolimus (Ridaforolimus) • PP242 • Torin 1 • GDC-0980 • Metformin • AICAR
Inhibitors of class I PI3K signaling	• CH5132799 • GDC-0980 • GDC-0941
Modulators of intracellular Ca_2^+	• Fluspirilene • Verapamil • Loperamide • Amiodarone • Thapsigargin
Proteasome inhibitors	• Bortezomib • NPI-0052 • MG-132
Histone deacetylase (HDACs) inhibitors	• Suberoylanilide hydroxamic acid (SAHA) • OSU-HDAC42 • Trichostatin A (TSA) • Valproic acid (VPA) • 5-Aza-cytidine (AZA)
Synthetic and plant-based chemotherapeutic agents	• Temozolomide (TMZ) • Tamoxifen • Resveratrol • Cannabinoids • β-Lapachone • Avicins • Betulinic acid derivative B10 • Plant lectins
Autophagy inhibitors	
Class III PI3K inhibitors blocks autophagy	• 3-Methyladenine (3-MA) • Wortmannin • LY294002 • Spautin • Vps34 inhibitors

(continued)

Table 9.1 (continued)

Microtubule modulators	• Vinblastine • Nocodazole • Cytochalasin B and D
Lysosomal inhibitors	• Chloroquine (CQ) • Hydroxychloroquine (HCQ) • Quinacrine • Lys05, a dimeric CQ • Monensin • Lucanthone • Matrine
Vacuolar H+-ATPase inhibitors	• Bafilomycin A1 • Concanamycin A • Azithromycin
Inhibitors of lysosomal hydrolases and proteases	• E64d • Pepstatin A
c-Jun N-terminal kinase (JNK) inhibitors	• SP600125

9.3 Measuring Autophagy Markers by Immunoblotting

In autophagy research, Western blot data are widely used as a semiquantitative method to analyze autophagic marker proteins in cells, animals, and in human tissues. When appropriate precautions are taken before and after sample preparation, Western blot provides useful information for monitoring autophagy in cancer research. Here we provide basic information of some well-known autophagic marker proteins and key points that should be considered when performing Western blots for the detection and analysis of autophagy markers.

(a) Microtubule-associated protein 1A/1B-light chain 3 (LC3)

Detecting LC3 by immunoblotting has become a reliable method for monitoring autophagy and autophagy-related processes. Readers are advised to refer Chap. 10 for details on LC3 immunoblotting. To assess autophagic flux using LC3, autophagy modulators are used to perturb autophagy and rationally conclude the effects on autophagy flux in the given system (see below).

(b) Other autophagy marker proteins

Depending on the cell types and the stimuli, the autophagic marker proteins are differentially regulated during autophagy induction. During autophagy, the ratio of LC3-II/LC3-I, or the amount of LC3-II, is generally increased, but other autophagy-related proteins, such as Beclin 1, Atg5–Atg12, Atg4, and Atg7, may or may not be increased.

9.3.1 p62 (SQSTM1/Sequestosome 1)

p62 is a ubiquitin- and LC3-binding protein. The analysis of p62 (also called as SQSTM1/sequestosome 1) protein levels along with LC3 can provide insights about autophagic flux in a tissue-dependent manner. Total cellular levels of p62 inversely correlate with autophagic activity in most conditions, because p62 directly binds to LC3 and gets selectively incorporated into autophagosomes and degraded by autophagy [17]. Thus, in a given condition, low autophagic flux can be determined by high basal levels of p62 and low LC3-II levels. Conversely, high flux can be inferred by high LC3-II and decreased p62 levels after autophagy stimulation. However, it should be noted that changes in p62 levels are also used to indicate a defect in the turnover of poly-ubiquitinated protein aggregates. Thus, to monitor autophagic flux, analysis of p62 protein levels should be used only in combination with other methods such as LC3-II turnover [18]. P62 is also regulated by oxidative stress and the NF-kB pathway. Therefore there are often discordant behaviors between autophagic flux and p62 levels. The interpretation of changes in p62 should therefore be made cautiously.

9.3.2 Beclin, ATG5, ATG7, and Other Core Autophagy Proteins

Beclin (ATG8) is monoallelically deleted in cancers which demonstrate a loss of the neighboring tumor suppressor gene BRCA1 [19]. Beclin levels have been used by some as a measure of autophagy, but this should be avoided. In all cases of Beclin allelic loss, the retained allele always harbors wild-type Beclin, and beclin levels can be transcriptionally increased to wild-type levels even in beclin heterozygous cells. ATG5 levels have been shown to be regulated by promoter methylation in melanoma cells [20]. The measurement of ATG proteins in general is not a reliable reflection of autophagic flux, unless the protein levels of these enzymes are close to zero, as would be the case in genetically engineered cell lines, or as mentioned epigenetically silenced cell lines. Even in these cases, confirmation of LC3 levels is necessary. In our experience >70 % knockdown of ATG5 in melanoma cells blunted but did not completely abrogate LC3 lipidation [21].

9.3.3 Phosphorylation Status of ULK

There are multiple ULK isoforms which exist in mammalian cells, including ULK1, ULK2, ULK3, ULK4, and ULK5. ULK1 may be the predominant isoform responsible for the initiation of autophagy. Phosphorylation of ULK1 on Ser 317 and Ser777 in certain contexts can serve as marker for autophagy activity [22]. One problem with the detection of phospho-ULK1 by western blot is the low abundance of endogenous ULK1 in many systems.

9.4 Monitoring the Number of Autophagosomes and Autophagy Flux by Western Blot

9.4.1 Measuring the Number of Autophagosomes by LC3-I to LC3-II Conversion

The number of autophagosomes observed at any specific time point is a function of the balance between the rate of their generation and the rate of their conversion into autolysosomes. Thus, a number of autophagosomes can be monitored simply by detecting the conversion of LC3-I to LC3-II by immunoblotting. Due to the association of LC3-II with the autophagosome membrane, the levels of LC3-II correlates with the number of autophagosome formation (the amount of autophagic membrane labeled with LC3-II). The conversion of LC3-I to LC3-II provides an indicator of autophagic process but not the activity [23], because LC3-II increases during early autophagy (autophagosome formation), but at later steps it decreases (due to self-degradation). Therefore, the amount of LC3-II does not reflect the activity of autophagy as shown in Fig. 9.2. Increased LC3-II levels in a cell line or tissue could be associated with any of the following reasons: (1) enhanced autophagosome synthesis, (2) reduced autophagosome turnover, (3) delayed lysosome trafficking, (4) reduction of fusion between compartments (lysosomes with autophagosomes), (5) impaired proteolytic activity in lysosomal compartment. The factors which affect the interpretation of the LC3 Western blot data are as follows: (1) differential affinities of antibodies for LC3-I compared to LC3-II, (2) different expression levels of LC3-I and LC3-II depending on cell line and tissue, (3) LC3-II itself is subject to autophagic degradation at the lysosome [24].

9.4.2 Monitoring Autophagic Flux Using the Bafilomycin Clamp Assay

Given the fact that measuring the conversion of LC3-I to LC3-II and/or LC3-II normalization with loading control (actin, tubulin, or GAPDH) is not always a good indicator of cellular autophagic activity, it is mandatory to discriminate whether or not LC3-II accumulation is due to induction of autophagy or due to the blockage in the later stages of autophagy by conducting "autophagic flux" assays in their

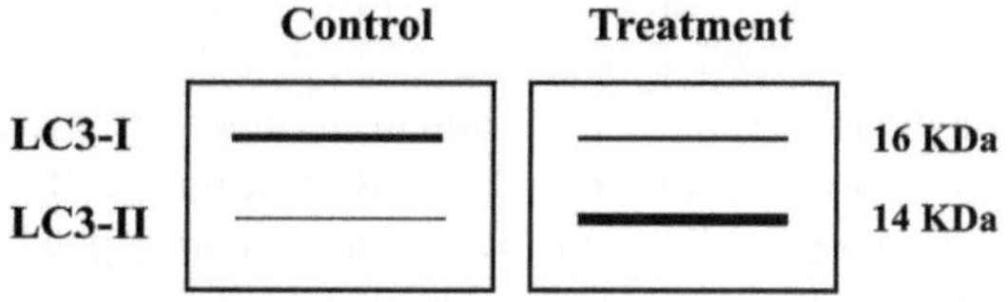

Fig. 9.2 Schematic representation of LC3-I to LC3-II conversion during a typical treatment condition

Table 9.2 Partial list of conditions and inhibitors commonly used to study autophagic flux

Category	Compounds
Starvation (induce autophagy)	• *Dulbecco's phosphate-buffered saline* (*DPBS*)—which lacks serum and all amino acids. • *Dulbecco's Modified Eagle Medium* (*DMEM*) medium—lacks serum and glutamine. • *Earle's Balanced Salt Solution* (*EBSS*)—without calcium/magnesium and sugars. • *Hank's buffered salt solution* (*HBSS*)—without calcium/magnesium.
Lysosomotropic agents	• *Ammonium chloride* • *Chloroquine* (*CQ*)—CQ is a weak base that accumulates in acidic organelles (lysosomes and late endosomes), where it gets trapped upon protonation [addition of a proton (H+)], leading to the alkalinization (increasing the pH) of these organelles. CQ prevents the degradation of autophagosomes before fusion with lysosome and inhibits lysosomal hydrolases and thereby prevents cargo degradation. • *Bafilomycin A1* (*Baf*)—is an inhibitor of vacuolar H^+-ATPase which inhibits Na^+ H^+ pump at the lysosome. Baf treatment for shorter time slows down the degradation of LC3-II within existing autolysosomes and impairs the fusion of autophagosomes with lysosomes (inhibit acidification) at longer incubation.
Lysosomal proteases	• *E-64-d* —is a cocktail of cathepsins B, H, and L. • *Pepstatin A* —inhibitor of cathepsins B.

experimental condition [25]. Here, we discuss how LC3 Western blot experiment can be designed and used to measure autophagic flux with some examples. LC3 turnover can be examined in a cell line or tissues by inducing starvation (amino acids depletion/serum) alone or in combination with inhibitors that inhibit degradation of autolysosome content. Table 9.2 gives a partial list of conditions and inhibitors commonly used to study autophagic flux.

To better understand and interpret the changes in levels of LC3-II processing (autophagic flux) in a given condition, we have provided an example (Fig. 9.3) where cells with low and high autophagic levels were cultured in regular nutrient-rich and starved media with or without inhibitor such as bafilomycin A1 (BafA1). As shown in Fig. 9.3, the differences in the level of LC3-II can be used to distinguish the autophagic rate between low (Cell Line A Fig. 9.3) and high (Cell Line B Fig. 9.3) autophagy cells under starvation/nonstarvation, with and without BafA1. Levels of LC3-II are elevated by treatment with BafA1 even under nutrient-rich condition in both cells lines [low (lane 2 vs. 1) and high (lane 6 vs. 5)]. Starvation induces LC3B processing in both cell lines when compared with nutrition-rich media [low (lane 3 vs. 1) and high (lane 7 vs. 5)] and treatment with BafA1 increased the amount of processed LC3B-II in both cell lines, but it is even higher in highly autophagic cells with lower autophagic capacity [low (lane 2) and high (lane 6)]. This finding would indicate that Cell Line B has a high basal rate of autophagy,

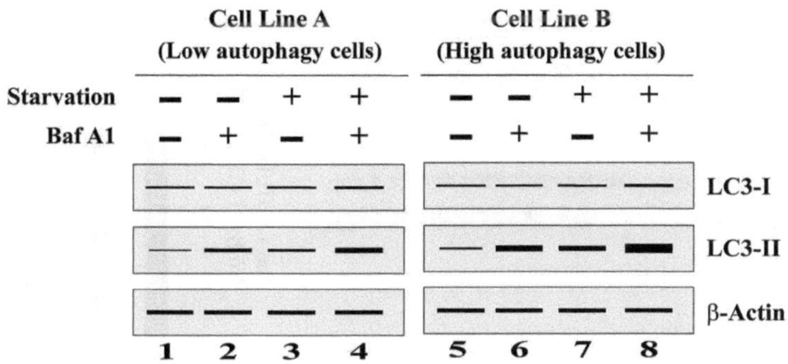

Fig. 9.3 A schematic representation of a Western blot after LC3 turnover assay to distinguish autophagy level in low and high autophagic cells. Cells were cultured in regular nutrition-rich media without Baf A1 (lane 1 and 5), regular nutrition-rich media with Baf A1 (lane 2 and 6), starvation media without Baf A1 (lane 3 and 7), and starvation media with Baf A1 (lane 4 and 8). *Baf A1* bafilomycin A1

which is further increased by starvation [low (lane 4) and high (lane 8)]. From the Western blot, we can interpret that accumulation of LC3-II positive autophagosomes in the presence of BafA1 would be evidence of efficient autophagic flux. Whereas if there was any failure in the increase of LC3-II protein during the presence of BafA1, this would indicate that there is a defect or delay in the early autophagic process (prior to degradation of LC3-II at autolysosome).

9.4.3 Discovery of New Autophagy Modulators via the Bafilomycin Clamp Assay

Even though several pharmacological compounds are known to inhibit autophagy in vitro, only CQ or its derivative hydroxychloroquine (HCQ) have been used in clinical trials. So, there is the clear need for more work on the development of selective inhibitors that target autophagy proteins directly. At the same time, careful consideration is needed when targeting these proteins; because some of the autophagic proteins are also involved in autophagy-independent functions (e.g., UVRAG inhibits translocation of Bax from the cytosol to mitochondria, thereby preventing apoptosis). Also, better methods or multiple methods should be combined in the discovery and screening of new specific small-molecule autophagy modulators, both inducers and inhibitors. For example we have previously reported that BRAF inhibitors induce autophagy in BRAF mutant melanoma. To ensure that BRAF inhibition was in fact inducing autophagy and not blocking distal clearance of AVs, a bafilomycin clamp experiment was conducted to determine how PLX4720 impacted autophagic flux (Fig. 9.4). A375P cells were treated with DMSO, PLX4720 1 μM, rapamycin 500 nM, or HCQ 10 μM, in the absence or presence of BafA1. At 24 h, PLX4720 or rapamycin (a proximal autophagy inducer) treatment resulted in a

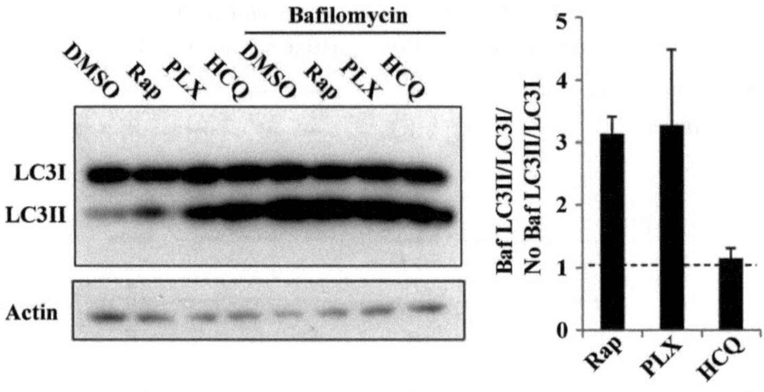

Fig. 9.4 A bafilomycin clamp demonstrates BRAF inhibitor-induced autophagy. Immunoblotting against LC3 was performed using A375 (BRAF mutant melanoma) cell lysate 24 h after treatment as indicated. Representative image of one out three experiments is shown. Quantification of the bands demonstrates that in the presence of Baf A1, LC3II levels increased with PLX treatment compared no Baf A1

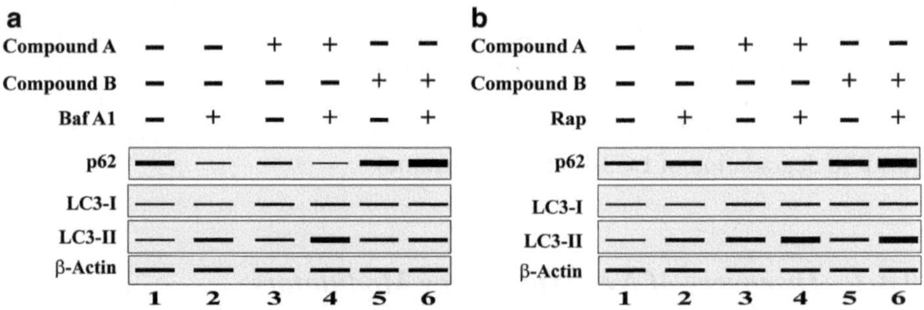

Fig. 9.5 A schematic representation of a Western blot to show how the results of LC3-I to LC3-II conversion in an bafilomycin clamp assay in the presence of (**a**) bafilomycin (Baf A1) or (**b**) rapamycin (Rap) and p62 degradation could be used to identify the mode of action of new autophagic modulators. Compound A (inducer) and compound B (Inhibitor)

threefold increase in the LC3II/LC3 ratio in Baf A1-treated cells compared to control cells whereas HCQ (distal autophagy inhibitor) did not demonstrate an increase in LC3II/LC3I ratio in Baf A1-treated cells compared to control, providing further evidence that BRAF inhibition induces autophagy.

Figure 9.5 shows another example of how to interpret the results of LC3-I to LC3-II conversion, the bafilomycin clamp assay, and integrate this information with the level of p62 when screening the efficacy of autophagy modulators (inhibitor and activator). To elucidate the mode of action of any modulators, one should do the bafilomycin clamp assay to compare the new modulators with known autophagy modulators such as BafA1 (inhibitor) or Rapamycin (inducer). As depicted in Fig. 9.5a, treatment of cells with BafA1 increased the level of LC3-II (lane 2) by blocking the late stage of autophagy. Both compound A (inducer) and compound B (inhibitor) increased LC3-II level (Fig. 9.5, lanes 3 and 5). However, co-incubation of these compounds with BafA1 showed drastic differences. Treatment of compound A along with BafA1 induced further accumulation of LC3-II (lane 4) when compared with LC3-II levels after treatment with BafA1 alone or compound A alone (lanes 2 and 3 respectively). This result suggests the increased level of LC3-II after treatment with compound A was further enhanced when autophagic flux was further blocked by BafA1, which confirms that compound A is an autophagy activator. On the other hand, no synergistic increase of LC3-II level was observed after co-incubation of compound B with BafA1 (lane 6) when compared with BafA1 alone treatment (lane 2) or compound B alone (lane 5). This confirms that compound B is neither an inducer nor an early stage inhibitor, because the LC3-II level induced by compound B was unaffected by the additional blockage of late-stage autophagic flux by BafA1. Here an additional experiment is needed to prove the mode of action of compound B (inhibitor). As shown in Fig. 9.5b, treatment of cells with rapamycin (Rap), an activator of autophagy (through mTOR inhibition), induced autophagy and accumulated the LC3-II level (lane 2). When compound B was co-incubated with Rap, it induced a greater increase in LC3-II (lane 6) than the LC3-II level of either Rap alone (lane 2) or compound B alone (lane 5), which denotes the compound B blocked autophagic flux. Interestingly, the compound A (activator) co-incubation with Rap induced a greater level of LC3-II (lane 4) when compared with either compound A alone (lane 3) or Rap alone (lane 2), even though both compounds activate autophagy.

When cells were treated with compound A as shown in Fig. 9.5a, it increased the level of LC3II and assisted the degradation of p62 whereas treatment with compound B also increased the level of LC3II, but inhibited the degradation of p62 level in the cells Fig. 9.5b. From the quantification of LC3II and p62 levels, we can tell that compound A acts as a autophagy inducer and compound B as inhibitor. This synergistic effect by compound A proves its effectiveness in activation of autophagy pathway. Therefore, in any experimental condition, one should be able to distinguish whether autophagosomes accumulation is due to autophagy induction or a block of the late stages by performing "autophagy flux" assays.

9.5 In Vivo Labeling by Acidotropic Dyes

9.5.1 Monodansylcadaverine (MDC) or Dansylcadaverine

MDC is a dye which emits a blue fluorescence and is thought to preferentially accumulate in autophagic vesicles but not in the early and late endosome. MDC accumulation in autophagic vesicles is exclusively due to a combination of ion trapping and specific interactions with vesicle membrane lipids. The mechanism of MDC accumulation is mainly dependent on the type of cells, condition, and whether it is fixed or non-fixed and so on. MDC's autofluorescent property (excitation wavelength at 365 nm) is due to the presence of a dansyl group conjugated to (diamine-pentane) cadaverine. MDC was initially characterized as a selective marker of autolysosomes

[26] and later as a marker of earlier autophagic compartments [27, 28]. Both in cultured cells and in animal tissues, accumulation of MDC-positive vesicles can be used as a marker to characterize autophagy by various different autophagy modulators. The size and number of MDC-fluorescent vesicles markedly increases or decreases in response to several autophagy modulators. For example, in cells subjected to a physiological or pharmacological stimulus of autophagy, such as amino acid deprivation or rapamycin treatment, the MDC-labeled compartments increases [28]. On the other hand, incorporation of MDC is almost completely inhibited when cells are treated with well-known inhibitors of autophagy, such as 3-methyladenine (3-MA) and wortmannin (WM). In addition to the morphological analysis of the autophagy pathway by fluorescence microscopy, autophagy modulation can be quantitatively monitored by flow cytometry. Therefore, MDC can be used as a good marker of autophagic vesicles; however in our experience MDC likely also accumulates in late endosomes and potentially other vesicular compartments. MDC fluorescence is variable and often not uniform across fields. Therefore MDC staining is not accepted as a stand-alone measurement of autophagy [29].

9.5.2 *Acridine Orange*

Acridine orange is a lysosomotropic green fluorescent dye that accumulates in acidic organelles in a pH-dependent manner. Within acidic vesicles (autolysosomes), acridine orange becomes protonated and trapped within the organelle and forms aggregates that emit bright red fluorescence, while in the nucleus acridine orange fluoresces bright green. At neutral pHs, Acridine Orange is a hydrophobic green fluorescent molecule. Thus, it is possible to track the formation of acidic vesicular organelles with acridine orange staining in any cultured cells [30]. But, it should be noted that acridine orange can also accumulate in other acidic nonlysosomal compartments such as endocytic vesicles and the trans-Golgi apparatus. Therefore, acridine orange staining should be used with other autophagic markers. Acridine orange labeled cells can be measured by flow cytometry or fluorescence microscopy. The advantage of labeling cells with acridine orange in this assay is not dependent on the availability of specific antibodies or probes. The precaution in using acridine orange is that one should not over-digest the cells with trypsin-ethylenediaminetetraacetic acid (EDTA) as EDTA will change the permeability of the cells and cause the cells to lose acridine orange staining.

9.5.3 *Bovine Serum Albumin Derivatives (DQ-BSAs)*

DQ Green BSA and DQ Red BSA dyes by Molecular Probes are self-quenching derivatives of bovine serum albumin (BSA) that are labeled with BODIPY® dyes, BODIPY FL and BODIPY TR-X. These fluorophores can be used to visualize a vesicular compartment known as amphisome, a combination of autophagic and endocytic pathways [31]. Subsequently, this compartment fuses with a lysosome, in which the trapped materials are degraded by lysosomal enzymes. After proteolytic digestion, DQ Green BSA and DQ Red BSA probes release fragments with excitation and emission maxima of ~505 nm and ~515 nm and ~590 nm and ~620 nm respectively [32]. Thus, these dyes can be used to analyze the convergence between autophagic compartments with a functional lysosome, determination of the intracellular proteolytic activity and the completion of the autophagic pathway in real time.

9.5.4 *Staining with LysoTracker and LysoSensor Probes*

Invitrogen's LysoTracker and LysoSensor probes are weakly basic amine based fluorescent dye; they selectively accumulate in the acidic subcellular compartments with low internal pH (below 5) of the cell by endocytosis. They are mainly used for labeling and tracing acidic organelles in live cells. LysoSensor reagents display a pH-dependent increase in fluorescence intensity upon acidification which is not seen in LysoTracker probes. LysoTracker staining can be used to detect abnormalities in vesicular pH [33] and efficiency of autophagosome/lysosome fusion in live cells [34]. The combination of fluorescently tagged LC3 and Lysotracker staining has been used to obtain insights about the fusion between autophagosomes and acidic endo/lysosomal compartments [35]. LysoSensor probes are mainly used to investigate the acidification of lysosomes and alterations of lysosomal function or trafficking that occur in cells. For example, tumor cells with lower pH [36] in their lysosomes can be compared with one having higher pH [37].

9.6 Autophagy Detection by Electron Microscopy

9.6.1 *Conventional Transmission Electron Microscopy (TEM)*

Analysis of autophagy by conventional transmission electron microscopy (TEM) is considered as a sensitive and reliable semiquantitative method, to show the increase in the number of autophagic vesicles (AV) in a given cell or tissue area. Also, it can be used for both qualitative and quantitative analysis of changes in various autophagic structures. At high magnification (20,000–25,000×) EM can potentially identify and distinguish autophagosomes from autolysosomes [38]. Double-membrane autophagosomes indicate immature AVs and degradative single-membrane autolysosomes are late AVs. The single-membrane autolysosomes mostly contain cytoplasmic material and/or organelles at various stages of degradation. Sometimes secretory vesicles (SV) are confused with AVs, because both morphology and size (500–1 mm) are similar in both. So the very important distinguishing feature that separates AV from SV is that the AV (autophagosomes) should have a clear double-membrane structure separated by an electron-lucent cleft, with encapsulated organelles (mitochondria) and undigested cytoplasmic contents (glycogen granules).

9.6.1.1 Key Steps in TEM Protocol for Cultured Cells

- The ideal number of cells for EM is enough cells to form a pellet in an Eppendorf tube when spun down.
- For tumor and nontumor tissue: a sesame seed size piece of tissue is ideal for fixation. Larger tissues may lead to fixation artifact.
- Fix the cells with a solution containing 3 % glutaraldehyde plus 2 % paraformaldehyde in 0.1 M cacodylate buffer.
- Most electron microscopy core facilities will process samples, embed, cut, and stain grids for EM imaging. Methods detailing this process can be found in [39].
- Examine the images in a transmission electron microscope at an accelerating voltage of 80 kV.

9.6.1.2 Quantification of Autophagic Vesicles in Clinical Trial Specimens

Quantitative EM to measure autophagic vesicles was incorporated into the first five clinical trials involving hydroxychloroquine for cancer patients [40–44]. In these studies peripheral blood mononuclear cells were used as a surrogate for tumor tissue. In one study of temsirolimus and hydroxychloroquine [41] tumor tissue was analyzed for AVs via EM. Successful translation of this assay into the clinic was demonstrated in these clinical trials where, for the first time, a formal pharmacokinetic-pharmacodynamic relationship between HCQ exposure and AV accumulation was made. The following methods were adapted from these papers, and demonstrate the feasibility of using an EM-based assay to obtain useful information even in a multi-institution clinical trial setting.

9.6.1.3 Quantification of AV in PBMC

1. Collect venous blood in cell preparation tubes with a ficoll gradient from patients before treatment and at specific time points on treatment. PBMCs isolated should be separated into 2–4 cell pellets. PBMC pellet one should be immediately fixed with 2 % glutaraldehyde and stored at 4 °C until embedding. Embedding can be performed as described above.
2. Image capture: High-powered micrographs (10,000–12,000×) of 20–25 mononuclear cells from multiple distinct low-powered fields in each sample should be obtained.

3. Scoring of Vesicles: Autophagy vesicles should be scored by two independent experienced investigators who are blinded to treatments and time points. Morphological criteria for AV include (1) circularity, (2) contrast with structures that were white or lighter than the cytoplasm, (3) vesicles with contents, (4) vesicles >200 in size and, (5) vesicles >200 nm interior to the plasma membrane. Vesicular structures with cristae characteristic of mitochondria in cross section should be excluded. The average of two investigators counts along with the standard deviation should be reported for vesicle counts.
4. PBMC pellets 2–4 can then be used for immunoblotting against LC3 as described in Chap. 10.
5. For tumor tissue a similar process can be used. Quantification of a number of AV per cell is much more challenging in tumor tissue if the sample is not well fixed because cell boundaries can be vague.

9.6.1.4 Disadvantage of TEM

1. Identifying and classifying structures need expertise and experience.
2. When quantifying AVs on a per cell basis, the magnification (8000–12,000×) usually precludes determination of whether or not candidate vesicles do in fact have a double membrane. Therefore there is an error rate with every count for labeling structures AV that upon much higher magnification (20,000×) would in fact be reclassified as another subcellular structure.
3. Ex vivo tissue should be fixed immediately and systematically across samples to avoid changes in autophagy that may occur simply due to elapsed time ex vivo.
4. EM pictures should also be taken over different times to ensure detection of autophagosomes. Artifacts may be easily generated during fixation and staining processes. Thus, repeating the processing of samples especially cutting and staining the grids ultimately used for visualization is often needed [45].
5. The cost and labor intensive nature of EM analysis is prohibitive.

9.6.2 Immuno-electron Microscopy (IEM)

The combination of EM and immunogold labeling can facilitate the identification of vesicles such as endosomes and golgi vesicles/tubules that are difficult to distinguish from AV in conventional EM. In IEM, an antibody against precisely defined subcellular proteins can be used to monitor AVs in both basal and stress conditions [46]. Table 9.3 shows a partial list of proteins whose antibodies which have been successfully used for IEM in autophagic research. Using the combination of classical TEM and IEM, different vesicular compartments (double membrane, multivesicular, multilamellar) and subpopulations of autophagic bodies

Table 9.3 Partial list of some key proteins which are commonly targeted for immunogold labeling

Protein	Conditions and interpretation
Beclin-1	• Under basal conditions, beclin-1 immunolabeling can be found as distinct cytoplasmic labeling. Also beclin-1 immunolabeling can be found in rough endoplasmic reticulum (RER) membranes and in the spaces between them. In the mitochondria, gold particles can be seen associated with the outer, as well as the inner, mitochondrial membrane. The cell nucleus will not be labeled. • During stress, immunogold beclin-1 translocalizes to AV and mainly localized to the autophagic bodies membranes. Sometime beclin-1 gold particles can also be found inside the vesicles lumen, because of the sequestering of mitochondria, membrane-like structures, or other degenerated material. • RER cisternae and the nucleus will have almost no gold markers.
Calnexin	• A small group of ER-resident chaperone protein anchored to the ER membrane by a transmembrane domain.
Protein disulfide isomerase (PDI)	• Enzyme of the endoplasmic reticulum.
Cathepsin D	• Strongly decorate lysosomal compartments.

(autophagosomes, autophagolysosomes, multilamellar bodies and dense residual bodies) can be identified by various morphologic and biochemical criteria as described elsewhere [47].

9.7 Monitoring Autophagy by Fluorescence Microscopy

Readers are kindly advised to refer Chap. 10 for details on imaging of LC3-GFP and Tandem RFP-LC3-GFP constructs (tfLC3) by fluorescence microscopy.

9.8 Quantitative Assay for Monitoring Autophagy in Live Cells Using Enzo's Cyto-ID® Autophagy Detection Kit

The Cyto-ID® Autophagy Detection Kit from Enzo Life Sciences can be used to visualize autophagic vacuoles and to monitor the autophagic flux in living cells using fluorescence microscopy and flow cytometry [48]. The probe is a cationic amphiphilic tracer (CAT) dye, selectively and rapidly labels autophagic vacuoles. When the dye enters into autophagy-associated vacuoles [pre-autophagosomes, autophagosomes, and autolysosomes (autophagolysosomes)], they show bright fluorescence, while it stains minimally within lysosomes. The Cyto-ID® dye specifically labels autophagic vacuoles independent of LC3 protein and eliminates the need for transfection. It is excluded from lysosomes as seen with other lysosomotropic dye-based assays such as MDC.

9.9 Immunohistochemical Analysis of Autophagy-Related Proteins

Recently, the role of autophagy in cancer development and progression has been investigated by many researchers using immunohistochemistry. Many antibodies are commercially available and are routinely used for immunohistochemistry against proteins involved in autophagy pathways such as LC3. Our group developed a novel staining method for analysis of LC3B in formalin-fixed, paraffin-embedded (FFPE) tissues, which uses light microscopy and quantitative immunofluorescence [automated quantitative analyses (AQUA)] [49]. AQUA analysis allowed for objective computer-assisted quantification of LC3 staining intensity and puncta. When applied to a tissue microarray of breast cancer and melanoma specimens, a linear correlation was made between LC3 staining intensity and LC3 puncta. Other groups have found that LC3 staining intensity does not correlate with LC3 puncta in other tumor types.

9.9.1 Assessment of LC3 Staining by AQUA

For analysis of LC3B in a multitumor tissue microarray (TMA), rabbit anti-LC3 B (1:5000, overnight at 4 °C) was used and rabbit horseradish peroxidase-conjugated secondary antibody and Cy5 tyramide signal amplification were used. The immunofluorescence intensity of LC3B was averaged for each pixel on the basis of the surrounding 15 pixels (~2 μm^2). Pixels with an LC3B expression level above the local mean were designated as "punctate" and the remaining pixels as "diffuse." Oversaturated pixels were excluded from the analysis. The expression of LC3B in each designation was then calculated as the percentage of pixels assigned to the punctate category. In a given tissue the AQUA program computes fluorescence-conjugated anti-LC3B staining patterns by designating pixels yellow for punctate and blue for diffuse LC3B staining. Other groups also have reported the LC3 punctate staining in FFPE of colorectal tumors, lymph node, and liver metastasis [50]. Also strong LC3 expression was observed in esophageal, gastric, colorectal cancers and correlated with high Ki-67 expression [51]. Taken together, it seems that the quantification of autophagic marker LC3 punctate is correlated with tumor cell proliferation, metastasis, high nuclear grade, and worse patient outcome [49] and the staining method described coupled with the AQUA system could be incorporated into clinical trials of drugs that are known to modulate autophagy. If AQUA is not available, quantification by traditional histological scoring has been successful as well [52].

9.10 Secreted Cytokines as Biomarkers of Autophagy Levels in Melanoma

So far in autophagic research, there are no quantitative preclinical assays that have been developed, which can be easily translated into clinics for testing the efficacy of autophagy modulators. In addition, it is not realistic to use traditional two-dimensional (2D) culture system for developing effective autophagy markers, because it does not accurately recapitulate the tumor microenvironment. In this regard, recently, we developed a three-dimensional (3D) cell culture system and a molecular profiling method to identify and quantitate autophagy-related secretion of proteins [53]. This 3D cell culture system appears to more faithfully reproduce autophagy dynamics found in the tumor microenvironment compared to traditional 2D culture.

9.10.1 Sample Acquisition for Secretome Analysis

Here we summarize the workflow of 3D culture and comparative secretome analysis of melanoma cells (Fig. 9.6). Genetically identical melanoma cell lines, WM793 (a primary melanoma) and 1205Lu (derived from WM793 metastases in vivo),

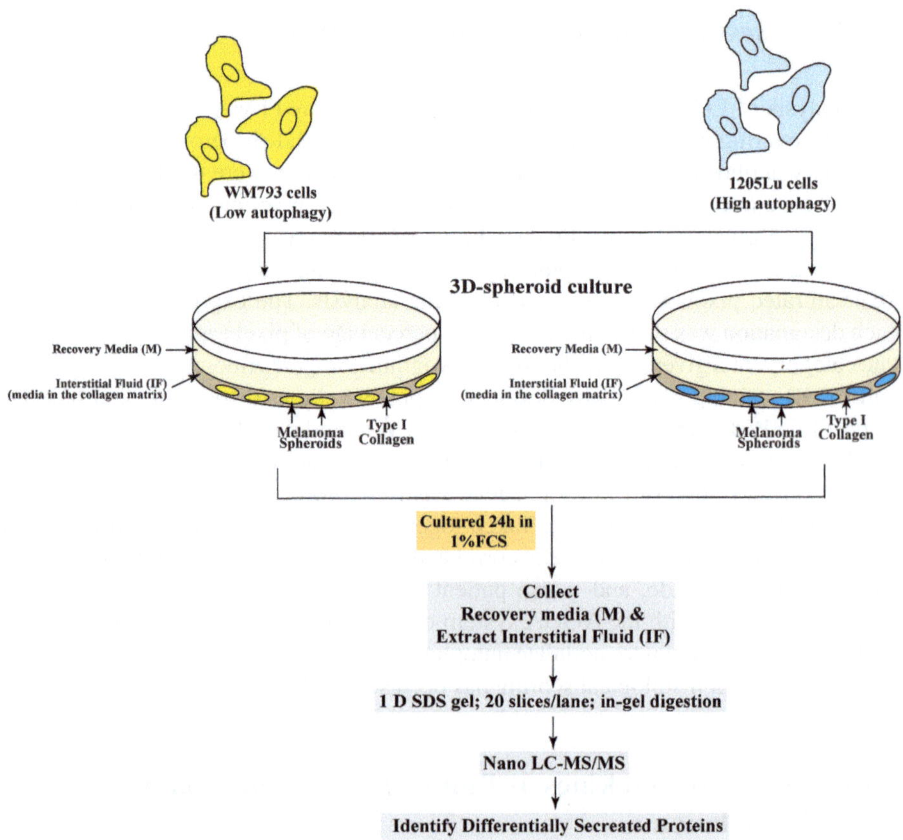

Fig. 9.6 Schematic workflow of 3D cell culture and sample (overlaying media and interstitial fluid) collection for comparative secretome analysis of melanoma cells

were used for the development of this method. Electron micrographs, fluorescent images of melanoma cells expressing tandem fluorescent tagged LC3 (mCherry-eGFP-LC3), and Western blot analysis on WM793 and 1205Lu show that 1205Lu (subclone of WM793) has higher autophagic flux than WM793 [53].

9.10.1.1 Uses of 3D Culture and Comparative Secretome Analysis

- By mass spectrometry (MS) analysis, there are 599 differentially secreted proteins identified across high- and low-autophagy cell lines, 571 were present at similar levels in both cell lines, 26 proteins were elevated in 1205Lu, and 2 proteins were elevated in WM793.
- After MS analysis, the proteins with minimum 6-fold increase in abundance were further characterized by ELISA. The proteins such as IL1B, CXCL8, LIF, FAM3C, and DKK3 were elevated in the media of high-autophagy cell lines.
- Consistent with the cell culture system, using commercially available ELISA kits, the above five candidate biomarkers were found to be significantly elevated in the serum of melanoma patients who had high-autophagy tumors compared to patients who had low-autophagy tumors as measured by EM [53].

This demonstrates that our comparative secretome analysis provides a unique window into how this method can be utilized to identify novel prognostic, predictive, or pharmacodynamic biomarkers of autophagy (Fig. 9.7). Development of such circulating markers of autophagy could enhance laboratory research in autophagy and eventually could aid cancer therapy decisions in melanoma or in any type of cancer. However, it needs to be validated in a larger number of patients and in other cancer types.

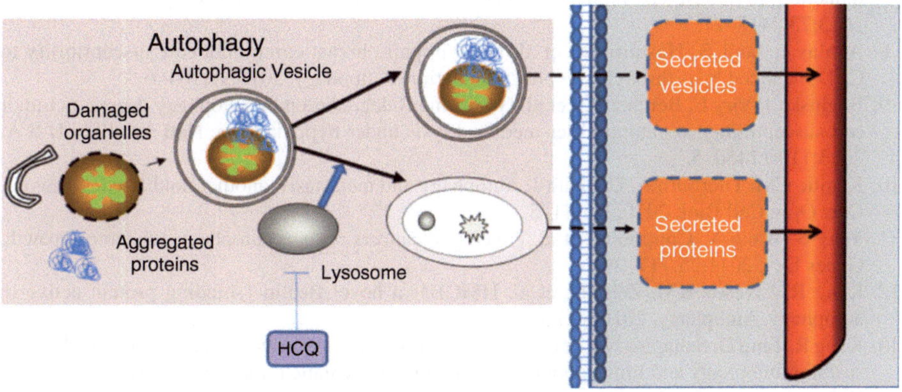

Fig. 9.7 Scheme of autophagic dynamics and the release of autophagy-related secreted proteins and vesicles in the circulation

9.11 Concluding Remarks and Future Perspectives

Due to the intense interest in the role of autophagy in human diseases, numerous methods have been developed in the past decade to monitor autophagy in mammalian cells. Even though we have discussed most of the currently available methods and techniques in autophagy detection, there are new methods being developed constantly. So readers are advised to keep up with these advances and must always consider the variables into account when designing the experiment and data interpretation. In addition, we recommend the use of more than one assay to measure autophagosomes number or to measure autophagic flux, whenever possible. In future, we look forward to the development of more quantitative noninvasive assays to measure autophagy within the tumor microenvironment. For instance with increased knowledge about the autophagic pathway, it may be possible to develop radiological technologies such as positron emission tomography that can detect autophagy for use in clinical medicine.

References

1. Chen Y, Klionsky DJ. The regulation of autophagy—unanswered questions. J Cell Sci. 2011; 124:161–70.
2. Noda NN, Inagaki F. Mechanisms of autophagy. Annu Rev Biophys. 2015;44:101–22.
3. Galluzzi L, Pietrocola F, Bravo-San Pedro JM, et al. Autophagy in malignant transformation and cancer progression. EMBO J. 2015;34:856–80.
4. Chen N, Debnath J. Autophagy and tumorigenesis. FEBS Lett. 2010;584:1427–35.
5. Schoenlein PV, Periyasamy-Thandavan S, Samaddar JS, et al. Autophagy facilitates the progression of ERalpha-positive breast cancer cells to antiestrogen resistance. Autophagy. 2009;5:400–3.
6. Yang ZJ, Chee CE, Huang S, et al. The role of autophagy in cancer: therapeutic implications. Mol Cancer Ther. 2011;10:1533–41.
7. Akalay I, Janji B, Hasmim M, et al. Epithelial-to-mesenchymal transition and autophagy induction in breast carcinoma promote escape from T-cell-mediated lysis. Cancer Res. 2013;73:2418–27.
8. Akalay I, Janji B, Hasmim M, et al. EMT impairs breast carcinoma cell susceptibility to CTL-mediated lysis through autophagy induction. Autophagy. 2013;9:1104–6.
9. Baginska J, Viry E, Berchem G, et al. Granzyme B degradation by autophagy decreases tumor cell susceptibility to natural killer-mediated lysis under hypoxia. Proc Natl Acad Sci U S A. 2013;110:17450–5.
10. Kenific CM, Thorburn A, Debnath J. Autophagy and metastasis: another double-edged sword. Curr Opin Cell Biol. 2010;22:241–5.
11. Yang S, Wang X, Contino G, et al. Pancreatic cancers require autophagy for tumor growth. Genes Dev. 2011;25:717–29.
12. Kang R, Livesey KM, Zeh HJ, et al. HMGB1: a novel Beclin 1-binding protein active in autophagy. Autophagy. 2010;6:1209–11.
13. Kang R, Tang D, Schapiro NE, et al. The receptor for advanced glycation end products (RAGE) sustains autophagy and limits apoptosis, promoting pancreatic tumor cell survival. Cell Death Differ. 2010;17:666–76.
14. Rubinsztein DC, Codogno P, Levine B. Autophagy modulation as a potential therapeutic target for diverse diseases. Nat Rev Drug Discov. 2012;11:709–30.

15. White E, DiPaola RS. The double-edged sword of autophagy modulation in cancer. Clin Cancer Res. 2009;15:5308–16.
16. Rebecca VW, Amaravadi RK. Emerging strategies to effectively target autophagy in cancer. Oncogene. 2015. doi:10.1038/onc.2015.99.
17. Pankiv S, Clausen TH, Lamark T, et al. p62/SQSTM1 binds directly to Atg8/LC3 to facilitate degradation of ubiquitinated protein aggregates by autophagy. J Biol Chem. 2007;282:24131–45.
18. Bjorkoy G, Lamark T, Pankiv S, et al. Monitoring autophagic degradation of p62/SQSTM1. Methods Enzymol. 2009;452:181–97.
19. Laddha SV, Ganesan S, Chan CS, et al. Mutational landscape of the essential autophagy gene BECN1 in human cancers. Mol Cancer Res. 2014;12:485–90.
20. Liu H, He Z, von Rutte T, et al. Down-regulation of autophagy-related protein 5 (ATG5) contributes to the pathogenesis of early-stage cutaneous melanoma. Sci Transl Med. 2013;5:202ra123.
21. Ma XH, Piao S, Wang D, et al. Measurements of tumor cell autophagy predict invasiveness, resistance to chemotherapy, and survival in melanoma. Clin Cancer Res. 2011;17:3478–89.
22. Egan DF, Shackelford DB, Mihaylova MM, et al. Phosphorylation of ULK1 (hATG1) by AMP-activated protein kinase connects energy sensing to mitophagy. Science. 2011;331: 456–61.
23. Tanida I, Minematsu-Ikeguchi N, Ueno T, et al. Lysosomal turnover, but not a cellular level, of endogenous LC3 is a marker for autophagy. Autophagy. 2005;1:84–91.
24. Mizushima N, Yoshimori T. How to interpret LC3 immunoblotting. Autophagy. 2007;3: 542–5.
25. Ni HM, Bockus A, Wozniak AL, et al. Dissecting the dynamic turnover of GFP-LC3 in the autolysosome. Autophagy. 2011;7:188–204.
26. Biederbick A, Kern HF, Elsasser HP. Monodansylcadaverine (MDC) is a specific in vivo marker for autophagic vacuoles. Eur J Cell Biol. 1995;66:3–14.
27. Iwai-Kanai E, Yuan H, Huang C, et al. A method to measure cardiac autophagic flux in vivo. Autophagy. 2008;4:322–9.
28. Munafo DB, Colombo MI. A novel assay to study autophagy: regulation of autophagosome vacuole size by amino acid deprivation. J Cell Sci. 2001;114:3619–29.
29. Pacheco CD, Kunkel R, Lieberman AP. Autophagy in Niemann-Pick C disease is dependent upon Beclin-1 and responsive to lipid trafficking defects. Hum Mol Genet. 2007;16:1495–503.
30. Han J, Burgess K. Fluorescent indicators for intracellular pH. Chem Rev. 2010;110:2709–28.
31. Klionsky DJ, Abdalla FC, Abeliovich H, et al. Guidelines for the use and interpretation of assays for monitoring autophagy. Autophagy. 2012;8:445–544.
32. Voss Jr EW, Workman CJ, Mummert ME. Detection of protease activity using a fluorescence-enhancement globular substrate. Biotechniques. 1996;20:286–91.
33. Eskelinen EL, Schmidt CK, Neu S, et al. Disturbed cholesterol traffic but normal proteolytic function in LAMP-1/LAMP-2 double-deficient fibroblasts. Mol Biol Cell. 2004;15:3132–45.
34. Gonzalez-Polo RA, Boya P, Pauleau AL, et al. The apoptosis/autophagy paradox: autophagic vacuolization before apoptotic death. J Cell Sci. 2005;118:3091–102.
35. Pierzynska-Mach A, Janowski PA, Dobrucki JW. Evaluation of acridine orange, LysoTracker Red, and quinacrine as fluorescent probes for long-term tracking of acidic vesicles. Cytometry A. 2014;85:729–37.
36. Chauhan SS, Liang XJ, Su AW, et al. Reduced endocytosis and altered lysosome function in cisplatin-resistant cell lines. Br J Cancer. 2003;88:1327–34.
37. Jiang LW, Maher VM, McCormick JJ, et al. Alkalinization of the lysosomes is correlated with ras transformation of murine and human fibroblasts. J Biol Chem. 1990;265:4775–7.
38. Eskelinen EL, Reggiori F, Baba M, et al. Seeing is believing: the impact of electron microscopy on autophagy research. Autophagy. 2011;7:935–56.
39. Yla-Anttila P, Vihinen H, Jokitalo E, et al. Monitoring autophagy by electron microscopy in Mammalian cells. Methods Enzymol. 2009;452:143–64.

40. Mahalingam D, Mita M, Sarantopoulos J, et al. Combined autophagy and HDAC inhibition: a phase I safety, tolerability, pharmacokinetic, and pharmacodynamic analysis of hydroxychloroquine in combination with the HDAC inhibitor vorinostat in patients with advanced solid tumors. Autophagy. 2014;10:1403–14.
41. Rangwala R, Chang YC, Hu J, et al. Combined MTOR and autophagy inhibition: phase I trial of hydroxychloroquine and temsirolimus in patients with advanced solid tumors and melanoma. Autophagy. 2014;10:1391–402.
42. Rangwala R, Leone R, Chang YC, et al. Phase I trial of hydroxychloroquine with dose-intense temozolomide in patients with advanced solid tumors and melanoma. Autophagy. 2014;10:1369–79.
43. Rosenfeld MR, Ye X, Supko JG, et al. A phase I/II trial of hydroxychloroquine in conjunction with radiation therapy and concurrent and adjuvant temozolomide in patients with newly diagnosed glioblastoma multiforme. Autophagy. 2014;10:1359–68.
44. Vogl DT, Stadtmauer EA, Tan KS, et al. Combined autophagy and proteasome inhibition: a phase 1 trial of hydroxychloroquine and bortezomib in patients with relapsed/refractory myeloma. Autophagy. 2014;10:1380–90.
45. Eskelinen EL. To be or not to be? Examples of incorrect identification of autophagic compartments in conventional transmission electron microscopy of mammalian cells. Autophagy. 2008;4:257–60.
46. Dunn Jr WA. Studies on the mechanisms of autophagy: maturation of the autophagic vacuole. J Cell Biol. 1990;110:1935–45.
47. Dunn Jr WA. Studies on the mechanisms of autophagy: formation of the autophagic vacuole. J Cell Biol. 1990;110:1923–33.
48. Chan LL, Shen D, Wilkinson AR, et al. A novel image-based cytometry method for autophagy detection in living cells. Autophagy. 2012;8:1371–82.
49. Lazova R, Camp RL, Klump V, et al. Punctate LC3B expression is a common feature of solid tumors and associated with proliferation, metastasis, and poor outcome. Clin Cancer Res. 2012;18:370–9.
50. Sato K, Tsuchihara K, Fujii S, et al. Autophagy is activated in colorectal cancer cells and contributes to the tolerance to nutrient deprivation. Cancer Res. 2007;67:9677–84.
51. Yoshioka A, Miyata H, Doki Y, et al. LC3, an autophagosome marker, is highly expressed in gastrointestinal cancers. Int J Oncol. 2008;33:461–8.
52. Ma XH, Piao SF, Dey S, et al. Targeting ER stress-induced autophagy overcomes BRAF inhibitor resistance in melanoma. J Clin Invest. 2014;124:1406–17.
53. Kraya AA, Piao S, Xu X, et al. Identification of secreted proteins that reflect autophagy dynamics within tumor cells. Autophagy. 2015;11:60–74.

Chapter 10
Methods: Using Three-Dimensional Culture (Spheroids) as an In Vitro Model of Tumour Hypoxia

Russell Leek, David Robert Grimes, Adrian L. Harris, and Alan McIntyre

Abstract Regions of hypoxia in tumours can be modelled in vitro in 2D cell cultures with a hypoxic chamber or incubator in which oxygen levels can be regulated. Although this system is useful in many respects, it disregards the additional physiological gradients of the hypoxic microenvironment, which result in reduced nutrients and more acidic pH. Another approach to hypoxia modelling is to use three-dimensional spheroid cultures. In spheroids, the physiological gradients of the hypoxic tumour microenvironment can be inexpensively modelled and explored. In addition, spheroids offer the advantage of more representative modelling of tumour therapy responses compared with 2D culture. Here, we review the use of spheroids in hypoxia tumour biology research and highlight the different methodologies for spheroid formation and how to obtain uniformity. We explore the challenge of spheroid analyses and how to determine the effect on the hypoxic versus normoxic components of spheroids. We discuss the use of high-throughput analyses in hypoxia

*These authors contributed equally.

R. Leek
Nuffield Division of Clinical Laboratory Sciences, Department of Oncology, University of Oxford, Oxford OX3 9DU, UK
e-mail: Russell.leek@oncology.ox.ac.uk

D.R. Grimes
Gray Laboratory, Cancer Research UK/MRC Oxford Institute for Radiation Oncology, University of Oxford,
Old Road Campus Research Building, off Roosevelt Drive, Oxford OX3 7DQ, UK
e-mail: davidrobert.grimes@oncology.ox.ac.uk

A.L. Harris
Department of Oncology, Weatherall Institute of Molecular Medicine, University of Oxford, Oxford OX3 9DS, UK
e-mail: aharris.lab@imm.ox.ac.uk

A. McIntyre (✉)
Cancer Biology, Division of Cancer and Stem Cells, University of Nottingham, QMC, D Floor, West Block, W/D/1374, Nottingham NG7 2UH, UK
e-mail: alan.mcintyre@nottingham.ac.uk

C. Koumenis et al. (eds.), *Tumor Microenvironment*, Advances in Experimental Medicine and Biology 899, DOI 10.1007/978-3-319-26666-4_10

screening of spheroids. Furthermore, we examine the use of mathematical modelling of spheroids to understand more fully the hypoxic tumour microenvironment.

Keywords Spheroids, 3D culture • Hypoxia • Carbonic anhydrase IX • pH

10.1 Introduction

Hypoxia is a state of low oxygen below pO_2 7 mmHg. Normal tissues have an oxygen level of pO_2 9 mmHg–pO_2 100 mmHg (1.2–13 % O_2) [1]. Hypoxia is an environmental stress induced in many pathological settings including wound healing, inflammation, ischemia and cancer [2]. Hypoxic regions of tumours are caused by high metabolic and proliferative rates and poor tumour vascularisation [3]. Hypoxia is a major physiological difference between normal and tumour tissues [4], associated with worse patient survival and chemotherapy [5] and radiotherapy resistance [6]. Hypoxia stabilises the transcription factors, hypoxia inducible factors, HIF1α and HIF2α, which dramatically change the hypoxic cell transcriptome as a key response to the hypoxic insult [2]. This triggers more aggressive tumour growth, survival, invasion and metastasis and increases the stem cell component of tumours through HIF1α and HIF2α regulated genes [7]. Because of the impact of hypoxia on tumour biology and therapy resistance it is a key area of research for improving anti-cancer therapy, and, it is crucial therefore to be able to model the hypoxic microenvironment effectively in vitro.

To examine the effect of reduced oxygen levels on cancer cells, the simplest model is to use a cell culture chamber with controllable oxygen levels to reduce oxygen levels to usually between 1 and 0.1 % O_2 (pO_2 7 mmHg and below). These are useful for examining effects of reduced oxygen levels on 2D cells with a range of outputs (gene and protein expression, growth and survival, etc.). However, conditions of low oxygen are associated with a variety of other physiological gradients in tumours including a reduction in the availability of nutrients and build up of lactate and acidic pH, which also impact upon tumour cell physiology [8].

Spheroids naturally produce gradients of oxygen concentration. Spheroid cultures are of intermediate complexity containing many elements found in tumours including regions of chronic hypoxia, extra-cellular matrix, cell–cell and cell–extra-cellular matrix interactions, metabolite/catabolite gradients, necrosis and pH gradients [8]. Furthermore the reduction in proliferation in hypoxic regions of tumours is modelled in spheroids [8, 9]. Reduced drug penetration has been identified in spheroids, which in combination with other modelled factors gives spheroids an in vivo like resistance to chemotherapy and radiotherapy [8, 10]. Utilising spheroids as an in vitro model of three-dimensional tumours for investigations of hypoxia has been key in our understanding of many aspects of tumour physiology and the impact or lack thereof of therapeutic drugs on this environment. Furthermore spheroids have facilitated in vitro selection of drugs before progression to more expensive in vivo preclinical modelling [8]. Conversely spheroids do not contain all aspects of the tumour microenvironment, they are avascular and monoculture spheroids lack the other normal cell infiltrate found in tumours. Many examples of co-culture spheroid modelling have been developed and have contributed to our understanding of cell–cell interactions and the impact of these on therapy and patient response [11–13]. It is important to differentiate between spheroids and cell aggregates, which are loosely packed cell cultures and lack the gradients found in spheroids. In spheroids, as in tissues, HIF1α is stabilised roughly 80 μm from the periphery (or functional blood vessel) [10] and thus spheroids with a diameter of greater than 160 μm in diameter should start to develop hypoxic cores, which as they grow larger to between 400 and 500 μm will become necrotic. However, the pattern of these features in spheroids is cell line specific and needs to be validated in the model of use.

With regards gene expression profiling 2D hypoxic culture can enable effective analysis of hypoxia on global expression patterns although evidence is emerging that additional factors found in the hypoxic microenvironment such as acidosis significantly attenuate some hypoxic gene induction [14]. Nutrient and pH gradients likely also impact hypoxic tumour metabolism. This is increasingly important as hypoxia motivated metabolic investigations utilising 2D cultured cells overlook shifts in proliferative rates and increasing concentrations of catabolites, for example lactate, which accumulate in the hypoxic region of spheroids and tumours [8, 15]. The physiological gradients, interactions between normoxic and hypoxic fractions and the impact of these fractions upon test situations can be difficult to interpret and the complexity of the model can require more analysis than just simple growth studies. Further detailed analysis can include examination of fixed embedded and sectioned or frozen material by immunohistochemistry, which enables regional variations of phenotypes such as apoptosis to be identified.

There are a number of different approaches to 3D cell culture. The main discussion in this chapter will be surrounding the use of spheroids. Other types of three-dimensional cultures include mammospheres [16], and organoids [17]; however, their lack of uniformity and often oxygen gradients preclude their use for many hypoxia related investigations. Here, we review the methodology of spheroid formation and discuss the range of spheroid analyses, which are critical for determining the effects of test compounds or gene knockdowns on spheroids and essentially the hypoxic cells within these. We evaluate the position of spheroids in hypoxia biology discovery screens, before examining the use of mathematical modelling of spheroids as a tool to investigate and understand the impact of oxygen gradients on tumour growth.

10.2 Spheroid Formation

It is possible to prepare multi-cell tumour spheroids in a number of ways depending on whether the aim is to produce large numbers of spheroids or to produce spheroids of a consistent size. To produce large numbers of spheroids, it is usual to use a

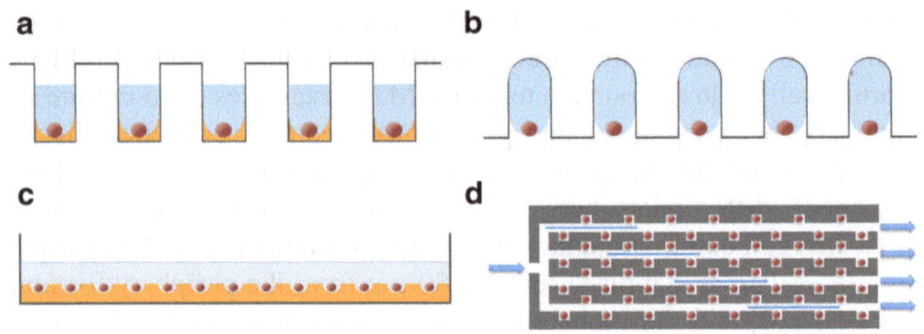

Fig. 10.1 Spheroid formation methods. Spheroids—*red*, agarose—*yellow*, culture medium—*blue*. (**a**) Multi-well spheroid culture. Cross section of a flat-bottomed multi-well plate. Individual spheroids are growing at the base of each well on a non-adherent agarose surface. Spheroids are covered with culture medium. (**b**) Hanging drop culture. Cross section of a round-bottomed inverted multi-well plate. Individual spheroids are suspended at the meniscus of each hanging drop of culture medium. (**c**) Microwell array. Spheroids grow in micrometre scale pits in an agarose surface with liquid overlay. (**d**) Micro-fluidic spheroid array, with continuous flow of culture medium. This figure was adapted with permission from Fennema et al. 2013 [19]

spinner flask system. To produce spheroids of a uniform size and shape, it is preferable to grow them individually either in a multi-well plate with a single spheroid in each well, or alternatively to grow the spheroid in a hanging drop or hanging drop array, spheroid array or, more recently, by using micro-fluidic techniques and nano-imprinted culture plates (NCP) (Fig. 10.1).

10.2.1 Individual Spheroids Grown in a Multi-well Plate

Initially the cell line being used to create spheroids is cultured normally in its usual growth medium in a 2D monolayer. The cells are harvested during their exponential growth phase in the appropriate way either by trypsinisation or cell scraping with disaggregation. The cells are counted with a haemocytometer and diluted appropriately in growth medium. The number of cells that are used to seed an individual well varies greatly, dependent upon the cell line being used in the experiment, but is usually between 1000 and 40,000 cells per well. Some optimisation of cell number per well is usually required before full-scale production of spheroids can be established. 96-Well tissue culture plates are usually used to grow individual spheroids and they can either be polyhema coated (50 μl 0.5 % polyhema in 95 % ethanol air-dried for 3 days at 37 °C for 3 days prior to use) [18] or ultra low-attachment round bottom plates or standard flat bottom plates with a non-adherent agarose gel layer. The advantage of using multi-well plate methods to grow spheroids is that the spheroids produced are of a consistent size and shape; also the spheroids can be grown over several weeks [19].

10.2.2 Initiating Spheroids Rapidly Using Ultra-Low-Attachment 96-Well Plates

This is a rapid method of initiating spheroids and is dependent upon using a high number of cells to seed each well (2000–40,000 cells per well). Sometimes it is necessary to add Matrigel to the initial cell mixture to aid in the aggregation process. Whether Matrigel is used or not is dependent on the cell line. When it is used, it is normally added to the culture medium at a dilution of 25–50 µl per ml of medium. However, this dilution may vary and should be optimised.

To initiate the spheroids, 200 µl of the growth medium (with or without Matrigel) and cell mix are added to each well. The cell mix is usually kept on ice before individual wells are seeded while the 96-well plate is on ice. The plate is then centrifuged at 1000 × *g* for 10 min at 4 °C. Cells initially form an aggregate at the base of each well of the plate and then establish their spheroid morphology after 24–48 h in culture [18].

10.2.3 Initiating Spheroids in Agar Coated 96-Well Plates

Using this method of spheroid culture requires preparation of agarose coated 96-well tissue culture plates. The agarose forms a hemi-spherical meniscus that prevents the spheroid from adhering to the well to produce a well-formed spherical structure. This method uses fewer cells than the rapid method above and allows the spheroid to grow naturally as the cells multiply, mirroring more accurately, the process of three-dimensional cell growth found in tumours in vivo [20]. To prepare the 96-well plates, a 1.5 % agarose solution in appropriate growth medium without FCS or glutamine is prepared. The powdered agarose is dissolved in the medium using a small beaker in a larger beaker filled with water on the verge of boiling. The solution is stirred while dissolving using a heated magnetic stirrer. Once dissolved, the agarose should be left in just boiling water for an additional 20 min to ensure the solution is sterile. The solution is then rapidly pipetted in 100 µl aliquots into the wells of the plate under sterile conditions and allowed to cool. Once cooled, the plates can be used immediately or stored in their original packaging at 4 °C for a few weeks. If refrigerated, the plates should be allowed to warm to room temperature before use.

To initiate spheroids, cells are harvested from monolayer culture and counted. Cells are seeded at a concentration of 2000 cells per well in their normal growth medium, although this number will vary depending on the cell line used. Once the spheroid culture has been initiated, the plate should be incubated at 37 °C and left undisturbed for 48 h as movement will disrupt the formation of the newly forming spheroids.

10.2.4 Feeding Spheroids

Spheroids that are grown in 96-well plates need to have their medium replaced every 1–3 days, a process referred to as feeding. To achieve this, 100–180 μl has to be aspirated from each well without disturbing the spheroid. The volume is then replaced with 100–180 μl of fresh medium using a multi-channel pipette.

10.2.5 Spinner Flask Culture

Culturing spheroids in spinner flasks is one of the original methods for growing spheroids and is useful when large numbers of spheroids are required [21]. With this technique cells are either inoculated directly into the spinner flasks, or are grown on non-adherent petri dishes first to make pre-formed aggregates that are then added to the spinner flask. Like the multi-well plate methods above, the cell line is first grown as a 2D monolayer culture and harvested by trypsinisation when the cells are in the exponential growth phase. If the cells are being pre-aggregated before being put into the spinner flasks they are counted and diluted in growth medium to a concentration of around 1,000,000 cells in 15 ml/100 mm in a non-adherent petri dish (this may vary). Aggregates are allowed to form in the non-adherent petri dishes for 3–4 days and then transferred to a 1 l spinner flask in 100 ml of the same growth medium (this step can be skipped if the spheroids are seeded directly into the flask). The spinner flask is usually run between 50 and 100 rpm in a 37 °C incubator and around 60 % of the medium should be replaced approximately every 24 h. The number of spheroids per flask should be reduced gradually with increasing spheroid size to maintain a relatively constant cell count of $\leq 2 \times 10^5$ cells/ml medium in the spinner flask. Spheroids in spinner culture can vary in size, a representative sample should be analysed for size as discussed in Sect. 10.4.1.

10.2.6 Hanging Drop Culture

For the hanging drop method [22, 23], predetermined concentrations of cell suspensions are suspended from the lids of culture dishes coated with poly-dimethylsiloxane. The easiest way to achieve this is to dispense 20–50 μl of cell suspension (usually 500–2000 cells per 100 μl growth medium) into each well of a 48- or 60-well tissue culture plate. The plate is quickly inverted and the hanging drops are formed by surface tension of the fluid and the hydrophobic nature of the plastic substrate of the culture plate. The inverted plates are then placed inside large tissue culture dishes which are either partially filled with sterile water or have smaller dishes of water in them, which prevents the hanging drops from drying out. The plates are then incubated as normal in a humidified 37 °C incubator. The cells gather at the liquid-air interface of the drop, where they aggregate and eventually form up into a spheroid after a few days. Spheroids initiated this way cannot be effectively fed with new medium and so the technique can only be run for a few days. However, this technique is considered to be suitable for initiating spheroids that are subsequently to be transferred to non-adherent multi-wall plates (described above) or producing spheroids that are destined to go into other 3D model systems such as implantation in 3D collagen gels or in vivo. More recently the hanging drop method has been further refined by the introduction of 384-well hanging drop array plates that are now commercially available [24].

10.2.7 Microwell Arrays

The concept of microwell arrays is similar to the method of growing individual spheroids in agarose coated multi-wall plates and is particular useful for producing large numbers of small but uniformly sized spheroids [25]. The difference between this method and the traditional multi-well system is that there are a much larger number of wells, in the micrometre scale, cast into an agarose gel or polyacrylamide hydrogel slab [26]. The cast is made using a wax, elastomer or poly-dimethylsiloxane (PDMS) micro-mould. The moulds can be created from 3D printed formers, but are also available commercially. Using this method it is possible to produce microwell arrays consisting of 900 wells of 500 μm diameter. The cast arrays are trimmed to fit into the wells of six-well culture plates and exposed to UV sterilisation.

To initiate the spheroids, the cell suspension in growth medium is added to the culture plate and the plate is shaken at 50 × *g* for 24 h in a tissue culture incubator at 37 °C allowing the cells to settle and begin aggregating in the microwells. The type of medium and cell concentration varies depending on cell type but is usually of the order of magnitude of 2000 cells per ml of medium. The culture medium should be replaced initially after 3–4 h and then every 24 h for the remainder of the experiment.

To harvest the spheroids, the array is detached from the tissue culture plate and soaked in phosphate buffered saline (various methods include having the PBS on ice, at room temperature or even at 37 °C). The array is gently shaken with a forceps to detach the spheroids and the solution is transferred to a conical bottomed tube to allow the spheroids to settle. They can then be processed as described above. Due to the small size of the spheroids required for the densities of these production techniques, it is unlikely that spheroids produced in this way will grow large enough to develop hypoxic cores. These smaller spheroids could be placed in hypoxic chambers; however, the model looses the elegance of the combined additional gradients in larger spheroids.

10.2.8 The Future of Spheroid Culture: Micro-fluidic Self-Assembly and NCP

Micro-fluidic self-assembly systems for spheroid production are still relatively new and technologically complex [27]. They depend on the ability to fabricate quite sophisticated micro-fluidic devices that incorporate micro-channels and wells that can be continuously streamed with new medium and treatments making them extremely useful for high-throughput screening of new drugs. The currents within the micro-fluidic environments trap the cells in channels, or specially designed wells, where they can spontaneously aggregate to form spheroids in great numbers. As they grow, the spheroids can be exposed to drugs and other changes in their environment, which are thought to closely mimic conditions found in in vivo cellular microenvironments [28]. Exciting possibilities also exist for incorporating such systems onto chips in the near future [29], enabling continuous monitoring of the spheroids as they grow and their real-time responses to changes in experimental conditions.

NCP are similar to the traditional 96-well plate method described above [30]. The key difference here is that the base of each well is imprinted with a nano-scale 3D grid. The grid is imprinted onto a transparent synthetic resin surface in either a square or honeycomb pattern. The result is a surface, which is neither adherent nor non-adherent, instead it is described as low binding. The surface allows cells to migrate and establish cell-to-cell interactions and consequently form into uniform spheroids that are lightly anchored to the surface. This is thought to increase cell viability by reducing cell-death induced when cells are separated from a substrate such as extra-cellular matrix. NCP have been used in high-throughput drug screening and are now commercially available [31].

10.3 Spheroid Co-cultures

As well as growing spheroids composed of a single cell line, several methods for growing spheroids as co-cultures of at least two cell lines have also been developed. Such spheroid co-cultures can be used to partially mimic in vitro the complex cellular heterogeneity found in tumours in vivo and are particularly useful for examining how tumour cells interact with the surrounding non-neoplastic cell population. There are basically four methods for co-culturing spheroids that are outlined below; the mixed mosaic spheroid, spheroid in cell suspension, spheroid on monolayer and confrontation culture methods. These methods are performed using multi-well plates, but some are amenable to the hanging drop or spinner flask methods.

10.3.1 Mixed Mosaic Spheroid Culture

Mixed mosaic (or hybrid) spheroids can be grown on multi-well plates, spinner flasks and bioreactors or in hanging drop culture. They are particularly useful for mixing different populations of tumour cell lines for studying drug resistance or therapy response [32] and for mixing tumour and fibroblast cell populations to examine tumour–stromal cell interactions [33]. Mostly two cell lines are used but it is possible to use more, although this increases the complexity of the culture technique. Two cell suspensions are mixed and used to seed spheroids in the usual way (Fig. 10.2a). The proportion of the two cell populations ideally would be equal, but due to differences in cell growth rates, intercellular adhesion, migration and survival between different cell types, the exact proportions must be optimised for the particular cell combinations. Depending on the cell lines used the spheroid will either differentiate into a mosaic of mixed cells, or alternatively may form a hybrid spheroid with incomplete mixing of the cell types.

10.3.2 Spheroids in Cell Suspension

With this method, single cell type spheroids are initiated as normal and after a period of maturation a cell suspension of the second cell type are added to the medium (Fig. 10.2b). Again, the maturation stage of the spheroid and the concentration of the cell suspension should be optimised around the particular cell lines and the experimental parameters. This technique is particularly suited to modelling the process of infiltration of stromal cells into tumour tissue and has been used to examine the infiltration of immune cells [34, 35] such as monocytes, macrophages, T-lymphocytes and natural killer cells. The technique can also be used to co-culture tumour spheroids with endothelial cells in suspension [36].

10.3.3 Spheroid on Monolayer

In this method, a normally prepared spheroid is transferred onto the surface of a monolayer culture (Fig. 10.2c). This approach has been used for looking at solid tumour–fibroblast interactions [37] and tumour vascular interactions [38] with tumour spheroids being placed on fibroblast or endothelial cell monolayers.

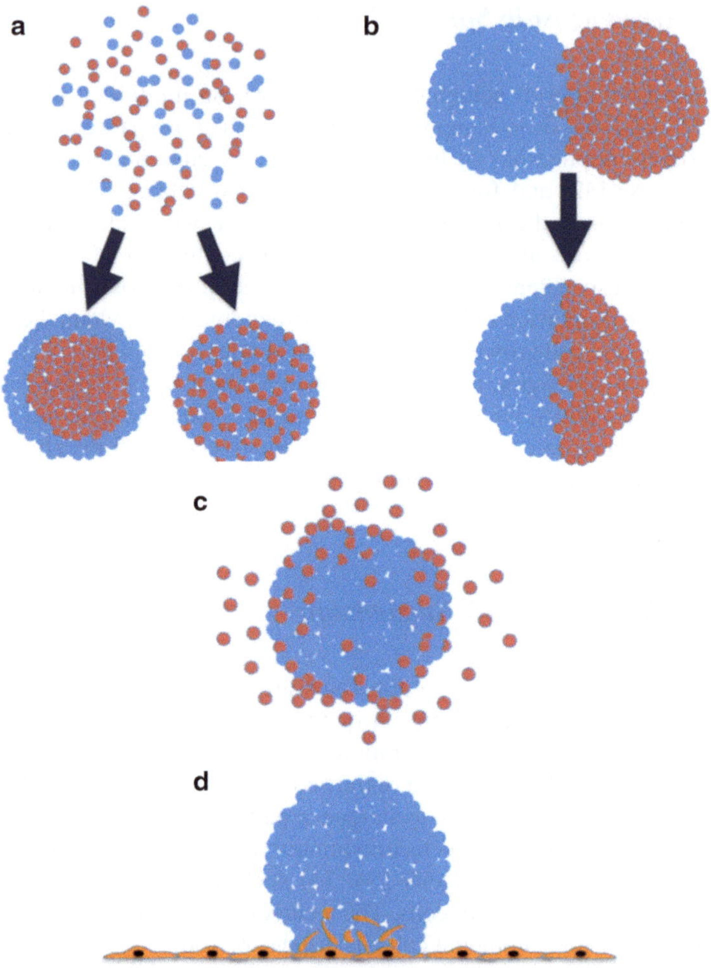

Fig. 10.2 Spheroid co-culture methods. (**a**) Mixed mosaic/hybrid spheroids. Cells coalesce and start to divide as mixed spheroid that either forms an admixed structure (*right*) or layered structure (*left*). (**b**) Confrontation culture. Fully formed spheroids merge to form one spheroid. (**c**) Spheroid in cell suspension. Cells in suspension migrate into fully formed spheroid. (**d**) Spheroid on monolayer. Monolayer and spheroid cells merge

10.3.4 Confrontation Culture

This technique involves culturing two formed spheroids together in a single non-adherent well. This method has been primarily used to examine the interactions between fibroblasts and tumour cell spheroids [39]. Fibroblasts are known to secrete growth factors that modulate the behaviour of tumour cells and this is an appropriate model to examine these interactions, in vitro. It also allows investigation of the migration and invasion of neoplastic cells into normal stroma.

10.4 Spheroid Analyses

10.4.1 Spheroid Growth Analysis

An important aspect of spheroid analysis is the ability to measure spheroid growth. This requires the repeated analysis of spheroid size over a time course. Phase contrast images of spheroids can be taken with camera mounted inverted microscopes. In situations of increased scale an automated imaging system can be used. However, care should be taken that the image is in focus so as to give a clear representation of the spheroid size. Images should be taken every 1–3 days depending upon spheroid growth kinetics. The number of images required will depend upon the uniformity of the spheroids. However, even in examples of high uniformity it is good practice for a minimum of six spheroid images to be analysed per condition. Once the representative spheroid images are taken, the downstream analysis will depend on which metric of size the researcher would wish to use for example, area, diameter or spheroid volume. A relatively automated method of analysing spheroids can be achieved in the ImageJ open source software (http://imagej.nih.gov/ij/) [9].

Spheroid images should be changed to 8-bit to enable thresholding (Image>Type>8-bit). Images should then be thresholded to enable image segmentation. This produces a binary image with the spheroid in black and the rest of the image in white (Image>Adjust>Threshold). The threshold level should be adjusted so that the area of the spheroid is highlighted but other areas on the image are not. The area of the spheroid can then be measured (Analyse>Measure). This analysis will give the area of the spheroid in pixels. Calibration of these analyses can be achieved by taking a picture of calibration slide or a haemocytometer and utilising the software to calculate the number of pixels in the area of one of the four corner squares, equal to 1 mm^2. By dividing spheroid area results by the number of pixels in 1 mm^2 the data is transformed to mm^2. From this the spheroid radius can be calculated ($r=\sqrt{(A/\pi)}$). From which the diameter ($d=2r$) and volume can be calculated ($v=(4/3)\pi\ r^3$). This enables spheroid growth rate in test versus control spheroids, which can be calculated by linear regression of log-transformed data [9]. A macro can be used to batch analyse spheroid images as below. Care should be taken that the threshold (user defined threshold, UDT) is set for each batch of spheroids and that the threshold requirements do not vary between spheroids. Similarly the minimum size (user defined minimum size, UDMS) of spheroids should be determined to prevent analysis of background imperfections. If the batch function is used, an output file is produced containing the outlines of the thresholded area. In the case of batch analysis, it is good practice for the outlines of the thresholded areas to be checked against the spheroid pictures to ensure accurate analysis.

An ImageJ macro for batch analysis of phase contrast spheroid images. (Process>Batch>Macro, with user defined input and output folders).

```
setAutoThreshold("Default");
//run("Threshold...");
setThreshold(0, UDT);
```

```
setOption("BlackBackground", false);
run("Convert to Mask");
run("Analyze Particles...", "size=UDMS-Infinity show=Outlines display summarize");
```

A more complex version of this for images with poor spheroid contrast has been published elsewhere [40].

10.4.2 Cell Viability

Representative spheroids can be analysed during a time course and/or at the assay end point by cell viability or cell counting. For cell counting, spheroids can be disaggregated by trypsin and the viable cells counted using an automated cell counter or haemocytometer. In addition, once dissociated, cells from within spheroids can be analysed by flow cytometry. Dual staining with a hypoxia marker such as CA9 (which has a half life of 38 h) [41] can be utilised to determine the investigated effect on the hypoxic versus normoxic fraction of cells from within the spheroid by flow cytometry.

Cell viability of intact spheroids can be an efficient method of analysis of a large number of conditions and can be analysed by a number of assays including Resazurin assay [40] MTT assay [42] and acid phosphatase assay [40, 43]. Resazurin reduction assay, acid phosphatase assay and cell counts can be carried out on the same spheroids sequentially as described in [40]. Similar assays have also been performed including the cell titre glo assay to measure ATP levels [31].

LDH isoenzyme release [44] can be analysed as a marker of cell damage. However, previous comparison has found that the MTT assay is a clearer determiner of effect on cell viability due to the high background of LDH isoenzyme release in spheroid culture [44]. For these assays, it is best practice to perform standard curve assays with known cell numbers to calculate the number of cells from the assays based on absorbance and determine the linear range of the assay for the cell lines tested.

10.4.3 Resazurin Assay

Resazurin (7-hydroxy-3*H*-phenoxazin-3-one 10-oxide) is a blue dye reduced in the mitochondria by NADPH or NADH to form the red fluorescent, pink coloured resorufin. To perform the resazurin assay on live undissociated spheroids, 60 μM resazurin is freshly prepared in appropriate culture medium. 150 μl/200 μl of spheroid medium is removed and replaced with 150 μl of resazurin solution. Spheroids are incubated for 4 h in a tissue culture incubator at 37 °C and 5 % CO_2. Spheroids are analysed utilising a fluorescent plate reader, excitation 405 nm emission 630 nm [40]. Comparison between the resazurin assay and cell counts, identified a significant correlation between the data sets for spheroids across a wide size range (up to 100,000 cell per spheroid)[40].

10.4.4 MTT Assay

The MTT assay quantifies cell viability by assaying NAD(P)H-dependent oxidoreductase enzyme activity in viable cells which reduce the soluble 3-(4,5-dimethylthi azol-2-yl)-2,3-diphenyltetrazolium bromide to formazan which is insoluble and has an absorption of between 500 and 600 nm, and is purple [45]. To perform the assay, medium is removed and spheroids washed with PBS. Cells are incubated with MTT in PBS at final a concentration of 1 mg/ml for 3–4 h. The contents of each well are removed and placed in 96-well flat bottom plates and centrifuged for 5 min at $1000 \times g$. Medium is removed and plates dried by blotting with paper towels. The produced aqueous insoluble Formazan is dissolved in 100 μl of DMSO and absorbance measured at 570–590 nm utilising an appropriate plate reader [44, 46].

10.4.5 Acid Phosphatase Assay

The acid phosphatase assay is based on quantification of cytosolic acid phosphatase activity. Viable cells are lysed and intracellular acid phosphatases hydrolyse-nitrophenyl phosphate to *p*-nitrophenol. *p*-Nitrophenol can be quantified at 405 nm [47]. To perform the assay, medium is removed from the spheroids and spheroids are washed carefully once with PBS. PBS is removed and replaced with a final volume of 200 μl of the acid phosphatase assay buffer (0.1 M sodium acetate, 0.1 % (v/v) Triton-X-100 and PBS in 3:2.5 ratio supplemented with 2 mg/l of *p*-nitrophenyl phosphate) and incubated at 37 °C for 90 min. After incubation 10 μl of 1 N NaOH is added to each well. Absorbance is immediately measured at 405 nm [47, 48].

10.4.6 LDH Isoenzyme Release

Cytotoxicity can be measured by analysing lactate dehydrogenase isoenzyme release from unviable cells [44]. This assay can be performed utilising the CytoTox 96® Non-Radioactive cytotoxicity assay kit (Promega, USA) according to the manufacturer's instructions. This assay is performed to enable the percentage of LDH release to be calculated based on the maximum amount that could be released from the cells in the assay. This is an important consideration as it controls for any differences in spheroid size that have occurred during the experiment. To enable the maximum LDH levels to be identified before the start of the assay, lysis solution is added to maximum LDH level controls for 45 min. Plates are centrifuged at $250 \times g$ for 4 min. 50 μl of supernatant from each condition is removed to a flat bottom 96-well plate and 50 μl of reconstituted substrate mix is added. The plate is incubated in the dark at room temperature for 30 min after which 50 μl of stop solution is added. Absorbance is recorded at 490 nm. Cytotoxicity was calculated as a percentage of maximum LDH release [44].

10.4.7 Clonogenic Assay

Spheroids are collected, counted, washed with PBS before dissociation with trypsin. Trypsinisation is quenched with appropriate cell culture medium and the cells collected by centrifugation and resuspended in appropriate cell culture medium so that the cells are dispersed evenly. Cells are counted and plated at 1000–2000 cells per 10 cm dish with 12 ml of medium. After 7–10 days, medium is removed and cells are simultaneously fixed and stained with 1 % methylene blue in 70 % Methanol:PBS for 1–2 h. Methylene blue solution is removed and plates are washed twice with tap water and then air-dried overnight at room temperature. The number of colonies is counted either by eye or using a colony counter such as the GelCount™ (Oxford Optronix, UK). Colony numbers are used to calculate the percentage of colony forming cells [49].

10.4.8 Radiation

Given the impact of hypoxia and tumour microenvironment on the efficacy of radiotherapy response, spheroids are an important tool to understanding these relationships in vitro. Spheroids can be analysed by one of the methods defined above examining cell viability in response to radiotherapy such as the acid phosphatase assay [48] and clonogenic assay [50]. These spheroid-based assays have also been used to investigate the effect of drug radiotherapy combination responses [48, 50].

10.4.9 Bioreporters

An additional method for investigating a defined output is using bioreporters. This requires the production of spheroids from cells stably selected with reporter expression cassettes. Reporter expression cassettes with GFP or luciferase expression under control of a promoter, which defines a specific output. For example, hypoxia response element regulated expression of GFP or luciferase would enable detection of the relative amount of hypoxic cells. Published examples of these include; the utilisation of luciferase under regulation of the vimentin promoter as a marker of EMT in spheroids [51] and; a GFP based glutathione-specific redox sensor that quantifies glutathione redox potential using structured illumination [52].

10.4.10 Quantifying Oxygen Levels and pH

A number of other technologies have been utilised to investigate spheroid physiology. The Seahorse machine can be used to analyse oxygen consumption and extracellular acidification rates [53]; however, these measurements are likely most greatly impacted by the non-hypoxic peripheral cells of the spheroid. Alternatively pH can be measured across the central plane of spheroids using confocal microscopy and the dual emission Fluoroprobe SNARF®-1 (Invitrogen, USA) [54]. Investigations of the intracellular and extra-cellular pH of spheroids has produced important data on the impact of carbonic anhydrase 9 (CA9) on pH in the 3D microenvironment [54]. This work utilised pH calibration of the dyes [54]. Similarly oxygen levels can be measured by a number of probe systems including the $NanO_2$ probe (Luxcel Biosciences) which enabled direct, real-time analysis of spheroid O_2 distribution using one-photon confocal PLIM imaging [55]. Alternatively, as a simple binary solution, the presence or absence of low oxygen levels in spheroids can be identified with the fluorescent hypoxia probe, LOX-1 (SCIVAX Life Sciences) [31]. However, this begins to fluoresce between 10 and 5 % O_2 concentration [56] well within the O_2 range of normal tissue. In the cell line investigated SCC-7, there was an increase in HIF1α stabilisation at these O_2 levels [56].

10.4.11 Spheroid Based Screening

Combining spheroid analysis with screening technologies is an important step forward in the utilisation of these techniques to investigate hypoxia tumour biology. It is documented that drugs/gene knockdowns may have effects in 2D but little effect in vivo [57] these false positive are mirrored by false negative results where targets are shelved due to poor 2D in vitro results which could have an impact in vivo such as CA9 [9] and β1-integrin [58]. However, utilising spheroid screens can be a complicated approach to analyse effects on the hypoxic fraction of cells, as it is difficult to differentiate between the effects on the normoxic and hypoxic fractions. For example, effects on cell proliferation or survival in the hypoxic fraction of spheroids can be masked by the proliferation of the normoxic cells.

There a number of important factors to consider before beginning a spheroid screen these are discussed in detail elsewhere [43]. However, when performing screens with investigations of hypoxia biology or hypoxia targeting as the main aim there are two key considerations. The first is spheroid size and the size of the hypoxic fraction, if it is an investigation of effects on the hypoxic fraction is the size of this within the spheroid large enough to see the effect expected. The second is the methodology. The methodology of drug or shRNA screening will be dependent entirely on what the endpoint analysis is. It is likely to include one or more of the techniques described in detail above. However, will the output provide enough detail about the hypoxic fraction?

A number of screens utilising spheroids have now been published. However, only a few of these were designed to identify genes required for, or drugs targeting, the hypoxic microenvironment in particular [31, 53, 59]. Although other studies have investigated hypoxia related phenotypes such as stem cells [60] and invasion [51] both of which are increased in response to hypoxia [7], these studies did not investigate the hypoxic role specifically.

These screens identify that methodology is in place to carry out spheroids screens. However, major issues remain. In each of the hypoxia focused screens, there is an issue with the size of the hypoxic fraction of spheroids or lack of evidence for the spheroid hypoxia. It is clear based on current technologies that corresponding work is generally required in 2D culture with cells in normoxia and hypoxia to help identify and validate specific events. This approach was used in the referenced hypoxia focused studies.

The second major issue with this approach is the lack of a high-throughput endpoint test that has hypoxic specificity, which is a major bottleneck in streamlining hypoxia based spheroid screening. It is also important to note that these hypoxia focused spheroid screens were drug-based and not using gene knockdown or knockout technologies. Spheroid based assays require time for the hypoxic fraction of spheroids to develop and this precludes the use of transfected siRNAs and therefore requires the use of lentiviral transduced shRNA or CRISPR systems.

10.5 Spheroid Immunohistochemistry

Size, growth and cell viability are important outputs for quantifying spheroid experiments; however, they do not differentiate between normoxic and hypoxic fractions of cells. It is key to understanding hypoxia biology to include additional analyses. Immunohistochemistry analysis of spheroids enables staining for markers of hypoxia alongside markers of apoptosis and proliferation. Furthermore it is important to identify the presence of hypoxia within the spheroids of investigation and identify the amount of hypoxia within these.

10.5.1 Paraffin Embedding and Processing of Spheroids

Spheroids can be carefully collected from plates by using either a Pasteur pipette or a 1000 μl pipette with the tip cut off are fixed overnight in 10 % formalin in a polypropylene disposable centrifuge tube. The next day the formalin is aspirated away, leaving the spheroids in the conical base of the tube. Molten 2 % w/v agarose dissolved in 10 % formalin at 60 °C is carefully pipetted over the spheroids in the tube and centrifuged briefly to ensure the spheroids remain in the conical base of the tube. Placing the tube on ice solidifies the agarose and, once solid, the agarose cone containing the spheroids is removed from the tube. The tip of the agarose plug containing the spheroids is cut off and placed within an embedding cassette. The spheroid agarose pellet is then wax infiltrated overnight in a tissue processor. The agarose pellets containing the spheroids can then be embedded in wax blocks the next day ready to be sectioned on a microtome. 4 μM sections can then be cut and placed onto histology slides ready for histochemical or immunohistochemical staining.

10.5.2 Immunohistochemical Analysis of Spheroids

There are several standard immunohistochemical stains that are more or less routinely applied to spheroid sections. Markers of proliferation, apoptosis and hypoxia are commonly used as well a simple haematoxylin and eosin stain to examine spheroid morphology. The type of primary antibody used will be dependent upon the species of the animal that donated the cell line used to grow the spheroid. Spheroids are usually made from either human or murine cell lines, so either a mouse monoclonal for human cell lines or rabbit polyclonal for mouse cell lines are used. The antibodies specified below are available from many different suppliers, which can be country specific (unless a specific supplier is noted). Detection methods will also vary between laboratories depending on whether staining is done manually or using an autostaining machine. Most of the antibodies below are in general use and are suitable for a range of standard visualisation methods.

10.5.3 Hypoxia Biomarkers

There are three methods for immunohistochemically identifying areas of hypoxia within spheroids. Two rely on the endogenous hypoxia regulated proteins CA9 and HIF1α. These can be very effective, if indirect, markers of hypoxia, but in some circumstances expression may be compromised if the hypoxia pathways are disrupted. An alternative is to use Pimonidazole, an exogenous marker.

There are several commercially available antibodies against CA9, but two that have been found to be effective in our hands are the rabbit polyclonal antibodies NB100-417 [61] from Novus and ab184006 [62] from Abcam (Fig. 10.3). Both are suitable for use on mouse and human cells. When studying hypoxia mechanisms in tumour spheroids there will often be a need to examine expression of the HIF1α. HIF1α can be identified immunohistochemically using the mouse monoclonal antibodies MOP1/Clone 54 (610958) [63] from BD Biosciences (for human HIF1α) and ESEE122 (ab8366) [64] from Abcam (suitable for human and mouse studies).

For pimonidazole analysis [65], spheroids are typically incubated for 1–2 h in the presence of pimonidazole at a concentration of between 100 and 200 μM. They are then harvested, fixed and processed into FFPE blocks in the usual way. In hypoxic conditions, pimonidazole forms covalently stable adducts with the thiol groups in proteins, peptides and amino acids. These thiol adducts can then be visualised immunohistochemically using a monoclonal antibody against them (Fig. 10.3). The most commonly used system for the pimonidazole IHC assay comes as a kit from a company called Hypoxyprobe (Chemicon International). The kit contains the pimonidazole HCl and the monoclonal antibody used to detect the thiol adducts in histological sections.

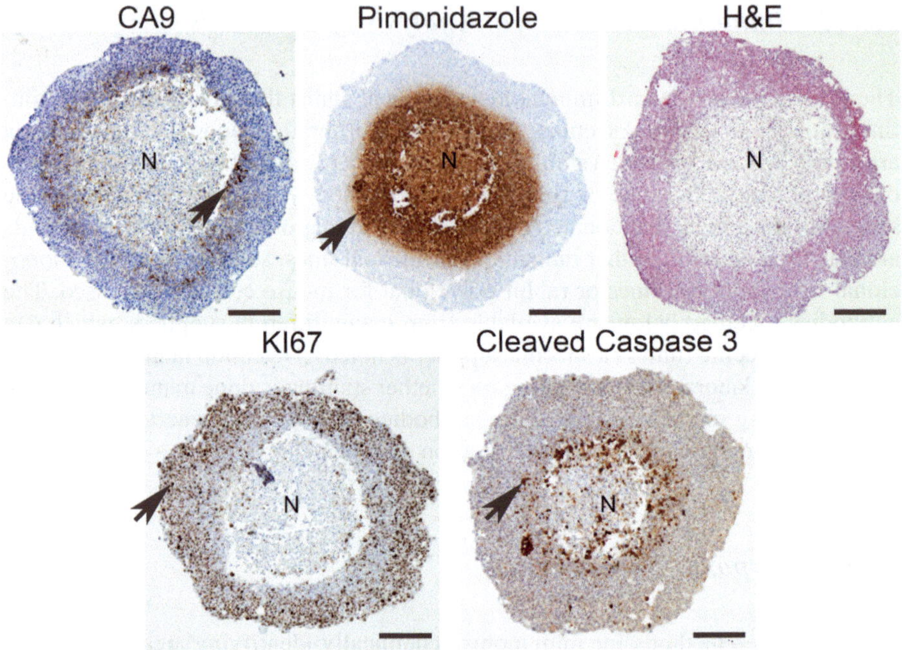

Fig. 10.3 Examples of immunohistochemistry analysis of HCT116 (colorectal cancer cell line) spheroids. Examples of spheroids stained for markers of hypoxia (carbonic anhydrase 9 (CA9) and pimonidazole), spheroid histology (hematoxylin and eosin H&E) a marker of proliferation (Ki67) and a marker of apoptosis (cleaved caspase 3). The scale bar denotes 200 μm, *arrows* point to the stained regions (DAB stain *dark brown*) and N = necrosis. CAIX (M75, Gift from J. Pastorek, Institute of Virology, Slovak Republic, 1:50); pimonidazole (hypoxyprobe-1; Chemicon International; 1:50); cleaved caspase-3 (RnD systems; 1:2000) and Ki67 (M7240; Dako; 1:50). Slides were incubated with the anti-rabbit/anti-mouse secondary antibody (Dako) for 30 min at room temperature. 3,3′-Diaminobenzidine (DAB; Dako) was applied to the sections for 7 min. The slides were counterstained by immersing in hematoxylin solution (Sigma–Aldrich)

10.5.4 Proliferation Biomarkers

The marker of proliferation of choice is Ki67, a nuclear protein expressed at all active stages of the cell cycle but absent in resting or quiescent cells. The most common monoclonal antibody used to stain for Ki67 in human tissue is MIB-1 [66]. Alternatively for mouse tissues, the mouse monoclonal MIB-5 can be used or the rabbit monoclonal SP6 has been shown to be effective [67] (Fig. 10.3).

10.5.5 Markers of Apoptosis

Apoptosis is commonly identified by caspase-3 cleavage [68]. There are several antibodies available for cleaved caspase-3. Antibody 9661 from Cell Signalling Technologies is a rabbit monoclonal antibody has been used extensively in our laboratory; another rabbit monoclonal from Cell Signalling Technologies is Antibody 9579 (D3E9). Both antibodies recognise human and mouse caspase-3 cleaved at asparagine 175 (Fig. 10.3).

10.6 Mathematical Modelling of Cellular Oxygen Consumption Rate in Spheroids

The tendency of tumour spheroids to yield naturally occurring regions of hypoxia mimics the behaviour of real avascular tumour growth. It has been long known that hypoxia has a significant effect of treatment prognosis and radiation sensitivity, with poorly oxygenated regions of tumour responding markedly worse to radiotherapy than corresponding well-oxygenated regions [69, 70]. Cancer spheroids have also shown potential as a proxy model for investigating FDG-positron emission tomography (PET) dynamics [71] in solid tumours. Imaging techniques, including PET, are increasingly used to monitor hypoxia in tumours and could potentially assist radiotherapy planning [72]. In order to effectively plan tumour irradiation based on macroscopic scale PET images, it is important to understand oxygen gradients within a tumour [72]. Because spheroid oxygen levels are readily obtained from theory and experiment, they can serve as a useful model of hypoxia and avascular oxygen dynamics for developing mathematical models of oxygen distribution [72]. Below we define the methodology of investigating tumour oxygen distribution in spheroids.

Spheroids also have some similarity to avascular tumours is in their growth dynamics; avascular growth has been examined by several authors [73–76] and remains an active topic in research. Conger and Ziskin [77] noted spheroids appeared to grow in three distinct stages; an initial exponential phase, followed by an approximately linear period before finally reaching a plateau. A similar type of growth was seen over 15 different tumour cell lines [78], and it was observed that this growth could be approximated to a Gompertzian curve, which described the approximate sigmoidal shape of the growth curves well. Gompertzian-type models have the advantage of being well suited to situations where empirical models are required, such as the optimisation of radiotherapy [76, 79, 80]. A hybrid "Gomp-ex" model [81] was also found to fit observed spheroid growth curves well [76]; in this model, initial growth is exponential, followed by a Gompertzian phase when the increasing cell volume reduces the availability of nutrients to tumour cells. While Gompertzian and other sigmoidal models of growth can fit tumour spheroids well, they are do not directly address the underlying mechanistic or biophysical processes and are used to capture the gross growth curves of spheroids rather than explain why this growth occurs.

Several more complex models of avascular growth, which can readily be applied to spheroids, have arisen from the field of applied mathematics. These models are typically systems of differential equations, which include terms for a wide array of intercellular processes [82–85]. These models have varying levels of mathematical elegance and sophistication, but numerous parameters make direct validation of such models difficult and are not always useful or suitable for in vitro data.

10.6.1 Analytical Modelling of Oxygen Distribution in Tumour Spheroids

From both a theoretical and experimental perspective, the oxygen consumption rate (OCR) of cells in a tumour spheroid is of significant interest, as the rate at which oxygen is consumed has implications for tumour growth and the effectiveness of metabolism modifying clinical compounds. Moreover, the OCR has significant consequences for spheroid composition, influencing the physical extent of hypoxia and the size of the anoxic core [72, 86]. A hypothetical spheroid with an anoxic core is illustrated in Fig. 10.4—as oxygen is diffusing throughout the spheroid whilst being consumed by cells in that mass, the problem can be analysed by the use of reaction-diffusion equations with appropriate spherical symmetry and boundary conditions. It is also possible to derive explicit analytical expressions relating the physical extent of the spheroid regions to OCR [72] and we shall outline this approach here. Initially when a spheroid forms it is generally small enough that oxygen can diffuse entirely throughout without being entirely consumed. In this case, all cells have an ample supply and there is no central anoxia. As the cells divide and the spheroid increases in radius, it will eventually achieve a critical radius where cells consume so much oxygen that the partial pressure is exactly 0 mmHg at the centre. The critical radius at which this occurs is given by

$$r_1 = \sqrt{\frac{6Dp_o}{a\Omega}} \tag{10.1}$$

where D is the diffusion constant for oxygen in water (typically $2\times10^{-9}\,\mathrm{m^2s^{-1}}$), p_o is the partial pressure at the spheroid external boundary so that $p(r_o) = p_o$ and a is the OCR in units of $\mathrm{m^3kg^{-1}s^{-1}}$. The constant Ω relates oxygen partial pressure to the

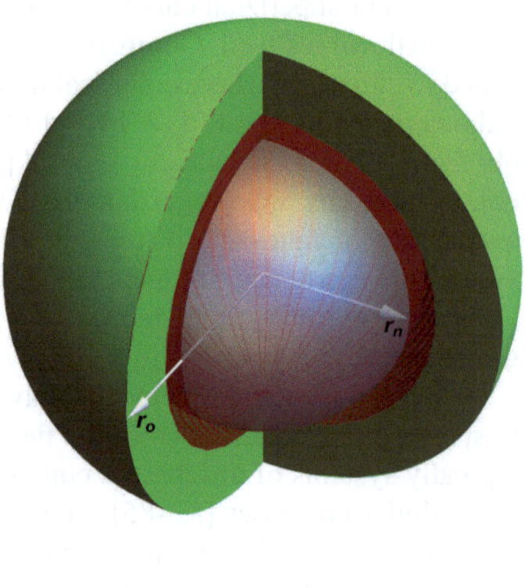

Fig. 10.4 A tumour spheroid with radius r_o and anoxic core of radius r_n. Well oxygenated regions are shown here in *green*, with regions of increasing hypoxia in *red*. At $r \leq r_n$, the spheroid is anoxic with a partial pressure of 0 mmHg at the core

volume of oxygen in tissue through, a consequence of Henry's law. At human body temperature (37 °C), it has a value of $\Omega = 3.0318 \times 10^7$ mmHg kgm^{-3}. At radii above the critical limit, an anoxic core of radius rn will form. The radius of the anoxic core is given by

$$r_n = r_o \left(\frac{1}{2} - \cos \left(\frac{\arccos(1 - \frac{2r_1^2}{r_o^2}) - 2\pi}{3} \right) \right). \tag{10.2}$$

This situation is illustrated in Fig. 10.4. The radius of the viable rim, r_c, is given by

$$r_c = r_o \left(\frac{1}{2} + \cos \left(\frac{\arccos(1 - \frac{2r_1^2}{r_o^2}) - 2\pi}{3} \right) \right). \tag{10.3}$$

We expect from the definition of the spheroid regions that $r_o = r_n + r_c$ and this is indeed the case of Eqs. (10.2 and 10.3) are summed. The partial pressure at any point within the viable rim (r_n " r" r_o) a distance r from the spheroid centre is given by

$$p(r) = p_o + \frac{a\Omega}{6D}\left(r^2 - r_o^2 + 2r_n^3 \left(\frac{1}{r} - \frac{1}{r_o} \right) \right). \tag{10.4}$$

It can also be shown through mathematical manipulation of the spheroid boundary conditions that the diffusion limit is related to a particular ratio of the spheroid radius r_o, thc anoxic radius r_n and the viable rim r_c [72]. This relationship is

$$a = \frac{6Dp_o r_o}{\Omega r_c^2 (r_o + 2r_n)} \tag{10.5}$$

The identity in Eq. (10.5) is valid for any spheroid with $r_n > 0$. For spheroids without an anoxic core, OCR can be estimated by manipulation of Eq. (10.4) provided that the oxygen partial pressure at some point r_p inside the spheroid is known ($p(r_p) = p$). Thus for spheroids with no anoxic core, the OCR is given by

$$a = \frac{6D(p_o - p)}{\Omega(r_o^2 - r_p^2)}. \tag{10.6}$$

10.6.2 Non-constant Oxygen Consumption

The identities established hold under the assumption that OCR stays approximately constant across the spheroid. If, however, we assume that oxygen consumption varies with oxygen concentration, the situation is somewhat more complicated. Indeed, some authors [72] assume that oxygen consumption falls in a hyperbolic manner with decreasing oxygen concentration, in a manner akin to Michaelis–Menten kinetics. In this case, denoting maximal oxygen consumption as a_o, consumption would take the form

$$a(p) = \frac{a_o p}{p + K_m}. \tag{10.7}$$

where K_m is the constant at which $a(p)$ is half maximal. For cellular oxygen consumption, this model is phenomenological and its sigmoidal form is intended to capture the possibility that the OCR in a given tissue might be lower under hypoxic conditions than under normoxia. In this case, the reaction-diffusion equations become analytically intractable and authors making this assumption tend to resort to numerical methods for solving spheroid related problems. However, it has been shown that a very close approximation [72] can be obtained from the parabolic nature of the function. From this, it is possible to yield an expression for oxygen at any point in the spheroid viable rim with an expression analogous to that in Eq. (10.4). Defining the anoxic radius in this situation as r_n^* and setting $k_r = \frac{K_m}{p_o}(r_o - r_n^*)^2$, the new expression for oxygen in the spheroid rim is

$$\begin{aligned} p(r) &= \frac{a_o \Omega}{6D}(r^2 - 3r_n^{*2} + \frac{2r_n^{*3} - 6k_r r_n^*}{r} + 6k_r - 3\sqrt{k_r}\pi r_n^* + 6\sqrt{k_r}\, r_n^* \arctan(\frac{\sqrt{k_r}}{r - r_n^*})) \\ &+ \frac{(6\sqrt{k_r}\, r_n^{*2} - 6k_r^{3/2})\arctan(\frac{r - r_n^*}{\sqrt{k_r}})}{r} + (\frac{6k_r r_n^*}{r} - 3k_r)\ln(\frac{(r - r_n^*)^2 + k_r}{k_r}). \end{aligned} \tag{10.8}$$

While the above expression is markedly more convoluted than that in Eq. (10.4), it reduces back to this form when $K_m = 0$. While the expression in Eq. (10.8) could be used with tumour spheroids, in practice it is not practical or necessary to do so—the same analysis from whence this equation was derived [72] shows that given the typically small values of the substrate constant in literature (K_m " 1mmHg) the assumption of constant consumption rate yields only very small differences from the more complex expression and assumption. In general, the form shown in Eq. (10.4) and the associated identities is suitable for spheroid analysis.

10.6.3 Experimental Measurement of OCR in Spheroids with an Anoxic Core

Given knowledge of the boundaries of a spheroid, Eq. (10.5) lends itself to OCR estimation for a spheroid with an anoxic core ($r_n > 0$) and Eq. (10.6) to OCR estimation when $r_n = 0$. Whilst it is possible to use oxygen sensitive electrodes to ascertain the oxygen concentration at any point in a spheroid [86], this can potentially disturb the gradient and isn't enough alone to determine the OCR. It is possible to stain the spheroids with various hypoxic and proliferation markers to find regions of a given oxygen tension without mechanically disturbing the gradient—this has been previously employed in a robust methods [72] for determination of oxygen consumption. In principle, if a spheroid with r_n is simply sectioned along through its central axis, then the ratio of the anoxic core to spheroid radius r_o can yield OCR by use of identity 5. In practice, spheroids are typically stained prior to sectioning, with markers such as Ki67, which binds to proliferating cells and EF5, which binds to cell with partial pressures between 0.8 and 10 mmHg. This is the situation depicted in Fig. 10.5, which depicts a dual stained DLD1 tumour spheroid sectioned through the spheroid centre. If this tumour can be sectioned accurately, then it is relatively straight-forward to determine the OCR with simple image analysis. A typical algorithm for determining OCR from a section image is outlined below.

1. Section the spheroid through its centre.
2. Use image analysis to determine the location of the spheroid centroid.
3. Use edge detection to find pixels corresponding to the outer spheroid radius.
4. Use edge detection to find pixels corresponding to the anoxic spheroid radius.
5. Calculate distance from spheroid centre to all pixels at r_o/r_n respectively.

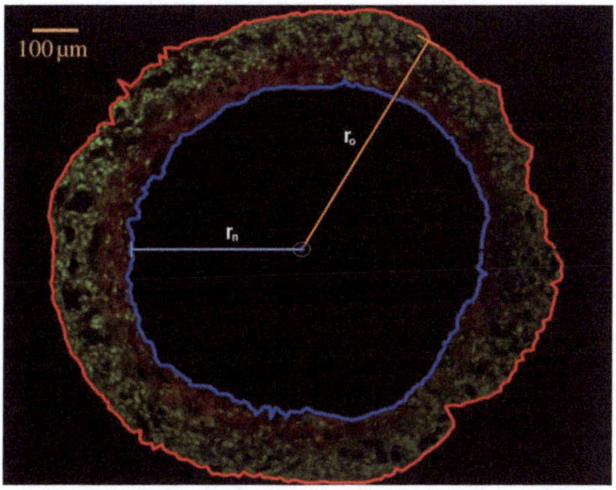

Fig. 10.5 A DLD1 tumour spheroid with radius r_o and anoxic core of radius r_n. Well oxygenated regions are shown here in *green* stained with the proliferation marker Ki67. Regions of increasing hypoxia ($p \leq 10$ mmHg) are stained with the hypoxia marker EF5, shown here in *red*. At $r \leq r_n$, the spheroid is anoxic with a partial pressure of 0 mmHg at the core

6. From this, determine average values and corresponding errors.
7. Employ Eq. (10.5) to estimate OCR.

If the spheroid maintains a roughly spherical shape after sectioning, the standard deviation on values of r_n and r_o is typically quite low, but it can increase significantly if spheroids are mechanically stressed and distorted into increasingly non-spherical shapes [72]. In Fig. 10.5, the image analysis algorithm depicts the boundary pixels at r_o in red and the pixels at r_n in blue. In practice, this analysis can be further strengthened by employing a further result from theory; it can be shown [72] that for any given partial pressure p in the spheroid, $0''\ p''\ p_o$, there is a corresponding radius r_p so that $p(r_p) = p$. This radius is given by

$$r_p = 2\sqrt{\frac{\phi(p)}{3}}\cos\left(\frac{1}{3}\arccos\left(-\sqrt{\left(\frac{3r_n^2}{\phi(p)}\right)^3}\right)\right) \quad (10.9)$$

where $\phi(p)$ is given by

$$\phi_p = r_o^2 + \frac{2r_n^3}{r_o} + \frac{6D(p - p_o)}{\Omega a}. \quad (10.10)$$

Thus, if the oxygen tension at which a given staining manifests is known, then it is entirely possible to use this information to estimate OCR or validate estimations. In the case of the spheroid illustrated in Fig. 10.5, the interface between the EF5 and Ki67 staining typically occurs at $p \sim 10$ mmHg [87]—this can be used to check OCR estimations if r_p is accurately determined.

10.6.4 Experimental Measurement of OCR in Spheroids Without an Anoxic Core

Spheroids without central hypoxia, such as the HCT116 spheroid illustrated in Fig. 10.6 require staining with a hypoxia marker to estimate hypoxia. In practice, multiple stains might be required to ascertain the value of r_p corresponding to a partial pressure of p. If one of the stains employed is EF5, the hypoxia binding dynamics are well established [87] and the interface between the EF5 stain and better oxygenated regions can be taken at approximately 10 mmHg. Different hypoxia binding agents will have different dynamics, but the principle remains the same. A similar image analysis protocol can be invoked, with the following steps.

1. Section the spheroid through its centre.
2. Use image analysis to determine the location of the spheroid centroid.
3. Use edge detection to find pixels corresponding to the outer spheroid radius.
4. Use edge detection to find pixels corresponding to $p(r_p) = p$.

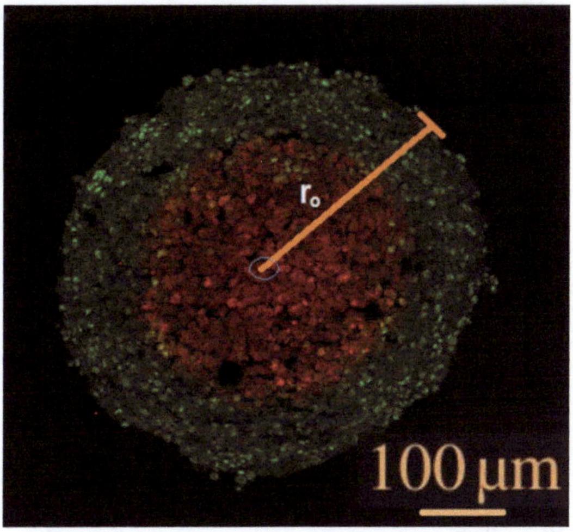

Fig. 10.6 A HCT116 tumour spheroid with radius r_o and no anoxic core. Well oxygenated regions are shown here in *green* and stained with Ki67, with regions of increasing hypoxia stained with EF5 in *red*

5. Calculate distance from spheroid centre to all pixels at r_o/r_p respectively.
6. From this, determine average values and corresponding errors.
7. Employ Eq. (10.6) to estimate OCR.

10.6.5 Oxygen Distribution in Tumour Spheroids

One of the benefits of estimating OCR is that it allows calculation of the anoxic radius and complete oxygen distribution for any spheroid radius r_o. For a known or experimentally determined value of OCR, a, then the diffusion limit r_l is readily calculated. For spheroids with $r_o > r_l$, the spheroid will have an anoxic core of radius r_n which can be readily determined from the equations established. Finally, oxygen tension throughout the entire spheroid can then be calculated by invoking Eq. 10.4, allowing rapid determination of the oxygen status of a spheroid given knowledge of its cellular OCR. Examples of oxygen distributions for tumour spheroids with $r_o = 500\,\mu m$ and varying values of OCR are shown in Fig. 10.7.

10.7 Conclusions

Spheroids are a valuable in vitro model of the hypoxic microenvironment. They enable analyses of the effects of physiological gradients such as pH or metabolites/catabolites and gene modulation and inhibitor investigations in these contexts. They are cheap and easy to produce and simple analyses such as growth or viability can be applied to high-throughput screen technologies. They form a bridge between

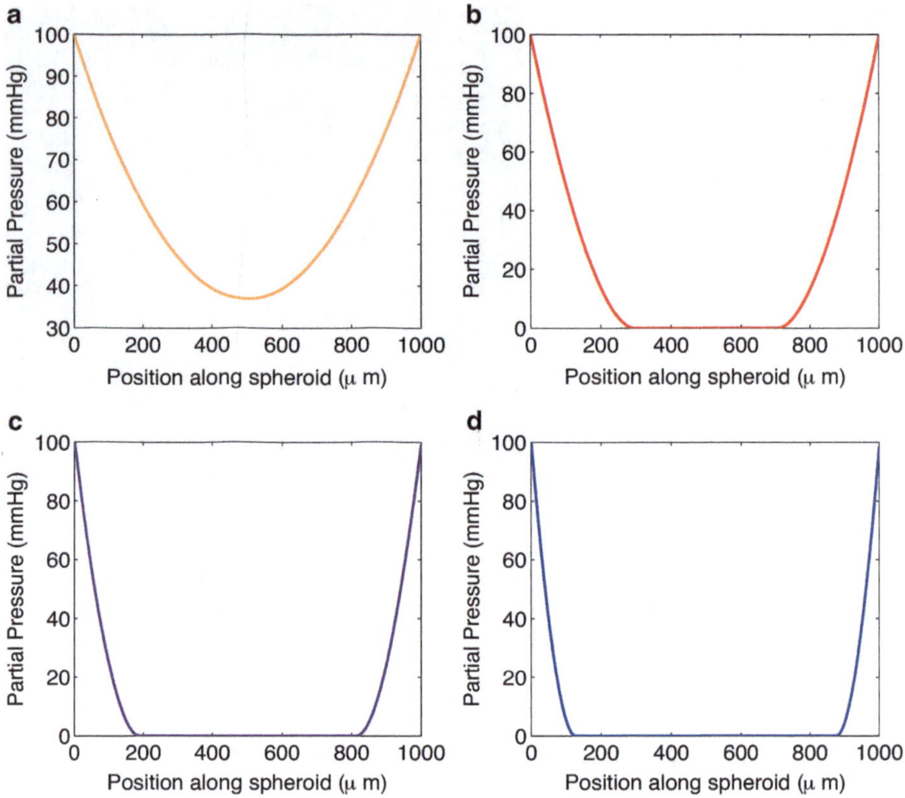

Fig. 10.7 Simulated oxygen tension along a spheroid of radius $r_o = 500$ μm with (**a**) $a = 1 \times 10^{-7}$ m^3 kg^{-1} s^{-1}, (**b**) $a = 2.5 \times 10^{-7}$ m^3 kg^{-1} s^{-1}, (**c**) $a = 5 \times 10^{-7}$ m^3 kg^{-1} s^{-1}, (**d**) $a = 1 \times 10^{-6}$ m^3 kg^{-1} s^{-1}

the less complex 2D cell culture and more complex in vivo xenograft experiments and can be used to increase the success rate in transfer between these. Because spheroids parameters such as oxygen levels and proliferation are readily observable from experimental data they serve as a bridge for the development of mathematical models to increase our understanding of tumour oxygen dynamics. The area that requires further development is the analysis of cell responses within the differential physiological gradients to facilitate high-throughput screening technologies. In particular, the lack of a high-throughput endpoint test that has hypoxic specificity is hindering the effectiveness of spheroids in hypoxia screening applications and will most likely be expedited by the utilisation of bioreporter assays to enable imaging of localised responses as an endpoint. Increased use of protocols developed for the successful growth of spheroids from primary patient tumour material may in future enable drug screening in a pretreatment patient spheroid model as a concept of personalised medicine [31].

References

1. Vaupel P. The role of hypoxia-induced factors in tumor progression. Oncologist. 2004;9(Suppl):510–7.
2. Choudhry H, Schodel J, Oikonomopoulos S, et al. Extensive regulation of the non-coding transcriptome by hypoxia: role of HIF in releasing paused RNApol2. EMBO Rep. 2014; 15(1):70–6.
3. Semenza GL. Oxygen sensing, hypoxia-inducible factors, and disease pathophysiology. Annu Rev Pathol. 2014;9:947–71.
4. Harris AL. Hypoxia—a key regulatory factor in tumour growth. Nat Rev Cancer. 2002; 2(1):38–47.
5. Rebucci M, Michiels C. Molecular aspects of cancer cell resistance to chemotherapy. Biochem Pharmacol. 2013;85(9):1219–26.
6. Multhoff G, Radons J, Vaupel P. Critical role of aberrant angiogenesis in the development of tumor hypoxia and associated radioresistance. Cancers (Basel). 2014;6(2):813–28.
7. McIntyre A, Harris AL. Metabolic and hypoxic adaptation to anti-angiogenic therapy: a target for induced essentiality. EMBO Mol Med. 2015;7(4):368–79.
8. Hirschhaeuser F, Menne H, Dittfeld C, et al. Multicellular tumor spheroids: an underestimated tool is catching up again. J Biotechnol. 2010;148(1):3–15.
9. McIntyre A, Patiar S, Wigfield S, et al. Carbonic anhydrase IX promotes tumor growth and necrosis in vivo and inhibition enhances anti-VEGF therapy. Clin Cancer Res. 2012;18(11): 3100–11.
10. Minchinton AI, Tannock IF. Drug penetration in solid tumours. Nat Rev Cancer. 2006; 6(8):583–92.
11. Bingle L, Lewis CE, Corke KP, et al. Macrophages promote angiogenesis in human breast tumour spheroids in vivo. Br J Cancer. 2006;94(1):101–7.
12. Ivanov DP, Parker TL, Walker DA, et al. In vitro co-culture model of medulloblastoma and human neural stem cells for drug delivery assessment. J Biotechnol. 2015;205:3–13.
13. Dolznig H, Rupp C, Puri C, et al. Modeling colon adenocarcinomas in vitro a 3D co-culture system induces cancer-relevant pathways upon tumor cell and stromal fibroblast interaction. Am J Pathol. 2011;179(1):487–501.
14. Tang XH, Lucas JE, Chen JLY, et al. Functional interaction between responses to lactic acidosis and hypoxia regulates genomic transcriptional outputs. Cancer Res. 2012;72(2):491–502.
15. Ellingsen C, Walenta S, Hompland T, et al. The microenvironment of cervical carcinoma xenografts: associations with lymph node metastasis and its assessment by DCE-MRI. Transl Oncol. 2013;6(5):607–17.
16. Grimshaw MJ, Cooper L, Papazisis K, et al. Mammosphere culture of metastatic breast cancer cells enriches for tumorigenic breast cancer cells. Breast Cancer Res. 2008;10(3):R52.
17. Koo BK, Stange DE, Sato T, et al. Controlled gene expression in primary Lgr5 organoid cultures. Nat Methods. 2012;9(1):81–3.
18. Ivascu A, Kubbies M. Rapid generation of single-tumor spheroids for high-throughput cell function and toxicity analysis. J Biomol Screen. 2006;11(8):922–32.
19. Fennema E, Rivron N, Rouwkema J, et al. Spheroid culture as a tool for creating 3D complex tissues. Trends Biotechnol. 2013;31(2):108–15.
20. Leek RD, Stratford I, Harris AL. The role of hypoxia-inducible factor-1 in three-dimensional tumor growth, apoptosis, and regulation by the insulin-signaling pathway. Cancer Res. 2005;65(10):4147–52.
21. Friedrich J, Ebner R, Kunz-Schughart LA. Experimental anti-tumor therapy in 3-D: spheroids—old hat or new challenge? Int J Radiat Biol. 2007;83(11-12):849–71.
22. Timmins NE, Nielsen LK. Generation of multicellular tumor spheroids by the hanging-drop method. Methods Mol Med. 2007;140:141–51.

23. Kelm JM, Timmins NE, Brown CJ, et al. Method for generation of homogeneous multicellular tumor spheroids applicable to a wide variety of cell types. Biotechnol Bioeng. 2003; 83(2):173–80.
24. Hsiao AY, Tung YC, Qu X, et al. 384 hanging drop arrays give excellent Z-factors and allow versatile formation of co-culture spheroids. Biotechnol Bioeng. 2012;109(5):1293–304.
25. Napolitano AP, Chai P, Dean DM, et al. Dynamics of the self-assembly of complex cellular aggregates on micromolded nonadhesive hydrogels. Tissue Eng. 2007;13(8):2087–94.
26. Shimizu K, Kusamori K, Nishikawa M, et al. Poly(N-isopropylacrylamide)-coated microwell arrays for construction and recovery of multicellular spheroids. J Biosci Bioeng. 2013; 115(6):695–9.
27. Torisawa YS, Chueh BH, Huh D, et al. Efficient formation of uniform-sized embryoid bodies using a compartmentalized microchannel device. Lab Chip. 2007;7(6):770–6.
28. Wu LY, Di Carlo D, Lee LP. Microfluidic self-assembly of tumor spheroids for anticancer drug discovery. Biomed Microdevices. 2008;10(2):197–202.
29. Torisawa YS, Takagi A, Nashimoto Y, et al. A multicellular spheroid array to realize spheroid formation, culture, and viability assay on a chip. Biomaterials. 2007;28(3):559–66.
30. Yoshii Y, Waki A, Yoshida K, et al. The use of nanoimprinted scaffolds as 3D culture models to facilitate spontaneous tumor cell migration and well-regulated spheroid formation. Biomaterials. 2011;32(26):6052–8.
31. Yoshii Y, Furukawa T, Waki A, et al. High-throughput screening with nanoimprinting 3D culture for efficient drug development by mimicking the tumor environment. Biomaterials. 2015;51:278–89.
32. Tofilon PJ, Arundel CM, Deen DF. Response to BCNU of spheroids grown from mixtures of drug-sensitive and drug-resistant cells. Cancer Chemother Pharmacol. 1987;20(2):89–95.
33. Djordjevic B, Lange CS. Cell-cell interactions in spheroids maintained in suspension. Acta Oncol. 2006;45(4):412–20.
34. Hauptmann S, Zwadlo-Klarwasser G, Jansen M, et al. Macrophages and multicellular tumor spheroids in co-culture: a three-dimensional model to study tumor-host interactions. Evidence for macrophage-mediated tumor cell proliferation and migration. Am J Pathol. 1993; 143(5):1406–15.
35. Gottfried E, Kunz-Schughart LA, Andreesen R, et al. Brave little world: spheroids as an in vitro model to study tumor-immune-cell interactions. Cell Cycle. 2006;5(7):691–5.
36. Timmins NE, Dietmair S, Nielsen LK. Hanging-drop multicellular spheroids as a model of tumour angiogenesis. Angiogenesis. 2004;7(2):97–103.
37. Vermeulen S, Van Marck V, Van Hoorde L, et al. Regulation of the invasion suppressor function of the cadherin/catenin complex. Pathol Res Pract. 1996;192(7):694–707.
38. Offner FA, Schiefer J, Wirtz HC, et al. Tumour-cell-endothelial interactions: free radicals are mediators of melanoma-induced endothelial cell damage. Virchows Arch. 1996;428(2): 99–106.
39. Kunz-Schughart LA, Heyder P, Schroeder J, et al. A heterologous 3-D coculture model of breast tumor cells and fibroblasts to study tumor-associated fibroblast differentiation. Exp Cell Res. 2001;266(1):74–86.
40. Ivanov DP, Parker TL, Walker DA, et al. Multiplexing spheroid volume, resazurin and acid phosphatase viability assays for high-throughput screening of tumour spheroids and stem cell neurospheres. PLoS One. 2014;9(8), e103817.
41. Rafajova M, Zatovicova M, Kettmann R, et al. Induction by hypoxia combined with low glucose or low bicarbonate and high posttranslational stability upon reoxygenation contribute to carbonic anhydrase IX expression in cancer cells. Int J Oncol. 2004;24(4):995–1004.
42. Yakymchuk OM, Perepelytsina OM, Dobrydnev AV, et al. Effect of single-walled carbon nanotubes on tumor cells viability and formation of multicellular tumor spheroids. Nanoscale Res Lett. 2015;10:150.
43. Friedrich J, Seidel C, Ebner R, et al. Spheroid-based drug screen: considerations and practical approach. Nat Protoc. 2009;4(3):309–24.

44. Ho WY, Yeap SK, Ho CL, et al. Development of multicellular tumor spheroid (MCTS) culture from breast cancer cell and a high throughput screening method using the MTT assay. PLoS One. 2012;7(9):e44640.
45. Mosmann T. Rapid colorimetric assay for cellular growth and survival: application to proliferation and cytotoxicity assays. J Immunol Methods. 1983;65(1-2):55–63.
46. Abuelba H, Cotrutz CE, Stoica BA, et al. In vitro evaluation of curcumin effects on breast adenocarcinoma 2D and 3D cell cultures. Rom J Morphol Embryol. 2015;56(1):71–6.
47. Friedrich J, Eder W, Castaneda J, et al. A reliable tool to determine cell viability in complex 3-d culture: the acid phosphatase assay. J Biomol Screen. 2007;12(7):925–37.
48. Senavirathna LK, Fernando R, Maples D, et al. Tumor SPHEROIDS as an in vitro model for determining the therapeutic response to proton beam radiotherapy and thermally sensitive nanocarriers. Theranostics. 2013;3(9):687–91.
49. Freyer JP, Sutherland RM. Proliferative and clonogenic heterogeneity of cells from EMT6/Ro multicellular spheroids induced by the glucose and oxygen supply. Cancer Res. 1986;46(7): 3513–20.
50. Roa WH, Miller GG, McEwan AJ, et al. Targeted radiotherapy of multicell neuroblastoma spheroids with high specific activity [125I]meta-iodobenzylguanidine. Int J Radiat Oncol Biol Phys. 1998;41(2):425–32.
51. Li Q, Chen C, Kapadia A, et al. 3D models of epithelial-mesenchymal transition in breast cancer metastasis: high-throughput screening assay development, validation, and pilot screen. J Biomol Screen. 2011;16(2):141–54.
52. Wittig R, Richter V, Wittig-Blaich S, et al. Biosensor-expressing spheroid cultures for imaging of drug-induced effects in three dimensions. J Biomol Screen. 2013;18(6):736–43.
53. Wenzel C, Riefke B, Grundemann S, et al. 3D high-content screening for the identification of compounds that target cells in dormant tumor spheroid regions. Exp Cell Res. 2014;323(1): 131–43.
54. Swietach P, Patiar S, Supuran CT, et al. The role of carbonic anhydrase 9 in regulating extracellular and intracellular ph in three-dimensional tumor cell growths. J Biol Chem. 2009;284(30):20299–310.
55. Dmitriev RI, Zhdanov AV, Nolan YM, et al. Imaging of neurosphere oxygenation with phosphorescent probes. Biomaterials. 2013;34(37):9307–17.
56. Zhang S, Hosaka M, Yoshihara T, et al. Phosphorescent light-emitting iridium complexes serve as a hypoxia-sensing probe for tumor imaging in living animals. Cancer Res. 2010;70(11):4490–8.
57. Kobayashi H, Man S, Graham CH, et al. Acquired multicellular-mediated resistance to alkylating agents in cancer. Proc Natl Acad Sci U S A. 1993;90(8):3294–8.
58. Abbott A. Cell culture: biology's new dimension. Nature. 2003;424(6951):870–2.
59. Herrmann R, Fayad W, Schwarz S, et al. Screening for compounds that induce apoptosis of cancer cells grown as multicellular spheroids. J Biomol Screen. 2008;13(1):1–8.
60. Mathews LA, Keller JM, Goodwin BL, et al. A 1536-well quantitative high-throughput screen to identify compounds targeting cancer stem cells. J Biomol Screen. 2012;17(9):1231–42.
61. Kang HJ, Kim IH, Sung CO, et al. Expression of carbonic anhydrase 9 is a novel prognostic marker in resectable hepatocellular carcinoma. Virchows Arch. 2015;466(4):403–13.
62. Tailor TD, Hanna G, Yarmolenko PS, et al. Effect of pazopanib on tumor microenvironment and liposome delivery. Mol Cancer Ther. 2010;9(6):1798–808.
63. Snell CE, Turley H, McIntyre A, et al. Proline-hydroxylated hypoxia-inducible factor 1alpha (HIF-1alpha) upregulation in human tumours. PLoS One. 2014;9(2):e88955.
64. Talks KL, Turley H, Gatter KC, et al. The expression and distribution of the hypoxia-inducible factors HIF-1alpha and HIF-2alpha in normal human tissues, cancers, and tumor-associated macrophages. Am J Pathol. 2000;157(2):411–21.
65. Durand RE, Raleigh JA. Identification of nonproliferating but viable hypoxic tumor cells in vivo. Cancer Res. 1998;58(16):3547–50.
66. Scholzen T, Gerdes J. The Ki-67 protein: from the known and the unknown. J Cell Physiol. 2000;182(3):311–22.

67. Birner P, Ritzi M, Musahl C, et al. Immunohistochemical detection of cell growth fraction in formalin-fixed and paraffin-embedded murine tissue. Am J Pathol. 2001;158(6):1991–6.
68. Gown AM, Willingham MC. Improved detection of apoptotic cells in archival paraffin sections: immunohistochemistry using antibodies to cleaved caspase 3. J Histochem Cytochem. 2002;50(4):449–54.
69. Gray LH, Conger AD, Ebert M, et al. The concentration of oxygen dissolved in tissues at the time of irradiation as a factor in radiotherapy. Br J Radiol. 1953;26(312):638–48.
70. Hall EJ, Giaccia AJ. Radiobiology for the radiologist. 6th ed. Philadelphia: Lippincott Williams & Wilkins; 2006.
71. Kelly CJ, Hussien K, Muschel RJ. 3D tumour spheroids as a model to assess the suitability of [18F]FDG-PET as an early indicator of response to PI3K inhibition. Nucl Med Biol. 2012;39(7):986–92.
72. Grimes DR, Kelly C, Bloch K, et al. A method for estimating the oxygen consumption rate in multicellular tumour spheroids. J R Soc Interface. 2014;11(92):20131124.
73. Burton AC. Rate of growth of solid tumours as a problem of diffusion. Growth. 1966; 30(2):157–76.
74. Boag JW (1977) Oxygen diffusion in tumour capillary networks. Bibl Anat(15 Pt 1):266–9.
75. Mcelwain DLS, Ponzo PJ. Model for growth of a solid tumor with nonuniform oxygen-consumption. Math Biosci. 1977;35(3-4):267–79.
76. Marusic M, Bajzer Z, Freyer JP, et al. Analysis of growth of multicellular tumour spheroids by mathematical models. Cell Prolif. 1994;27(2):73–94.
77. Conger AD, Ziskin MC. Growth of mammalian multicellular tumor spheroids. Cancer Res. 1983;43(2):556–60.
78. Freyer JP. Role of necrosis in regulating the growth saturation of multicellular spheroids. Cancer Res. 1988;48(9):2432–9.
79. Steel GG. Growth kinetics of tumours : cell population kinetics in relation to the growth and treatment of cancer. Oxford: Clarendon Press; 1977.
80. Swan GW. Role of optimal control theory in cancer chemotherapy. Math Biosci. 1990;101(2):237–84.
81. Wheldon TE. Mathematical models in cancer research. Bristol: Hilger; 1988.
82. Roose T, Chapman SJ, Maini PK. Mathematical models of avascular tumor growth. SIAM Rev. 2007;49(2):179–208.
83. Sherratt JA, Chaplain MAJ. A new mathematical model for avascular tumour growth. J Math Biol. 2001;43(4):291–312.
84. Ward JP, King JR. Mathematical modelling of avascular-tumour growth. IMA J Math Appl Med Biol. 1997;14(1):39–69.
85. Jones AF, Byrne HM, Gibson JS, et al. A mathematical model of the stress induced during avascular tumour growth. J Math Biol. 2000;40(6):473–99.
86. Muellerklieser W. Method for the determination of oxygen-consumption rates and diffusion-coefficients in multicellular spheroids. Biophys J. 1984;46(3):343–8.
87. Koch CJ, Evans SM, Lord EM. Oxygen dependence of cellular uptake of Ef5 [2-(2-Nitro-1h-Imidazol-1-Yl)-N-(2,2,3,3,3-pentafluoropropyl)acetamide]—analysis of drug adducts by fluorescent-antibodies vs bound radioactivity. Br J Cancer. 1995;72(4):869–74.

Chapter 11
Isolation of Glioma-Initiating Cells for Biological Study

Jing Hu, Geoffrey Markowitz, and Xiao-Fan Wang

Abstract Glioblastoma multiforme (GBM, WHO grade IV astrocytoma) is the most common and lethal primary brain tumor in adults, with an average survival of slightly more than 1 year after initial diagnosis. GBMs display significant heterogeneity within the tumor mass, among which a subpopulation of cells called glioma-initiating cells (GICs) is responsible for tumorigenesis and resistance to conventional therapies. Therefore, understanding the mechanism underlying the biological properties of GICs would help develop better therapies to target this population for GBM treatment. This protocol provides detailed procedures to isolate GICs and non-GICs from patient's specimen and glioma xenografts, which serves as the first step for the biological studies of GICs. Upon separation of GICs and non-GICs, a series of studies, such as expression profiling and functional screen, etc., can be performed to identify signal pathways responsible for the malignant nature of GICs. Besides, translational studies can also be conducted to examine drug responses of GICs. In sum, isolation of GICs with reliable methods will provide the basis for the further biological studies.

Keywords Glioblastoma • Glioma-initiating cells • CD133 • CD15

11.1 Introduction

Glioblastoma (GBM, WHO grade IV astrocytoma) is the most common and aggressive primary brain tumor in adults with an average survival of slightly more than 1 year past the initial diagnosis [1]. GBMs exhibit significant heterogeneity within the tumor mass, among which a subpopulation of cells named glioma-initiating cells (GICs) or cancer stem cells has been demonstrated to account for the fatal nature of GBM. GICs display stem-like properties usually associated with the neural stem cells,

The authors have declared that no conflict of interest exists.

J. Hu • G. Markowitz • X.-F. Wang (✉)
Department of Pharmacology and Cancer Biology, Duke University School of Medicine, Duke University Medical Center, C218 LSRC, Box 3813, Durham, NC 27710, USA
e-mail: xiao.fan.wang@duke.edu

C. Koumenis et al. (eds.), *Tumor Microenvironment*, Advances in Experimental Medicine and Biology 899, DOI 10.1007/978-3-319-26666-4_11

including self-renewal illustrated by their abilities to form neurospheres when cultured in the serum-free media in serial passages, expression of stemness markers (CD133, Sox2, Oct4, BMI1, etc.), and differentiation into multiple cell lineages such as astrocyte and oligodendrocyte. However, the regulatory program for its properties to self-renewal and differentiation is out of control so as to generate the aggressive tumor [2, 3]. Notably, GICs are responsible for the resistance to chemotherapy and radiotherapy [4–6]. Therefore, the biological properties of GICs are critical for GBM occurrence and recurrence. Many studies are aimed to elucidate the detailed mechanisms regulating the properties in GICs and ultimately develop the specific therapies targeting GICs and non-GICs.

To investigate the malignant nature of GICs, the first and most essential step is to isolate this small population of cells from the heterogeneous tumor mass. This protocol provides detailed procedures from multiple commonly used methods to enrich GICs and non-GICs, including isolation by cell surface markers and enrichment by specific culturing conditions. Upon separation of GICs and non-GICs, various biological studies could be performed on these cells. For instance, expression profiling of genes and noncoding RNAs can be examined in GICs and non-GICs, to investigate the regulatory networks responsible for the intrinsic biological features of GICs or maintenance of GICs in specific tumor microenvironment. With this approach, we have compared expression levels of microRNAs in GICs and non-GICs, and identified miR-33a mediated Notch and PKA pathways that are important for the GIC self-renewal [7]. Similarly, through microRNA profiling in GICs cultured under hypoxia which is an essential niche for this population, we revealed the HIF-miR-215-KDM1B signal axis that mediates GICs adaptation to hypoxia through modulating multiple critical pathways [8]. A series of oncogenes/suppressors have been uncovered using a similar approach [9, 10]. In addition, other studies including epigenetic profiling and functional screening and testing of drug responses could be designed to explore different aspects of GIC biology. Ultimately, findings from these biological studies would help reveal drug-targetable pathways in GICs and improve therapeutic application.

11.2 Protocol

11.2.1 Materials

1. Sterilized razor blades, scissors, and forceps.
2. Cell culture dishes with standard tissue culture treated surface: 60 mm, 10 cm, and 15 cm.
3. Petri dishes with untreated surface.
4. Papain Dissociation System (Worthington Biochemical, Cat. No. LK003150): Vial 1, Sterile Earle's Balanced Salt Solution (EBSS) with calcium, magnesium, bicarbonate and phenol red, 100 ml; Vial 2, Papain containing L-cysteine and EDTA, 100 U per vial; Vial 3, Deoxyribonuclease I (DNase), 1000 U per vial;

Vial 4, Ovomucoid protease inhibitor with bovine serum albumin, 320 mg ovomucoid inhibitor and 320 mg albumin.

5. Cell strainer, 40 μm (Fisher Scientific, Cat. No. 22363547).
6. Neurobasal media (Invitrogen, Cat. No. 21103-049).
7. Improved MEM Zinc Option (Invitrogen, Cat. No. 10373017).
8. B27 Supplement (50×), without vitamin A (Invitrogen, Cat. No. 12587-010).
9. Fibroblast Growth Factor basic Protein, Human recombinant (Millipore, Cat. No. GF003).
10. Epidermal Growth Factor Protein, Human recombinant (Millipore, Cat. No. GF144).
11. Sodium Pyruvate (100 mM) (Life technologies, Cat. No. 11360-070).
12. L-Glutamine (200 mM) (Life technologies, Cat. No. 25030-081).
13. Trypsin–EDTA (0.05 %), phenol red (Life technologies, Cat. No. 25300-120).
14. StemPro® Accutase® Cell Dissociation Reagent (Life technologies, Cat. No. A11105-01).
15. CD133 MicroBead Kit (Miltenyi Biotech, Cat. No. 130-050-801).
16. CD15 MicroBead Kit, Human (Miltenyi Biotech, Cat. No. 130-046-601).
17. Dead Cell Removal Kit (Miltenyi Biotech, Cat. No. 130-090-101).
18. Anti-Human CD15 FITC, HI98 (eBioscience, Cat. No. 11-0159).
19. CD133/2-PE (293C3), human (Miltenyi Biotech, Cat. No. 130-098-046).
20. Anti-FcR (anti-CD16/32 for mouse, Fc Receptor Binding Inhibitor for human).
21. LS Columns (Miltenyi Biotech, Cat. No. 130-042-401).
22. LD Columns (Miltenyi Biotech, Cat. No. 130-042-901).
23. MACS Separator.
24. FACS buffer: phosphate-buffered saline (PBS), pH 7.2, 0.5 % bovine serum albumin (BSA) and 2 mM EDTA.
25. 2 % Paraformaldehyde in PBS (Optional).
26. Antibiotic–Antimycotic (100×) (Life technologies, Cat. No. 15240-062).
27. Fetal Bovine Serum (FBS).
28. Round-bottom tubes.
29. Conical tubes (15, 50 ml).

11.2.2 Procedures

There are three methods commonly applied for isolating GICs—Separation of GICs by cell surface markers CD133, CD15 and isolation of GICs by specific culturing condition. Cell samples can be stained for the stem cell surface marker of interest to either collect the population of interest or validate the purity of the positively selected population. If samples are for sorting, perform all steps in an appropriate tissue culture hood and utilize sterile reagents. If samples are for validation of purity of a positively selected population, the protocol may be performed outside of a laminar flow hood.

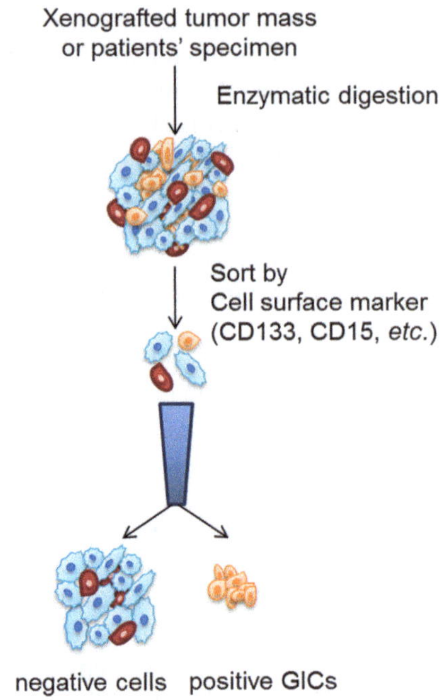

Fig. 11.1 Isolation of GICs and non-GICs by the cell surface markers. Xenografted tumors or patients' specimens are firstly dissociated by enzyme such as papain, then stained by the antibodies against specific cell surface markers (CD133, CD15), and finally separated by magnetic microbeads or flow cytometry to obtain GICs and non-GICs

11.2.2.1 Isolation of GICs by Cell Surface Marker CD133

CD133 is a cell surface glycoprotein that is expressed in hematopoietic stem cells [11], endothelial progenitor cells [12], neuron stem cells [13], and cancer stem cells [14]. As CD133 is highly expressed in GICs compared to non-GICs, one protocol is using CD133 to enrich GICs from patient's specimen or from glioma lines that are originally isolated from patients' specimens and maintained through serial passages in athymic BALB/v nu/nu mice as subcutaneous xenografts. This is an established experimental procedure that has been validated for the isolation of GICs in the previous studies from our laboratory and many other groups [2, 3, 7, 8]. Figure 11.1 shows the general steps of this approach.

1. Freshly harvest patients' specimens or patient-derived xenografted tumors with sterilized scissors and forceps. Transfer the tumors or specimen into 60 mm dish, and cut the tissue thoroughly until completely mashed using two razor blades that are placed side by side tightly.
2. Dissociate tumor tissues. Papain Dissociation System (Worthington Biochemical, Cat. No. LK003150) is used to dissociate tumors/specimen. Usually one vial of papain and DNase will be used to dissociate one tumor that is 0.3–0.4 cm^3 in volume.

   (a) According to the manufacturer's instructions in detail, 5 ml of EBSS (vial 1) is added into papain (vial 2), making a solution with 20 U of papain per ml in 1 mM L-cysteine and 0.5 mM EDTA. In the meantime, 0.5 ml of EBSS (vial 1) is added into DNase I (vial 3) to make a solution with 2000 U DNase I per ml. Briefly incubate the solutions to make sure full solubility. Avoid vigorous mixing. Add papain and DNase I solutions into mashed tumor tissues, mix, and incubate in 37 °C incubator with 5 % CO_2 for 30 min.

(b) 32 ml of EBSS (vial 1) is added into ovomucoid protease inhibitor (vial 4) to make a solution of 10 mg ovomucoid protease inhibitor and 10 mg albumin per ml. Equilibrate with sterile O_2:CO_2 before each use. After incubation with papain, add 5 ml of ovomucoid inhibitor into dissociated tissue, transfer into 50 ml tube through a cell strainer to remove aggregates. Wash the plate with Neurobasal medium without supplements, and transfer the medium into the same 50 ml tube through the cell strainer.

(c) Centrifuge the cell pellet with 1000 rpm for 5 min.

(d) Aspirate the supernatant carefully without disrupting the cell pellet. Add 10 ml PBS, mix, and add 30 ml sterilized distilled water into the cells to get rid of the blood cells. Quickly spin down the cells with 1500 rpm for 3 min. Avoid vigorous mixing after adding the water.

(e) Aspirate the supernatant. Improved MEM Zinc Option (with 10 % FBS and Antibiotics) is added into the cell pellet, followed by mixing and transferring into a new 50 ml tube through a new cell strainer.

(f) Centrifuge the cell pellet with 1000 rpm for 5 min.

(g) Aspirate the supernatant. Add a media mixture with 30 % of Improved MEM Zinc Option (with 10 % FBS and Antibiotics) and 70 % of Neurobasal media (supplemented with B27, 2 mM L-glutamine, 1 mM sodium pyruvate, 10 ng/ml bFGF, 10 ng/ml EGF and Antibiotics), mix, and plate the cells into cell culture plate.

3. Change media every other day. When cells are growing in confluent, dissociate the cells using trypsin–EDTA (0.05 %) for 10 min in 37 °C incubator with 5 % CO_2. Neutralize the trypsin with Improved MEM Zinc Option (10 % FBS and Antibiotics) and maintain the cells in the media with 30 % of Improved MEM Zinc Option and 70 % of Neurobasal media as described in Step 1(g) of Sect. 11.2.2.1.
4. Remove dead cells.

(a) Within 3 days of primary culture, dissociate the cells with trypsin–EDTA (0.05 %) and neutralize with Improved MEM Zinc Option (10 % FBS and Antibiotics).

(b) Transfer the dissociated cells into 15 or 50 ml tube. Centrifuge with 1000 rpm for 5 min.

(c) Aspirate the supernatant. Resuspend the cells with Neurobasal media (supplemented with B27, 2 mM L-glutamine, 1 mM sodium pyruvate, 10 ng/ml bFGF, 10 ng/ml EGF and Antibiotics). Plate the cells into petri dishes with untreated surface to reduce cell attachment on the plate. Depending on the cell numbers, plate the cells with appropriate density to avoid cell clumping. Incubate the cells in 37 °C incubator with 5 % CO_2 for 3–4 h.

(d) Mix the cells several times using pipet to destroy cell-cell attachment. Harvest and transfer the cells into 50 ml tubes through cell strainer to get rid of cell aggregates.

(e) Spin down the cells with 1000 rpm for 5 min. Remove supernatant completely.
(f) Dead cell removal kit (Miltenyi Biotech) is used to remove dead cells. According to manufacturer's instructions, prepare 1× binding buffer by diluting 20× binding buffer with sterile, double-distilled water. Resuspend cell pellet with 100 μl Dead Cell Removal Microbeads per 10^7 cells. Mix well and incubate for 10–15 min in room temperature.
(g) Use positive selection column, such as LS column (up to 10^8 dead cells and 2×10^9 total cells). Place the column in the magnetic field of the MACS Separator.
(h) Rinse the LS column with 3 ml 1× binding buffer.
(i) Add 5 ml 1× binding buffer into cell-microbeads mixture. Apply cells suspension onto the column to let the negative cells pass through. Rinse with 3 ml 1× binding buffer for four times. Collect effluent as live cell fraction.

5. Using CD133 microbead to separate CD133+ GICs and CD133– cells.

(a) Spin down the cells with 1000 rpm for 5 min. Remove supernatant completely.
(b) To avoid cell clumping, make Neurobasal Medium with 0.5 % BSA and 2 mM EDTA for magnetic labeling.
(c) Wash the cell pellets with Neurobasal Medium (0.5 % BSA and 2 mM EDTA). Determine cell number. Centrifuge and remove supernatant.
(d) Resuspend cell pellet in 300 μl Neurobasal Medium (0.5 % BSA and 2 mM EDTA) per 10^8 total cells.
(e) Add 100 μl FcR blocking reagent and 100 μl CD133 microbeads per 10^8 total cells.
(f) Mix well and incubate in room temperature for 50 min. Gently mix the cells every 10 min.
(g) Wash cells with 30 ml Neurobasal Medium (0.5 % BSA and 2 mM EDTA). Centrifuge with 1000 rpm for 5 min. Remove supernatant completely.
(h) Resuspend the cells with 5 ml Neurobasal Medium (0.5 % BSA and 2 mM EDTA). Gently mix the cells.
(i) Use LS column to positively select for the CD133+ cells. Place the column in the magnetic field of the MACS Separator.
(j) Rinse the column with 3 ml Neurobasal Medium (0.5 % BSA and 2 mM EDTA). Always wait until the column reservoir is empty before applying media/cell suspension.
(k) Apply cell suspension onto column.
(l) Rinse the column with 3 ml Neurobasal Medium (0.5 % BSA and 2 mM EDTA) for three times.
(m) Collect the effluent for depletion later.
(n) Remove the LS column from the MACS Separator and put on a collection tube.
(o) Add 5 ml Neurobasal media (supplemented with B27, 2 mM L-glutamine, 1 mM sodium pyruvate, 10 ng/ml bFGF, 10 ng/ml EGF and Antibiotics)

onto the column. Immediately flush out the magnetically labeled cells by pushing the plunger into the column.

(p) Repeat the previous step one more time. The cells collected are CD133+ GICs. Determine the cell numbers and maintain the CD133+ GICs in 37 °C incubator with 5 % CO_2. Cells will form spheres in culture.

(q) Prepare the LD columns for depletion. Put the column onto magnetic field of MACS Separator. Rinse column with 2 ml Neurobasal Medium (0.5 % BSA and 2 mM EDTA).

(r) Spin down the cells that are harvested from Step 5(m) of Sect. 11.2.2.1 with 1000 rpm for 5 min. Remove the supernatant completely.

(s) Resuspend the cells with 3 ml Neurobasal Medium (0.5 % BSA and 2 mM EDTA) and apply onto LD column.

(t) Collect unlabeled cells that pass through the column. Those cells are the CD133- cells. Centrifuge and remove the supernatant.

(u) Resuspend the cells in Improved MEM Zinc Option (10 % FBS and Antibiotics). Determine the cell numbers and maintain the CD133− cells in tissue culture plate in 37 °C incubator with 5 % CO_2. Cells will attach to the plate.

(v) Calculate the percentage of CD133+ and CD133− cells among the total cells before separation.

6. Evaluate the purity of CD133+ and CD133− cells separated by microbeads.

   (a) Prepare samples: for confirmation of positive selection of CD133+ cells and negative selection of CD133− cells, prepare an unstained control, a population from the nonselected cells, a population from the positively selected cells, and a population from the negatively selected cells.

   (b) Count negative and positive populations with Trypan Blue for staining dead cells, and suspend each sample at 2×10^7 viable cells/mL in 100 μl buffer.

   (c) Vortex sample briefly. Incubate with Anti-FcR diluted at a volume of 1:100 at room temperature for 15 min after a brief vortex to mix.

   (d) Vortex sample briefly. Add 10 μl CD133/2-PE (293C3); incubate at 2–8 °C for 30 min in the dark after a brief vortex to mix. If confirming positive selection, be sure to utilize an antibody specific for an epitope not used for the selection.

   (e) Add 1 mL of FACS buffer. Vortex sample briefly. Centrifuge at 1500 rpm for 5 min to wash sample.

   (f) Aspirate excess buffer. Add 1 mL of FACS buffer. Vortex sample briefly. Centrifuge at 1500 rpm for 5 min to wash sample a second time.

   (g) For immediate analysis, aspirate excess buffer and resuspend cells at 1×10^7 viable cells/mL in FACS buffer. Vortex briefly; incubate on ice until analysis. For later analysis, aspirate excess buffer and resuspend cells in 100 μL 2 % paraformaldehyde in PBS for 30 min at room temperature in the dark. Vortex briefly. After fixation, wash twice with 1 mL of FACS buffer as in Steps 6(e) and (f) of Sect. 11.2.1, and subsequently aspirate excess buffer and resuspend cells at 1×10^7 viable cells/mL in FACS buffer. Vortex briefly.

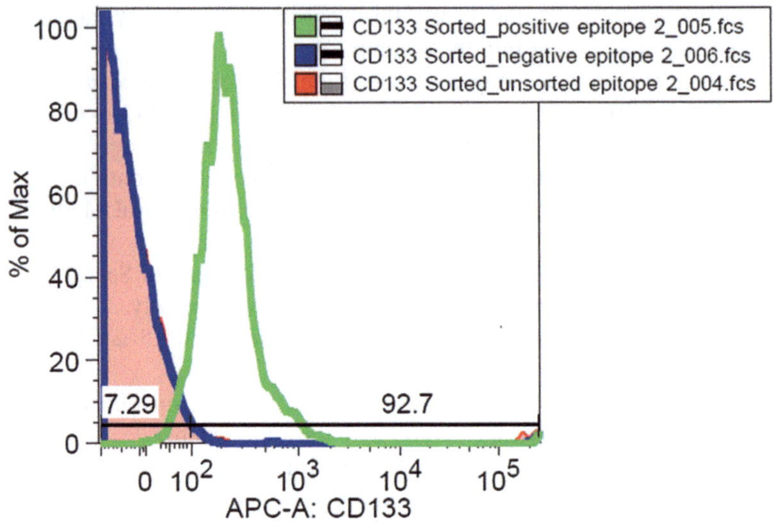

GateName	SampleName	Freq. of Parent
CD133+	CD133 Sorted_unsorted epitope 2_004.fcs	1.38
CD133-	CD133 Sorted_unsorted epitope 2_004.fcs	98.6
CD133+	CD133 Sorted_negative epitope 2_006.fcs	1.15
CD133-	CD133 Sorted_negative epitope 2_006.fcs	98.8
CD133+	CD133 Sorted_positive epitope 2_005.fcs	92.7
CD133-	CD133 Sorted_positive epitope 2_005.fcs	7.29

Fig. 11.2 Purity of CD133+ and CD133− cells separated by microbeads. Unsorted cells, cells positively sorted by CD133-microbeads, and cells negatively depleted by CD133-microbeads were stained with CD133/2-PE (293C3) as described in the protocol. The percentage of CD133+ and CD133− cells was analyzed by flow cytometry. The *table* shows the percentage of CD133+ and CD133− cells in each group (unsorted cells, positively sorted cells, negative depleted cells)

Incubate at 4 °C in the dark until analysis. Perform analysis utilizing the unstained control for calibration and to choose fluorescence gates. As shown in Fig. 11.2, the percentage of CD133+ cells measured by FACS is usually more than 90 % after microbeads separation, suggesting a positive separation by this method.

7. Alternative method: Using fluorescence-activated cell sorting to sort out CD133+ GICs and CD133− cells. Prepare an unstained control and the samples stained with 10 μl CD133/2-PE (293C3)/10^7 cells for sorting. Resuspend cells at 1×10^7 viable cells/mL in FACS buffer. Vortex briefly. Incubate on ice until sorting. Perform sorting under sterile conditions, utilizing the unstained control for calibration and to choose fluorescence gates.

With this approach, 5–15 % of the tumor cells were found to be CD133+ from multiple glioma lines in our lab, with the percentage of those cells increased modestly along with passage number of the xenografted tumors [7]. Consistently, studies from multiple groups also show that proportion of CD133+ cells ranged from 3 to 29 % in glioma patient samples [2, 3]. Although there might be impurity in the isolated populations, for example CD133– GICs in the CD133– cells, the biological properties between CD133+ and CD133– differ dramatically. Isolated CD133+ cells possess higher abilities to form neurospheres and intracranial tumors when limited number of cells were tested, compared to the CD133– cells [7], indicating that this method is valid for enriching GICs.

11.2.2.2 Isolation of GICs by Cell Surface Marker CD15

CD133– GICs have been identified from several reports [15–17], suggesting that CD133 may not be a universal marker to enrich GICs. CD15, also called SSEA-1, is a cell surface molecule that is highly expressed in pluripotent stem cells, cancer stem cells of medulloblastoma and glioblastoma. As an alternative approach to CD133, CD15 is also commonly used for isolating GICs [7–8, 17–19].

1. Freshly harvest tumor specimen and dissociate tumor tissues (same with Steps 1 and 2 of Sect. 11.2.2.1).
2. Maintain primary culture of cancer cells and remove dead cells (same with Steps 3 and 4 of Sect. 11.2.2.1).
3. Using CD15 microbeads to separate CD15+ GICs and CD15– cells. Similarly with 1.5, cells are incubated in 80 μl Neurobasal medium (0.5 % BSA, 2 mM EDTA) and 20 μl CD15 microbeads per 10^7 total cells in 2–8 °C according to manufacturer's instructions. The cell suspension is applied to the LS column, followed by wash with three times for positive selection of CD15+ GICs. LD column is used to negatively select CD15– cells. Flow cytometry analysis is performed to analyze the purity of CD15+ and CD15– cells after microbeads separation. Cells before and after separation are incubated with 5 μl (0.125 μg) anti-Human CD15 FITC (eBioscience) in a final volume of 100 μl in 4 °C for 10–15 min, followed by the flow cytometry analysis.
4. Alternative method: Using flow cytometry to sort out CD15+ GICs and CD15– cells. Incubate 10^7 cell suspension with 5 μl (0.125 μg) anti-Human CD15 FITC in a final volume of 100 μl in 4 °C for 30 min, followed by the flow cytometry sorting to separate CD15+ and CD15– cells. Figure 11.3 shows examples of separation of CD15+ and CD15– cells from three different glioma xenografts.

With this method, 2–50 % of the tumor cells were found to be CD15+ from multiple glioma lines in our lab. Consistently, 2–70 % of CD15+ GICs have been identified in a separate study [17]. Interestingly, CD15 has been reported to enrich specifically the PN/CIMP– subclass of GICs [20]. Similar with CD133+ cells, CD15+ cells also possess higher ability to self-renew, examined by expression of stemness genes and neurosphere formation, as well as initiate intracranial tumors, suggesting that it's a valid approach to enrich GICs [17].

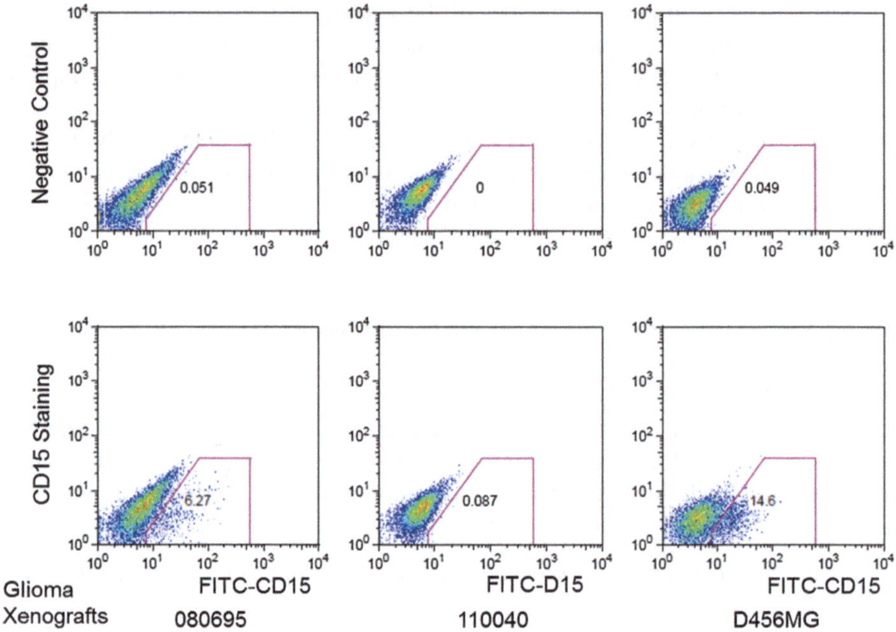

Fig. 11.3 Separation of CD15+ and CD15- cells by flow cytometry. As described in the protocol, cells dissociated from multiple glioma xenografts (080695, 110040, D456MG) were stained with CD15 antibody. CD15+ and CD15- cells were sorted by flow cytometry. The *numbers* showed the percentage of CD15+ cells

11.2.2.3 Isolation of GICs by Specific Medium

Besides the cell surface markers mentioned above, studies have been reported that specific culturing condition that is optimal for maintaining and propagating normal neural stem cells (NSC) can generate neurosphere cultures of self-renewing GICs with both CD133+ and CD133– populations [16, 21].

1. Same with Steps 1 and 2 of Sect 11.2.2.1, freshly harvest tumor specimen and dissociate tumor tissues.
2. Maintain and propagate GICs in Neurobasal media (supplemented with B27, 2 mM L-glutamine, 1 mM sodium pyruvate, 10 ng/ml bFGF, 10 ng/ml EGF and Antibiotics) to generate neurosphere cultures.
3. Maintain the non-GICs in Improved MEM Zinc Option (10 % FBS and Antibiotics).

Studies from our lab and other groups have compared the properties between the neurosphere cultures and the cells cultured with serum. Consistent results have been obtained that neurosphere cultures maintain stem cell features including expression of stemness genes, self-renewal, and initiating intracranial tumors [7, 16, 21].

11.3 Troubleshooting

1. Impure population of CD133+/– (or CD15+/–) cells after microbeads separation.

   (a) False positive population after positive separation. Cancer cells are very sticky and easily form cell aggregates during the procedure of recovering from trypsin (Step 4(c) of Sect. 11.2.2.1) and antibody incubation (Step 5(f) of Sect. 11.2.2.1). These cell clumps including both CD133+ (CD15+) and CD133– (CD15-) cells may be stuck in the LS column and flushed out in the positive selection, resulting in false positive selection. If this happens, lots of cell aggregates can be detected under the microscope after flushed out from the column. Re-separate the cells to increase purity. To avoid cell clumping, be sure to add EDTA in the buffer and mix the cells well during the procedures. In addition, lower the cell density in Steps 4(c) and 5(f) of Sect. 11.2.2.1.

   (b) False negative population after negative selection. It is most possible that the CD133 (CD15) microbeads are detached from the cells, probably because of vigorous wash and suspension of cells after staining in step 5(f–h) of Sect. 11.2.2.1. Mix more gently. Record the percentage of CD133+ GICs and CD133– cells among the total unseparated cells every time and compare with previous separations for the same glioma xenograft. If there is dramatically lower percentage of CD133+ and higher percentage of CD133– cells, there might be false negative selection and separation needs to be re-performed.

2. No viable cells after tumor dissociation. The qualities of different tumor specimens vary differently. In general, glioma-xenografted tumors may need more harsh conditions to dissociate (longer incubation time, more papain, etc.), compared to GBM specimens from patients. Overdissociation may be harmful for the cells from the patients' specimens. Optimize the condition with less papain and shorter incubation time (less than 30 min). If the GBM tissues from patients are mainly from the necrotic region, it is common that few viable cells can be successfully dissociated.
3. No differences in the biological properties of self-renewal and tumor initiation comparing CD133+ (CD15+) with CD133– (CD15–) cells. There are several possibilities. Firstly, CD133 and CD15 may not be the universal marker in the cells dissociated from the specific patient's specimen. If this is the case, use other separation marker such as α_6-integrin [22], side population assay [23], and the specific neurosphere culture to separate the two populations. Second, it's possible that examination of the biological properties is performed long time after separating and culturing the cells in vitro. GICs tend to differentiate and lose the stemness after in vitro culture for many passages. In the meantime, non-GICs may be selected to grow aggressively during in vitro culture. Therefore, for biological studies, we normally maintain the primary culture for 3 days after dissociation from the tumor; culture GICs within a month and non-GICs within 1 week

after separation from the tumor mass. Furthermore, it's important to maintain the glioma lines as xenografted tumors in mice which possess many features of the parental tumors even after a long series of passages. Dissociate cells from the tumor or patients' specimens freshly and separate GICs and non-GICs immediately after primary culture. Don't separate GICs and non-GICs from the frozen cells and never freeze GICs and non-GICs for the future study. Based on our experience, non-GICs separated from the frozen cells or frozen non-GICs showed dramatically enhanced abilities to form neurospheres compared to non-GICs separated from the fresh tumor for the same glioma xenograft, possibly because that DMSO in the frozen media or other frozen conditions could stimulate the aggressiveness in non-GICs.

11.4 Conclusion

Isolation of GICs and non-GICs is the initial step for biological studies to investigate mechanisms underlying the malignant nature of GICs and GBM. This protocol provides detailed procedures to separate GICs and non-GICs from GBM patients' specimens and glioma-derived xenografted tumors. Three commonly used approaches are elaborated. As there is no universal marker for GICs and non-GICs currently, neither of these methods is sufficient to isolate the pure population of GICs or non-GICs. Therefore, it's necessary to apply multiple approaches for enrichment of GICs and verification of the experimental results.

References

1. Ostrom QT, et al. CBTRUS statistical report: primary brain and central nervous system tumors diagnosed in the United States in 2007–2011. Neuro Oncol. 2014;16 Suppl 4:p. iv1–63.
2. Singh SK et al. Identification of human brain tumour initiating cells. Nature. 2004;432(7015):396–401.
3. Bao S et al. Glioma stem cells promote radioresistance by preferential activation of the DNA damage response. Nature. 2006;444(7120):756–60.
4. Bao SD et al. Glioma stem cells promote radioresistance by preferential activation of the DNA damage response. Nature. 2006;444(7120):756–60.
5. Eramo A et al. Chemotherapy resistance of glioblastoma stem cells. Cell Death Differ. 2006;13(7):1238–41.
6. Chen J et al. A restricted cell population propagates glioblastoma growth after chemotherapy. Nature. 2012;488(7412):522–6.
7. Wang H et al. miR-33a promotes glioma-initiating cell self-renewal via PKA and NOTCH pathways. J Clin Investig. 2014;124(10):4489–502.
8. Hu J et al. MiR-215 is induced post-transcriptionally via HIF-Drosha complex and mediates glioma-initiating cell adaptation to hypoxia by targeting KDM1B. Cancer Cell. 2016;29(1): 49–60.
9. Ernst A et al. Genomic and expression profiling of glioblastoma stem cell-like spheroid cultures identifies novel tumor-relevant genes associated with survival. Clin Cancer Res. 2009;15(21):6541–50.

10. Schraivogel D et al. CAMTA1 is a novel tumour suppressor regulated by miR-9/9*in glioblastoma stem cells. EMBO J. 2011;30(20):4309–22.
11. Yin AH et al. AC133, a novel marker for human hematopoietic stem and progenitor cells. Blood. 1997;90(12):5002–12.
12. Peichev M et al. Expression of VEGFR-2 and AC133 by circulating human CD34(+) cells identifies a population of functional endothelial precursors. Blood. 2000;95(3):952–8.
13. Uchida N et al. Direct isolation of human central nervous system stem cells. Proc Natl Acad Sci U S A. 2000;97(26):14720–5.
14. Medema JP. Cancer stem cells: the challenges ahead. Nat Cell Biol. 2013;15(4):338–44.
15. Beier D et al. CD133(+) and CD133(-) glioblastoma-derived cancer stem cells show differential growth characteristics and molecular profiles. Cancer Res. 2007;67(9):4010–5.
16. Chen R et al. A hierarchy of self-renewing tumor-initiating cell types in glioblastoma. Cancer Cell. 2010;17(4):362–75.
17. Son MJ et al. SSEA-1 is an enrichment marker for tumor-initiating cells in human glioblastoma. Cell Stem Cell. 2009;4(5):440–52.
18. Read TA et al. Identification of CD15 as a marker for tumor-propagating cells in a mouse model of medulloblastoma (vol 15, pg 135, 2009). Cancer Cell. 2009;16(3):267–7.
19. Suva ML et al. Reconstructing and reprogramming the tumor-propagating potential of glioblastoma stem-like cells. Cell. 2014;157(3):580–94.
20. Bhat KP et al. Mesenchymal differentiation mediated by NF-kappaB promotes radiation resistance in glioblastoma. Cancer Cell. 2013;24(3):331–46.
21. Lee J et al. Tumor stem cells derived from glioblastomas cultured in bFGF and EGF more closely mirror the phenotype and genotype of primary tumors than do serum-cultured cell lines. Cancer Cell. 2006;9(5):391–403.
22. Lathia JD et al. Integrin Alpha 6 regulates glioblastoma stem cells. Cell Stem Cell. 2010;6(5):421–32.
23. Kondo T, Setoguchi T, Taga T. Persistence of a small subpopulation of cancer stem-like cells in the C6 glioma cell line. Proc Natl Acad Sci U S A. 2004;101(3):781–6.

[illegible]

Chapter 12
Isolation of Mouse and Human Tumor-Associated Macrophages

Luca Cassetta, Roy Noy, Agnieszka Swierczak, Gaël Sugano, Harriet Smith, Lisa Wiechmann, and Jeffrey W. Pollard

Abstract The tumor microenvironment is a complex network of cells that support tumor progression and malignancy. It has been demonstrated that tumor cells can educate the immune system to promote a tumor-friendly environment. Among all these immune cells, tumor-associated macrophages (TAMs) are well represented and their presence in mouse models has been shown to promote tumor progression and metastasis. These effects are through the stimulation of angiogenesis, enhancement of tumor cell invasion and intravasation, immunosuppression, and at the metastatic site tumor cell extravasation and growth. However, the precise mechanisms are not fully understood. Furthermore there is limited information on TAMs derived from human cancers. For this reason it is important to be able to extract TAMs from tumors in order to compare their phenotypes, functions, and transcriptomes with normal resident tissue macrophages. Isolation of these cells is challenging due to the lack of markers and standardized protocols. Here we show an optimized protocol for the efficient isolation and extraction of resident macrophages and TAMs from

L. Cassetta • A. Swierczak • G. Sugano
MRC Centre for Reproductive Health, Queen's Medical Research Institute,
The University of Edinburgh, Edinburgh EH16 4TJ, UK
e-mail: Luca.Cassetta@ed.ac.uk; A.Swierczak@ed.ac.uk; gsugano@staffmail.ed.ac.uk

R. Noy
Department of Developmental and Molecular Biology, , New York, NY 10461, USA
e-mail: roy.noy@einstein.yu.edu

H. Smith
Department of Obstetrics and Gynecology and Women's Health, New York, NY 10461, USA
e-mail: hasmith@montefiore.org

L. Wiechmann
Department of Surgery, Albert Einstein College of Medicine, New York, NY 10461, USA
e-mail: lisawiechmann@gmail.com

J.W. Pollard (✉)
MRC Centre for Reproductive Health, Queen's Medical Research Institute,
The University of Edinburgh, Edinburgh EH16 4TJ, UK

Department of Developmental and Molecular Biology, , New York, NY 10461, USA
e-mail: Jeff.Pollard@ed.ac.uk

C. Koumenis et al. (eds.), *Tumor Microenvironment*, Advances in Experimental Medicine and Biology 899, DOI 10.1007/978-3-319-26666-4_12

human and mouse tissues by using multicolor flow cytometry. These protocols allow for the extraction of thousands of macrophages in less than 5 h from tissues as small as half a gram. The isolated macrophages can then be used for both "omics" and in vitro studies.

Keywords Tumor-associated macrophages • Macrophages • TAM • Breast cancer • Flow cytometry • Tissue • Mouse • Human

12.1 Introduction

Whole tissues are highly complex environments comprised of extracellular matrix and many cells types whose diversity depends on the organ but always includes epithelial cells and cells of mesenchymal origin such as blood vessels and fibroblasts as well as a diversity of immune cells. In solid cancers the epithelial cells are transformed and subsequently progress to malignancy that can lead to metastasis. The tumor cells recruit around them a specialized microenvironment that is often characterized by an intense infiltration of cells of the immune system such as T and B cells, neutrophils, and macrophages. These tumors resemble organs but with an overall lack of organization and thus have been referred to as "outlaw organs." In both tissues and tumors stromal cells can carry out a myriad of functions and different cell types within tissues can have opposing roles.

Most cancer studies have assessed whole tumor tissues but recent work has shown that isolating stromal cells can be more effective for identifying prognostic markers [1]. Hence it is important to study these cell types individually to better understand how they are involved in tumor progression. Indeed, in most cases, high macrophage density correlates with poor prognosis [2–10]. Tumor-associated macrophages (TAMs) have been shown to regulate many critical processes associated with malignancy including promotion of tumor cell migration [11–13], invasion and metastasis [14, 15], induction of the angiogenesis [16, 17], and seeding of metastatic cells, and support of their growth, at distant sites [18–20].

There are a number of methods to assess macrophage and TAM function and phenotype; these include (1) gene expression analysis [21–23]; (2) functional studies; (3) assessment of cytokine and chemokine production [24, 25]; and (4) analysis of protein expression and cell surface markers [26]. In order to carry out these analyses macrophages/TAMs must first be isolated from the tissue.

The most common methods to isolate macrophages include (1) magnetic bead-conjugated antibody cell isolation [27], (2) density gradient separation [28], (3) laser capture microdissection [29], and (4) digestion followed by fluorescence-activated cell sorting (FACS) [21]. Magnetic cell isolation is a relatively fast technique but is limited in regard to how many markers can be used to separate macrophages and TAMs from the other stromal cell types. Many immune cells share the same markers and it is rare to find only one marker that labels a particular immune cell type. While the density gradient method is cheap, it relies on differences in cell size and density to separate the cells leading to problems with purity. Laser capture microdissection, although allowing for isolation of cells according to spatial position and morphology, can only utilize 2–3 markers, requires the fixation of cells, is very slow, and yields low numbers of cells. These methods are a particular problem for macrophages as they are extremely heterogeneous and express a range of cell surface markers as well as being easily damaged. Therefore, FACS is particularly useful for isolating resident macrophages and TAMs as it allows for the use of multiple cell surface markers simultaneously; this not only leads to a higher purity of the isolated macrophages/TAMs but also allows for phenotypic analysis. Commonly used markers for mouse macrophage isolation are CD11b, F4/80, and Ly6G/C antigens [30, 31] while CD14, CD11b, HLA-DR, CD163, and CX3CR1 antigens are used to identify human resident macrophages and TAMs [32–34].

The first step to isolating macrophages and TAMs from tissues is to digest the tissue to get a single-cell suspension. A number of different digestion methods exist that involve different incubation periods, agitation speeds, and enzymes [35–37], but no protocol so far has been optimized for primary macrophage isolation. Moreover some digestion methods can result in loss of cell surface markers [38–40]; therefore we have developed a protocol where the cell surface markers remain intact. In this chapter we review the FACS methods developed in our laboratory over the last few years for isolation and analysis of macrophages and TAMs from mouse and human normal mammary tissue and breast tumors.

12.2 Protocol for Isolation of Resident Macrophages and TAMs from Mouse and Human Tumors

12.2.1 Before You Start

1. Mouse care and husbandry—all mouse work must be performed after approval and according to in-house institute protocols and appropriate national guidelines.
2. Human clinical samples—clinical samples must be collected following local ethics regulations and only after appropriate approval from the institution.
3. This protocol has been used extensively for the isolation of TAMs from mouse mammary tumors (PyMT model, [41]) and human breast tumors, but it can be used for isolation of TAMs from other solid tumors; this protocol has been optimized for 150–750 mg tumors and therefore volume adjustments need to be made for analysis of smaller or larger tumors (see troubleshooting).
4. It is recommended to use tumor-bearing mice that are within normal parameters in all other aspects including weight, injury, necrotic tissue, and infection.
5. For cellular assays and in vivo experiments sterile conditions must be maintained. The protocols must be carried out in a biohazard level 2 hood and all buffers must be filtered using 0.22 μm filters.

6. For multicolor staining, fluorescence compensation is required; we recommend using compensation beads (see troubleshooting).
7. This protocol is optimized for the identification and the isolation of resident tissue macrophages and TAMs; therefore we included only a set of basic extracellular markers; additional TAM markers, cytokines, and transcription factors or extracellular markers may be incorporated to the basic protocol in order to identify TAM subpopulations or particular functions.
8. Analysis of rare immune cell populations requires the collection of at least 5–10,000 events of the smallest population in order to ensure statistical power for analysis.
9. In addition to the experimental samples, negative unstained controls, isotype controls, and FMOs (fluorescence minus one) must be prepared (see troubleshooting).
10. This protocol requires 4–5 h of time.

12.2.2 Materials

- 60 and 100 mm petri dishes (Thermoscientific)
- Razor blades
- Forceps and surgical scissors for animal dissection (Fine Surgical Tools)
- DMEM (Gibco)
- 15 and 50 ml tubes (Falcon)
- 2 ml DNase and RNase-free collection tubes (Simport)
- 5 ml Polypropylene tubes (with and without filter cap) (Falcon)
- 10× Red blood cell (RBC) lysis buffer (eBioscience)
- Enzymes: Liberase TL and Liberase DL (Roche)
- DNase I (Sigma)
- Phosphate-buffered saline (PBS) (Gibco)
- Bovine serum albumin (BSA) (Sigma)
- 100 μm Cell strainers (Corning)
- Ethanol (EtOH)
- Isoflurane
- Blocking antibody (Ab) CD16/CD32 (eBioscience)
- Antibodies (Abs) for flow cytometry (see Tables 12.1 and 12.2)
- DAPI (eBioscience)
- Human AB serum (Lonza)
- Penicillin/streptomycin (Gibco)

12.2.3 Lab Equipment

- Vortex
- Lab centrifuge (TX-1000 rotor, 290 mm radius)
- Lab bench centrifuge (FA 45-30-11 rotor)

- Lab scale
- Flow cytometer
- Flow sorter
- Pipetman
- Pipettes

12.2.4 Solutions

- Staining buffer: PBS 2 % w/v BSA.
- Sorting buffer: PBS 0.1 % w/v BSA.
- Collection medium: DMEM 10 % v/v FBS, 1 % penicillin/streptomycin.
- 1× RBC lysis buffer: Dilute 10× RBC buffer in distilled water.
- Enzymes: Resuspend the lyophilized powder following the manufacturer's instructions. Make aliquots and avoid freeze and thawing.

12.2.5 Isolation of Resident Macrophages and TAMs from Mouse Primary Tissue

Tissue type: mouse mammary carcinomas, normal mammary gland
Average tissue weight: 0.5–1 g
Macrophages isolated with this protocol: resident tissue macrophages and TAMs

12.2.5.1 Tissue Extraction and Digestion

1. Anesthetize mice using CO_2 or isoflurane, followed by cervical dislocation.
2. In the case of mammary tumors gently remove the abdominal skin without tearing the peritoneal cavity (for other solid tumors remove the tumor according to an appropriate protocol).
3. Locate the local draining lymph node and remove it using forceps.
4. Gently separate the tumor from the skin using forceps and surgical scissors.
5. Transfer the tumor to a 60 mm petri dish and record the tumor weight.
6. Add 1 ml of medium without serum (if more than one tumor is processed keep on ice until further use; it is not recommended to keep the tumors at room temperature for any period of time).
7. Using a razor blade cut the tumor into small pieces (the efficiency of the digestion is dependent on how well the tumor is minced; large pieces will not digest properly and may need extra digestion time) (Fig. 12.1a).
8. Transfer the tumor lysates into a 15 ml tube using a P1000 pipette (cut the top of the tip in order to be able to take all the tissue) and adjust the volume to 4 ml of serum-free PBS.

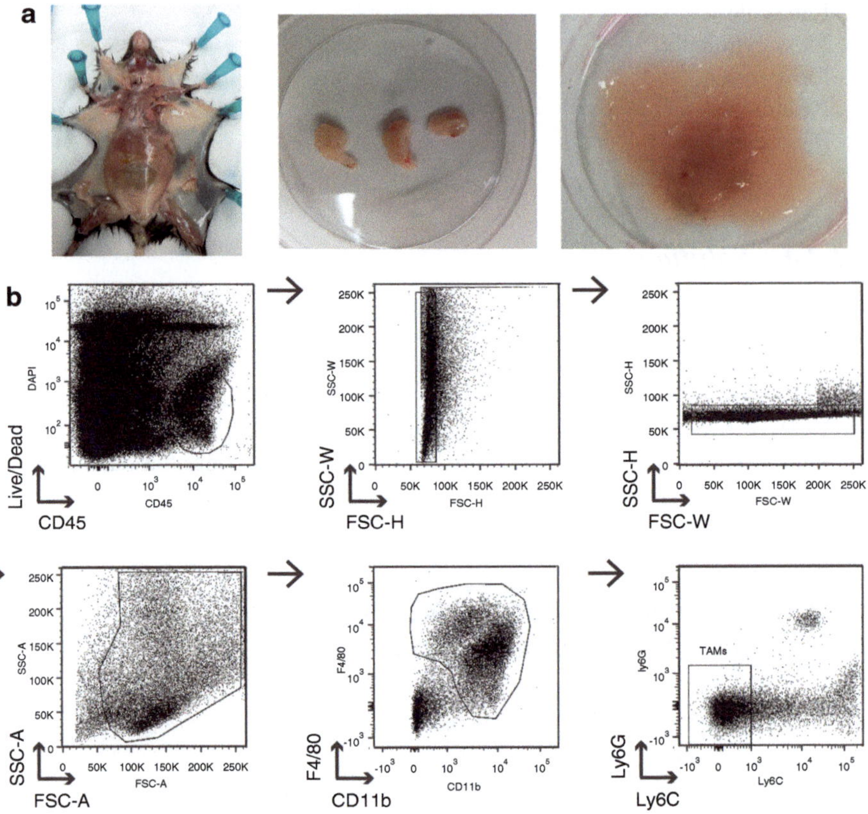

Fig. 12.1 Isolation of TAMs from mouse mammary tumors. (**a**) Representative images of mouse mammary tumor excision and processing; tumor-bearing mouse is euthanized and mammary tumors are exposed, and draining lymph nodes removed with forceps (*left panel*); tumors are excised from the skin using forceps and surgical scissors and transferred in a 60 mm petri dish (*central panel*); 1 ml of serum-free medium is added and tumor is cut into small pieces using a razor blade (*right panel*). (**b**) Representative gating strategy for the identification of TAMs in mouse tumors. TAMs are defined as $DAPI^-$, $CD45^+$, $CD11b^+$, $F4/80^+$, $Ly6C^-$, and $Ly6G^-$. First cells that are viable (DAPI negative) and are CD45 positive (to exclude nonimmune cells) are selected. All cells that are $CD11b^+$ and $F4/80^+$ are then selected (both markers are expressed by macrophages). In this particular analysis we gated also some $CD11b^+$ $F4/80^-$ in order to show the $Ly6G^+$ granulocyte population. Finally cells that are Ly6G- and Ly6C- (markers that are not expressed by mature macrophages, but mainly on monocytes and granulocytes) are selected

9. Add 40 μl of Liberase DL stock solution 28U/ml (Roche), 80 μl of Liberase TL stock solution 14 U/ml (Roche), and 40 μl of DNase I (15 mg/ml stock solution Sigma 100×). Mix using a vortex and incubate for 45 min at 37 °C under continuous rotation.
10. Check the sample visually; the cell suspension should look smooth (if the cell suspension still contains tissue fragments digest for an additional 15 min).

If after 15 min there are still tissue fragments remaining this is connective tissue that will not digest and there is no need for further digestion.

11. To end the enzymatic digestion add 10 ml PBS 1 % w/vBSA (staining buffer).
12. Filter the cells using a 100 μm cell strainer in a 50 ml tube and adjust the volume to 20 ml with staining buffer.
13. Centrifuge for 7 min at 500 rcf and 4 °C. Discard the supernatant.
14. Proceed to red blood cell lysis (Sect. 12.10.2.5.2).

12.2.5.2 Red Blood Cell Lysis

1. Add 3 ml of 1× RBC lysis buffer to the tumor pellet from Step 1.14, mix well, and incubate on ice for 10 min.
2. Add 30 ml of staining buffer.
3. Centrifuge for 7 min at 500 rcf and 4 °C. Discard the supernatant and resuspend the pellet in 1 ml of staining buffer.
4. Transfer to a 5 ml polypropylene tube.
5. Proceed to blocking (Sect. 10.2.5.3).

12.2.5.3 Blocking

1. Add 2 μl (1:500) of blocking Ab CD16/CD32 (clone 93), mix well, and incubate on ice for a minimum of 30 min (mix every 10 min).
2. Add 4 ml of staining buffer and centrifuge for 5 min at 500 rcf and 4 °C. Discard the supernatant, resuspend the pellet in 1 ml of staining buffer, and proceed to FACS staining for analysis (Sect. 10.2.5.4) or FACS staining for sorting (Sect. 10.2.5.5).

12.2.5.4 FACS Staining and Analysis

1. Count the cells (trypan blue exclusion method) and adjust the number to $1\text{–}2 \times 10^6$ cells/ml.
2. Transfer 1 ml into a 5 ml polystyrene tube.
3. Centrifuge for 5 min at 500 rcf and 4 °C. Discard the supernatant and resuspend the pellet in 100 μl of staining buffer.
4. Add the antibody master mix (see Table 12.1).

Table 12.1 Antibody master mix for FACS analysis and sorting, mouse tissue

Antigen and fluorochrome	Clone
CD45 APC	30-F11
CD11b eFluor 605	M1/70
F4/80 PerCp-Cy5.5	BM8
Ly6C PE-Cy7	HK1.4
Ly6G APC-Cy7	1A8
DAPI	

5. Incubate on ice for 1 h protected from the light.
6. Add 4 ml of staining buffer.
7. Filter using filter top 5 ml polystyrene tubes (40 μm) to prevent clogging the machine.
8. Centrifuge for 5 min at 500 rcf and 4 °c.
9. Resuspend the pellet in 2 ml of staining buffer.
10. Analyze using flow cytometer using the gating strategy (shown in Fig. 12.1b).

12.2.5.5 FACS Staining and Cell Sorting

1. After blocking add 9 ml of staining buffer and centrifuge for 7 min at 500 rcf and 4 °C. Discard the supernatant and resuspend the pellet in 100 μl of staining buffer.
2. Add the antibody master mix (see Table 12.1).
3. Incubate for 1 h on ice protected from light (mix every 10 min).
4. Wash once with a large volume of staining buffer, around 30–40 ml.
5. Centrifuge for 7 min at 500 rcf and 4 °C.
6. Discard the supernatant and resuspend the pellet in 2–5 ml (depending on the initial tumor size) of sorting buffer.
7. Sort TAMs as DAPI-, CD45+, CD11b+, F4/80+, Ly6C-, Ly6G-, CD3-, CD19-, and NK1.1-.
8. Sort cells into collection tubes that contain 1–2 ml of collection medium.
9. Sorted cells can be used for DNA, RNA, and protein extraction, in vitro experiments such as migration analysis, angiogenesis, T cell activation, or suppression, etc.

12.2.6 Isolation of TAMs and Resident Macrophages from Human Breast Tumor and Normal Adjacent Tissue

Tissue type: needle biopsies, surgical surplus
Tissue weight: 0.5–1 g
Macrophages isolated with this protocol: resident tissue macrophages and TAMs

Before starting: collect tissue in collection medium and keep it/store it at 4 °C.

12.2.6.1 Tissue Processing and Digestion

1. Transfer the tumor to a 60 mm petri dish, remove all medium with a pipette, and measure the tumor weight (Fig. 12.2a).
2. Add 1 ml of serum-free PBS (if more than one tumor is processed keep on ice until further use; it is not recommended to keep the tumors at room temperature for any time).

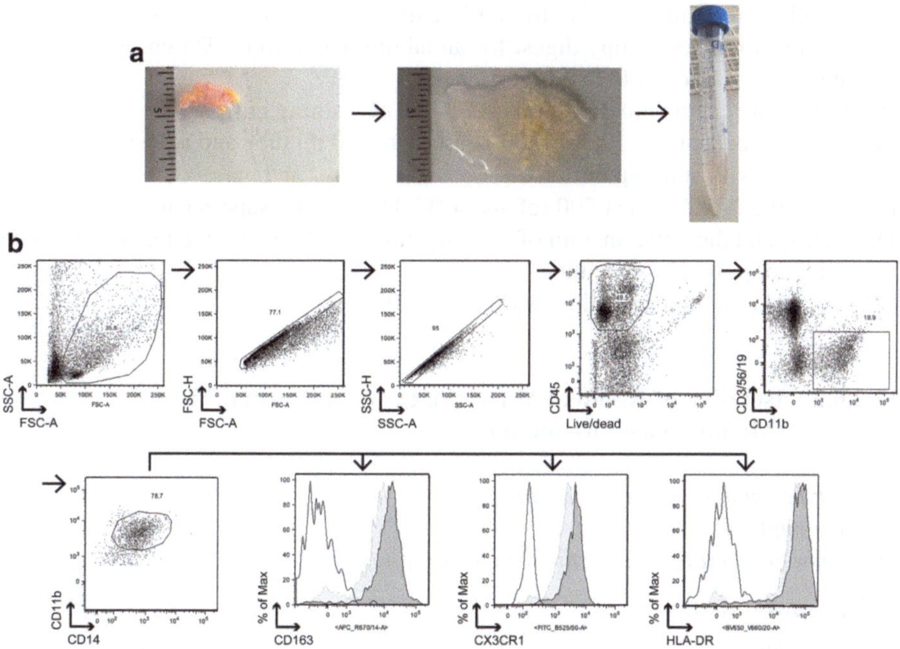

Fig. 12.2 Isolation of TAMs from human mammary tumors. (**a**) Representative images of human mammary tumor processing; after sample collection, medium is completely removed and the tumor is transferred in a 60 mm petri dish (*left panel*); 1 ml of serum-free PBS is added and tumor is cut into small pieces using a razor blade (*right panel*); after the digestion the mixture should look cloudy and >80 % of tissue fragments should be dissolved (*right panel*). (**b**) Representative gating strategy for the identification of resident and tumor-associated macrophages from human tissue. Tissue macrophages are defined as DAPI$^-$, CD45$^+$, CD11b$^+$, HLA-DR$^+$ CD14$^+$, CD3$^-$, CD19$^-$, and CD56$^-$. In addition, TAMs are CD163^{high} and CX3R1^{High} as shown in the histograms (*black-lined empty histogram*=isotype control, *light grey-colored histogram*=resident macrophages from normal mammary tissue, *dark grey-colored histogram*=TAMs from breast tumor). After adding a gate based on physical parameters (size and granularity) and after doublet removal, cells that are viable and CD45 positive are selected. A gate on CD11b$^+$ cells and negative for CD3 (T cells), CD56 (NK cells), and CD19 (B cells) identifies the myeloid cell populations in the tumor (granulocytes and macrophages mainly). Cells that are CD11b$^+$CD14$^+$CD163$^+$CX3CR1$^+$HLA-DR$^+$ are defined as macrophages

3. Using a razor blade cut the tumor into small pieces (the efficiency of the digestion is dependent on how well the tumor is minced, large pieces will not digest properly and may need more digestion time).
4. Transfer the tumor lysates to a 15 ml tube using a P1000 pipette (cut the top of the tip in order to be able to take all the tissue) and adjust the volume to 3 ml of serum-free PBS.
5. Add 30 μl of Liberase DL stock solution 28 U/ml (Roche), 120 μl of Liberase TL stock solution 14 U/ml (Roche), and 30 μl of DNase I (15 mg/ml stock solution Sigma 100×).
6. Mix using a vortex and incubate for 45 min at 37 °C applying continuous rotation or, if using a thermomixer, at 700/800 rpm.

7. Check digestion visually; the cell suspension should look smooth (if cell suspension is too lumpy digest for an additional 15 min). Do not incubate for more than 1 h to avoid overdigestion.
8. To end the enzymatic digestion add 10 ml of staining buffer.
9. Filter the cells using 100 μm cell strainer in a 50 ml tube and adjust the volume to 40 ml with staining buffer.
10. Centrifuge for 5 min at 500 rcf and 4 °C. Discard the supernatant.
11. Resuspend the pellet in 1 ml of staining buffer and transfer the residual volume to a 5 ml polypropylene tube.
12. Proceed to red blood cell lysis (Sect. 12.10.2.6.4)

12.2.6.2 Isolation of Resident Macrophages from Normal Tissue (Mammoplasty Reductions)

Tissue type: mammoplasty reductions
Tissue weight: 15–20 g
Macrophages isolated: resident tissue macrophages

Before you start:

1. Collect the tissue into collection medium and keep it/store it at 4 °C.
2. Sterilize the razor blades and forceps with ETOH, then rinse, and cool in a 100 cm dish of PBS.

12.2.6.3 Tissue Processing and Digestion

1. Transfer the breast tissue to a 100 cm dish and wash several times with serum-free PBS.
2. Transfer the tissue several times to fresh 100 mm dishes, washing with serum-free PBS each time. The goal is to remove all traces of blood. Be generous with the PBS: use the entire 500 ml bottle if needed.
3. Once the washes are complete, place the tissue into a dry 100 mm dish (some PBS carryover is preferred).
4. Using the forceps in one hand (to hold the tissue in place) and your other hand to hold the razor blade or scalpel, gently divide the tissue into three parts and place each part into a fresh 100 cm dish in order to be able to cut easily.
5. Using a razor blade cut the tissue into small pieces (the efficiency of the digestion is dependent on how well the tissue is minced; large pieces will not digest properly and may need more digestion time). This procedure can take a considerable amount of time. Keep the dishes on ice at all times.
6. Combine the tissues fragment and then separate into two 50 ml tubes. Make up the volume to 50 ml with serum-free PBS and centrifuge for 5 min at 500 rcf and 4 °C.
7. Due to the nature of the specimen, there will be a pellet as well as an upper layer of yellow fat. Use forceps to transfer the yellow fat layer to a new 50 ml Falcon tube.

8. Discard the supernatant and resuspend the pellet in 25 ml of serum-free DMEM together with the fat.
9. Add 10 μl of Liberase DL stock solution 28 U/ml, 20 μl of Liberase TL stock solution 14 U/ml, and 10 μl of DNase I (15 mg/ml stock solution 100×) per ml of solution.
10. Wrap the top of the tube and the cap with parafilm, mix using a vortex, and incubate for 10–18 h at 37 °C, applying continuous rotation.
11. Check the digestion status. After the incubation, the mixture should look like a greasy, brown broth. If >80 % of the tissue is digested add 25 ml of staining buffer. If not then continue digestion for an additional hour and check the digestion status again.
12. Filter the entire volume through a 100 μm cell strainer into a new 50 ml tube.
13. Centrifuge for 7 min at 500 rcf and 4 °C (if there is a lot of fat floating, discard it and take ONLY the pellet).
14. Discard the supernatant and proceed to red blood cell lysis (Sect. 12.10.2.6.4).

12.2.6.4 Red Blood Cell Lysis

1. Resuspend the pellet in 3 ml of 1X RBC lysis buffer, mix well, and incubate on ice for 10 min.
2. Add 30 ml of staining buffer.
3. Centrifuge for 5 min at 500 rcf and 4°c. Discard the supernatant and resuspend the pellet in 900 μl of staining buffer.
4. Proceed to blocking (Sect. 10.2.6.5).

12.2.6.5 Blocking

1. Add 10 % (100 μl in PBS; total volume of 1 ml) of human AB serum, mix well, and incubate on ice for a minimum 30 min (mix every 10 min).
2. Add 5 ml of staining buffer, filter using filter top 5 ml polystyrene tubes (40 μm) to prevent clogging the machine.
3. Centrifuge for 5 min at 500 rcf and 4°c. Discard the supernatant and resuspend the pellet in 1 ml of staining buffer.
4. Proceed to FACS staining for analysis (Sect. 10.2.6.6) or FACS staining for sorting (Sect. 10.2.6.7).

12.2.6.6 FACS Staining and Analysis

1. Count the cells, adjust the number to $1–2 \times 10^6$ cells/ml, and transfer 1 ml to a 5 ml polystyrene tube.
2. Centrifuge for 5 min at 500 rcf and 4°c.
3. Discard the supernatant and resuspend the pellet in 100 μl of staining buffer.
4. Add the antibody master mix (see Table 12.2).

Table 12.2 Antibody master mix for FACS analysis and sorting, human tissue

Antigen and fluorochrome	Clone
CD45 PE-Texas Red	HI30
CD11b BV605	ICRF44
CD14 BV510	M5E2
CD163 APC	GHI/61
CX3CR1 FITC	2A9-1
HLA-DR BV650	L243
CD3 BV711	OKT3
CD19 BV711	HIB19
CD56 BV711	HCD56
DAPI	

5. Incubate for 1 h on ice.
6. Add 4 ml of staining buffer.
7. Centrifuge for 5 min at 500 rcf and 4°c.
8. Resuspend the pellet in 350 μl staining buffer.
9. Analyze using a flow cytometer using the gating strategy shown in Fig. 12.2b.

12.2.6.7 FACS Staining and Cell Sorting

1. Count the cells in order to adjust antibodies' quantity accordingly.
2. Add 4 ml staining buffer.
3. Centrifuge for 5 min at 500 rcf and 4°c. Discard the supernatant and resuspend the pellet in 100 μl of staining buffer.
4. Add the antibody master mix (see Table 12.2).
5. Incubate for 1 h on ice protected from light (mix every 10 min).
6. Add 5 ml of staining buffer.
7. Centrifuge for 5 min at 500 rcf and 4°c. Discard the supernatant and resuspend in 2–5 ml (depending on the initial tumor size) sorting buffer.
8. Sort TAMs as DAPI-, CD45+, CD11b+, CD14+, CD163+, CX3CR1+, HLA-DR+, CD3-, CD19-, and CD56-.
9. Sorted cells can be used for DNA, RNA, and protein extraction, in vitro experiments such as migration analysis, angiogenesis, T cell activation or suppression, in vivo assays, etc.

12.2.7 Expected Cellular Yield

As shown in Fig. 12.3a, left panel, the weights of the mammoplasty reductions were generally higher than those of the tumor samples. However, we were able to sort significantly higher number of TAMs per gram of tumor tissue compared to resident macrophages (Fig. 12.3a, right panel). Our data confirmed that the density of TAMs is significantly higher than normal resident tissue macrophages. As expected there

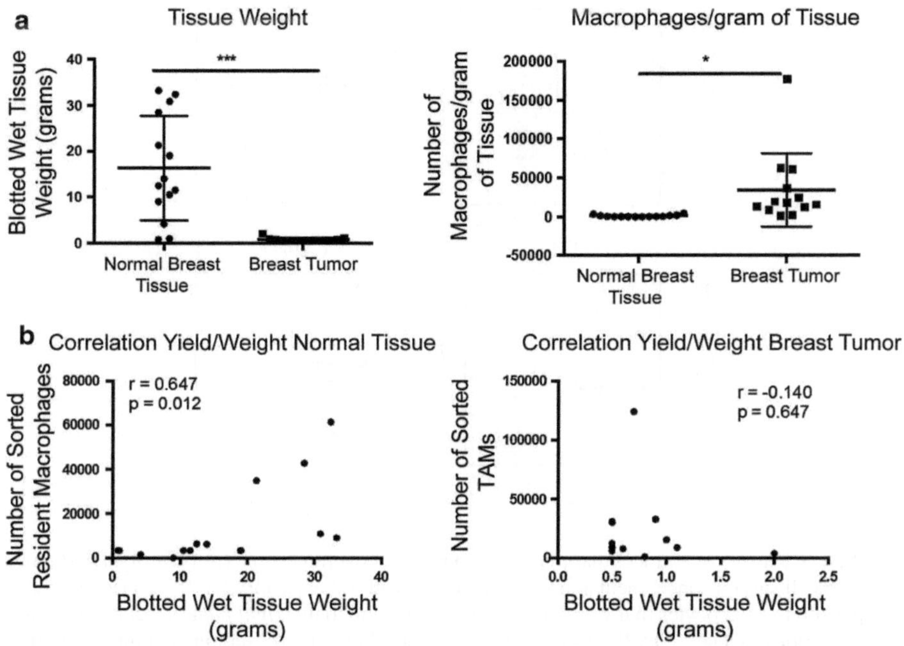

Fig. 12.3 TAM and resident macrophage yield from tumor and normal tissue. (**a**) *Left panel* represents the individual blotted wet tissue weights of normal mammary tissue and tumor samples collected ($N = 15$); *right panel* shows the number of macrophages extracted per gram of tissue in normal mammary tissue and tumor samples ($N = 15$). $* = p < 0.01$, $*** = p < 0.0001$, Student's T test. (**b**) Correlation between blotted wet tissue weight and cellular yield in normal tissue (*left panel*) and tumor tissue (*right panel*). Pearson correlation coefficient was calculated using Graphpad prism software. Each *dot* represents one sample. ($N = 15$, r = correlation coefficient, p = statistical value)

was a significant correlation between dry tissue weight and the number of cells extracted in normal tissue. However there was no such correlation in tumor samples, due to the extreme variability of tumor tissue composition (Fig. 12.3b, left and right panels, respectively).

12.2.8 Troubleshooting/Useful Tips

As with any scientific protocol there are caveats and important considerations to take into account, in order to avoid artifacts and the generation of unreliable results.

12.2.8.1 Tissue Digestion

Most TAM extracellular markers are stable and sustain enzymatic digestion, but it is fundamental to optimize the digestion protocol before starting.

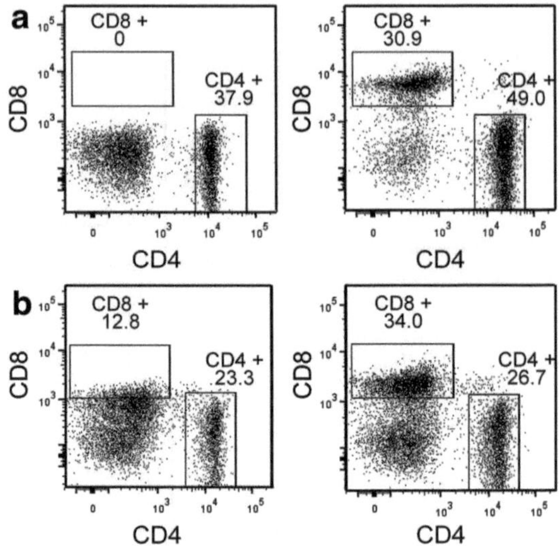

Fig. 12.4 Cleavage of extracellular markers as a result of overdigestion. (**a**) Loss of CD8 staining in single-cell suspensions—incubation of splenocytes with Liberase mix for 45 min (*left panel*) in comparison to splenocytes that were incubated with medium only (*right panel*). Data is presented after selection of $CD45^+$, $DAPI^-$, $F4/80^-$, $CD3^+$ cells. (**b**). Loss of CD8 staining in tumors—tumors were digested with a high concentration (twice higher than recommended, *left panel*) or with the recommended concentration (*right panel*) of Liberase mix for 45 min. Data is presented after selection of $CD45^+$, $DAPI^-$, $F4/80^-$, $CD3^+$ cells

In this protocol we use Liberase enzyme blends (HPLC-purified blend); other compounds using collagenase mixtures are available but they may contain additional proteases that can cleave extracellular markers. In addition, long digestion times and impurities of the enzyme mix can degrade extracellular markers of other immune cell populations such as T and B cells (see Fig. 12.4).

Excess enzymes can also degrade/cleave certain surface markers, leading to artifacts. An example of this is reported in Fig. 12.4; CD8 is rapidly lost on the surface of splenocytes and T cells from mouse mammary tumors if high concentrations of enzymes are used [40].

Take-home message: Check your markers and do not overdigest the samples; carefully select the digestion enzymes that suit your experiment. If you are worried about marker degradation reduce the enzyme concentration and digestion time accordingly.

12.2.8.2 FACS Staining

Multicolor flow cytometry requires a number of internal controls and optimization steps that are necessary for the performance of a valid experiment.

For general information about flow cytometry staining:

https://www.bdbiosciences.com/us/support/training/s/itf_launch

Compensation: It is important that each individual fluorochrome is well compensated against all the other fluorochromes. Make sure that you have a validated compensation matrix before starting the experiment.

Internal controls: We suggest to use isotype antibody controls and FMO controls in order to verify the specificity of the signal for each cell surface marker. It is extremely important that all antibodies are titrated before their use in the multicolor panel.

Make sure that at least 5–10,000 events of the smallest population are acquired, in order to ensure statistical power for the analysis.

Choice of fluorochromes: This is an important choice, even if sometimes limited by the antibodies available on the market. Our protocol shows examples of fluorochromes for a typical seven-color experiment. We suggest using the brightest and most common fluorochromes for the markers that are expected to have a low density, and to use the remaining fluorochromes for highly expressed markers. Particular attention must be given to tandem dyes, including the Brilliant Violet ones, because they are more prone to degradation or nonspecific binding if left in a mix for a prolonged time prior to analysis. Moreover the Brilliant Violet dyes, if used in combination, will require a specific staining buffer to be added to the antibody mix.

Blocking: Myeloid cells, macrophages especially, express high levels of Fc receptors. Make sure to use an effective blocking reagent (serum or CD16/CD32 antibodies) before antibody staining.

Staining: For multicolor staining we suggest to prepare an antibody master mix (if possible) rather than adding single-antibody aliquots to all samples; this procedure will avoid potential mistakes and will reduce experimental bias.

Sample filtration: Primary digested tissues are particularly prone to clogging the machines. Before analysis we strongly recommend filtration of all the samples using a 40 μm filter cap polypropylene tube.

Take-home message: Make sure to carefully titrate your antibodies, check your compensation, and choose your fluorochromes wisely based on cytofluorimeter laser settings.

12.2.8.3 Cell Sorting

Sorting TAMs from primary tissue can be very difficult, as the amount of tissue available is the limiting step.

Sample concentration: Resuspend the sample in sorting buffer and do not exceed the optimal sorting concentration (1×10^6 cells/ml) in order to avoid clogging of the instrument.

Nozzle: It is important that a 100 μm nozzle is used to sort primary macrophages; smaller nozzles (85, 70 μm) can reduce the cellular yield and cell viability.

Sorting temperature: If possible, perform cell sorting at 4 °C.

Flow rate: Monitor the flow rate and sheer pressure constantly; if the flow rate is too high you will lose cells and cell viability will be reduced.

Sort protocol: Based on your experiment you may be interested in maximizing cellular yield or purity; to do so you will need to choose the optimal in-built sorting protocol of the machine. If the final goal is to perform "omics" studies, the "purity-001" or "two-way purity" protocols are preferable (BD Facs Aria II and III).

Sorting purity check: Make sure to perform a sorting purity check during setup of the sorting protocol settings; after sorting the population take an aliquot of cells and acquire it to verify the purity level of your sort.

Collection tubes: You can use 15, 5, and 1.5 ml collection tubes. Make sure to put an adequate volume of serum-containing medium. Importantly, the sides of the collection tubes need to be coated with medium to avoid drying out the sorted cells; to do this vortex the collection tubes just prior to sorting. For small-cell populations we suggest to use V-bottom 2 ml collection tubes filled with at least 750 μl of medium. At the end of sorting the vial should be spun using a lab bench centrifuge for 10 min at 450 G_{av} and 4 °C. Make sure to draw a line on the border of the vial before centrifugation in order to identify the pellet later (sometimes it is almost invisible). Remove the supernatant without touching the pellet, and resuspend the pellet in complete medium for tissue culture or lysis buffer for RNA or DNA extraction.

Take-home message: Check cell concentration, use 100 μm nozzle, sort at 4 °C, check purity of sorted cells, and adjust sort protocol (yield vs. *purity).*

12.2.9 Macrophage Plasticity and Tissue Extraction

One of the main hallmarks of macrophages is plasticity, i.e., the ability to respond to stimuli and to rapidly adapt to changes in the tissue microenvironment [42]. Pathological conditions such as cancer, inflammation, and infection can profoundly modify macrophage phenotype and function [18, 43], but any external stimulus (mechanical, physical, and chemical) introduced during their extraction from tissue could rapidly introduce additional changes not related to the microenvironment they were extracted from. For these reasons particular attention should be paid when macrophage extraction from tissue is performed, in order to minimize any extraction-induced bias.

Isolation method. Gene expression profiling of different leukocyte subsets recently demonstrated that FACS sorting is the recommended method for isolation of leukocyte subsets for gene expression studies since this method results in the purest subset populations and does not appear to induce a stress response [44]. This is the best available isolation method at the moment for human tissue macrophage extraction. However mouse tissue macrophages can also be extracted using specific genetic labeling (fluorescent macrophages) and mechanical tissue disruption [21].

Temperature. Another important aspect to consider is the temperature; prolonged incubations of samples at 37 °*C* and room temperature can introduce modification in macrophage phenotype as cellular transcriptional machinery is on and RNase, DNase, and proteases are active. It is recommended to keep the samples at 4 °*C* where possible.

Fresh isolation. It is recommended to extract tissue macrophages from fresh tissue in order to increase cellular yield and viability; we do not recommend cultivating macrophages in vitro if the purpose of the study is to characterize their pathological associated phenotype or transcriptome as this step will likely modify their activation status.

Matched controls. It is important that the phenotype and the transcriptome of macrophages extracted from human tissues are compared with matched controls, ideally from the same tissue type; in vitro monocyte-derived macrophages, frequently used as normal negative controls, are an heterogeneous population of macrophages with different phenotypes and functions [45] and do not represent optimal controls for these kind of studies.

12.3 Conclusion

In conclusion this chapter explains the best protocol currently available for the isolation of resident and tissue-associated macrophages from human and mouse samples. The main limitations are related to the amount of starting material and the availability of matched normal controls, especially for human samples.

Currently the lack of specific TAM-associated markers renders the identification of this population a real challenge, especially for human samples where it is not possible to genetically label this population. For this reason there is the need to identify new markers unique to TAMs that we hope will be discovered in a near future.

Acknowledgments We would like to thank Dr Lisa Coussens, OHSU, for valuable discussions. This work was supported by Wellcome Trust (101067/Z/13/Z) and NIH R01CA172451 to JWP and Department of Defense (DOD W81XWH-111-0702) to Dr Lisa Coussens and JWP.

References

1. Finak G, Bertos N, Pepin F, Sadekova S, Souleimanova M, Zhao H, et al. Stromal gene expression predicts clinical outcome in breast cancer. Nat Med. 2008;14:518–27.
2. Yuan ZY, Luo RZ, Peng RJ, Wang SS, Xue C. High infiltration of tumor-associated macrophages in triple-negative breast cancer is associated with a higher risk of distant metastasis. Onco Targets Ther. 2014;7:1475–80.
3. Yang L, Wang F, Wang L, Huang L, Wang J, Zhang B, et al. CD163+ tumor-associated macrophage is a prognostic biomarker and is associated with therapeutic effect on malignant pleural effusion of lung cancer patients. Oncotarget. 2015;6:10592–603.

4. Wang B, Liu H, Dong X, Wu S, Zeng H, Liu Z, et al. High CD204+ tumor-infiltrating macrophage density predicts a poor prognosis in patients with urothelial cell carcinoma of the bladder. Oncotarget. 2015;6(24):20204–14.
5. Wang H, Li P, Wang L, Xia Z, Huang H, Lu Y, et al. High numbers of CD68+ tumor-associated macrophages correlate with poor prognosis in extranodal NK/T-cell lymphoma, nasal type. Ann Hematol. 2015;94(9):1535–44.
6. Nabeshima A, Matsumoto Y, Fukushi J, Iura K, Matsunobu T, Endo M, et al. Tumour-associated macrophages correlate with poor prognosis in myxoid liposarcoma and promote cell motility and invasion via the HB-EGF-EGFR-PI3K/Akt pathways. Br J Cancer. 2015;112:547–55.
7. Oishi K, Sakaguchi T, Baba S, Suzuki S, Konno H. Macrophage density and macrophage colony-stimulating factor expression predict the postoperative prognosis in patients with intrahepatic cholangiocarcinoma. Surg Today. 2015;45:715–22.
8. Richardsen E, Uglehus RD, Johnsen SH, Busund LT. Macrophage-colony stimulating factor (CSF1) predicts breast cancer progression and mortality. Anticancer Res. 2015;35:865–74.
9. Smith HO, Anderson PS, Kuo DY, Goldberg GL, DeVictoria CL, Boocock CA, et al. The role of colony-stimulating factor 1 and its receptor in the etiopathogenesis of endometrial adenocarcinoma. Clin Cancer Res. 1995;1:313–25.
10. Zhang QW, Liu L, Gong CY, Shi HS, Zeng YH, Wang XZ, et al. Prognostic significance of tumor-associated macrophages in solid tumor: a meta-analysis of the literature. PLoS One. 2012;7, e50946.
11. Condeelis J, Pollard JW. Macrophages: obligate partners for tumor cell migration, invasion, and metastasis. Cell. 2006;124:263–6.
12. Wyckoff J, Wang W, Lin EY, Wang Y, Pixley F, Stanley ER, et al. A paracrine loop between tumor cells and macrophages is required for tumor cell migration in mammary tumors. Cancer Res. 2004;64:7022–9.
13. Wyckoff JB, Wang Y, Lin EY, Li JF, Goswami S, Stanley ER, et al. Direct visualization of macrophage-assisted tumor cell intravasation in mammary tumors. Cancer Res. 2007; 67:2649–56.
14. Kitamura T, Qian BZ, Pollard JW. Immune cell promotion of metastasis. Nat Rev Immunol. 2015;15:73–86.
15. Qian BZ, Li J, Zhang H, Kitamura T, Zhang J, Campion LR, et al. CCL2 recruits inflammatory monocytes to facilitate breast-tumour metastasis. Nature. 2011;475:222–5.
16. Yeo EJ, Cassetta L, Qian BZ, Lewkowich I, Li JF, Stefater JA, et al. Myeloid WNT7b mediates the angiogenic switch and metastasis in breast cancer. Cancer Res. 2014;74:2962–73.
17. De Palma M, Naldini L. Angiopoietin-2 TIEs up macrophages in tumor angiogenesis. Clin Cancer Res. 2011;17:5226–32.
18. Porta C, Riboldi E, Totaro MG, Strauss L, Sica A, Mantovani A. Macrophages in cancer and infectious diseases: the 'good' and the 'bad'. Immunotherapy. 2011;3:1185–202.
19. Biswas SK, Allavena P, Mantovani A. Tumor-associated macrophages: functional diversity, clinical significance, and open questions. Semin Immunopathol. 2013;35:585–600.
20. De Palma M, Lewis CE. Macrophage regulation of tumor responses to anticancer therapies. Cancer Cell. 2013;23:277–86.
21. Ojalvo LS, King W, Cox D, Pollard JW. High-density gene expression analysis of tumor-associated macrophages from mouse mammary tumors. Am J Pathol. 2009;174:1048–64.
22. Chittezhath M, Dhillon MK, Lim JY, Laoui D, Shalova IN, Teo YL, et al. Molecular profiling reveals a tumor-promoting phenotype of monocytes and macrophages in human cancer progression. Immunity. 2014;41:815–29.
23. Pucci F, Venneri MA, Biziato D, Nonis A, Moi D, Sica A, et al. A distinguishing gene signature shared by tumor-infiltrating Tie2-expressing monocytes, blood "resident" monocytes, and embryonic macrophages suggests common functions and developmental relationships. Blood. 2009;114:901–14.
24. Luo Y, Zhou H, Krueger J, Kaplan C, Lee SH, Dolman C, et al. Targeting tumor-associated macrophages as a novel strategy against breast cancer. J Clin Invest. 2006;116:2132–41.

25. Sica A. Role of tumour-associated macrophages in cancer-related inflammation. Exp Oncol. 2010;32:153–8.
26. Qian B, Deng Y, Im JH, Muschel RJ, Zou Y, Li J, et al. A distinct macrophage population mediates metastatic breast cancer cell extravasation, establishment and growth. PLoS One. 2009;4, e6562.
27. Kusmartsev S, Gabrilovich DI. STAT1 signaling regulates tumor-associated macrophage-mediated T cell deletion. J Immunol. 2005;174:4880–91.
28. Lin EY, Li JF, Bricard G, Wang W, Deng Y, Sellers R, et al. Vascular endothelial growth factor restores delayed tumor progression in tumors depleted of macrophages. Mol Oncol. 2007;1:288–302.
29. Trogan E, Fisher EA. Laser capture microdissection for analysis of macrophage gene expression from atherosclerotic lesions. Methods Mol Biol. 2005;293:221–31.
30. Franklin RA, Liao W, Sarkar A, Kim MV, Bivona MR, Liu K, et al. The cellular and molecular origin of tumor-associated macrophages. Science. 2014;344:921–5.
31. Rose S, Misharin A, Perlman H. A novel Ly6C/Ly6G-based strategy to analyze the mouse splenic myeloid compartment. Cytometry A. 2012;81:343–50.
32. Ruffell B, Au A, Rugo HS, Esserman LJ, Hwang ES, Coussens LM. Leukocyte composition of human breast cancer. Proc Natl Acad Sci U S A. 2012;109:2796–801.
33. Lau SK, Chu PG, Weiss LM. CD163: a specific marker of macrophages in paraffin-embedded tissue samples. Am J Clin Pathol. 2004;122:794–801.
34. Zheng J, Yang M, Shao J, Miao Y, Han J, Du J. Chemokine receptor CX3CR1 contributes to macrophage survival in tumor metastasis. Mol Cancer. 2013;12:141.
35. Broz ML, Binnewies M, Boldajipour B, Nelson AE, Pollack JL, Erle DJ, et al. Dissecting the tumor myeloid compartment reveals rare activating antigen-presenting cells critical for T cell immunity. Cancer Cell. 2014;26:638–52.
36. Mroue R, Bissell MJ. Three-dimensional cultures of mouse mammary epithelial cells. Methods Mol Biol. 2013;945:221–50.
37. Smalley MJ, Kendrick H, Sheridan JM, Regan JL, Prater MD, Lindeman GJ, et al. Isolation of mouse mammary epithelial subpopulations: a comparison of leading methods. J Mammary Gland Biol Neoplasia. 2012;17:91–7.
38. Hines WC, Su Y, Kuhn I, Polyak K, Bissell MJ. Sorting out the FACS: a devil in the details. Cell Rep. 2014;6:779–81.
39. Hines WC, Yaswen P, Bissell MJ. Modelling breast cancer requires identification and correction of a critical cell lineage-dependent transduction bias. Nat Commun. 2015;6:6927.
40. Autengruber A, Gereke M, Hansen G, Hennig C, Bruder D. Impact of enzymatic tissue disintegration on the level of surface molecule exprcssion and immune cell function. Eur J Microbiol Immunol (Bp). 2012;2:112–20.
41. Lin EY, Jones JG, Li P, Zhu L, Whitney KD, Muller WJ, et al. Progression to malignancy in the polyoma middle T oncoprotein mouse breast cancer model provides a reliable model for human diseases. Am J Pathol. 2003;163:2113–26.
42. Sica A, Mantovani A. Macrophage plasticity and polarization: in vivo veritas. J Clin Invest. 2012;122:787–95.
43. Cassol E, Cassetta L, Alfano M, Poli G. Macrophage polarization and HIV-1 infection. J Leukoc Biol. 2010;87:599–608.
44. Beliakova-Bethell N, Massanella M, White C, Lada SM, Du P, Vaida F, et al. The effect of cell subset isolation method on gene expression in leukocytes. Cytometry A. 2014;85:94–104.
45. Eligini S, Crisci M, Bono E, Songia P, Tremoli E, Colombo GI, et al. Human monocyte-derived macrophages spontaneously differentiated in vitro show distinct phenotypes. J Cell Physiol. 2013;228:1464–72.

[illegible]

Chapter 13
Mouse Models of Brain Metastasis for Unravelling Tumour Progression

Manuel Sarmiento Soto and Nicola R. Sibson

Abstract Secondary tumours in the brain account for 40 % of triple negative breast cancer patients, and the percentage may be higher at the time of autopsy. The use of in vivo models allow us to recapitulate the molecular mechanisms potentially used by circulating breast tumour cells to proliferate within the brain.

Metastasis is a multistep process that depends on the success of several stages including cell evasion from the primary tumour, distribution and survival within the blood stream and cerebral microvasculature, penetration of the blood–brain barrier and proliferation within the brain microenvironment. Cellular adhesion molecules are key proteins involved in all of the steps in the metastatic process. Our group has developed two different in vivo models to encompass both seeding and colonisation stages of the metastatic process: (1) haematogenous dissemination of tumour cells by direct injection into the left ventricle of the heart, and (2) direct implantation of the tumour cells into the mouse brain.

This chapter describes, in detail, the practical implementation of the intracerebral model, which can be used to analyse tumour proliferation within a specific area of the central nervous system and tumour–host cell interactions. We also describe the use of immunohistochemistry techniques to identify, at the molecular scale, tumour–host cell interactions, which may open new windows for brain metastasis therapy.

Keywords Brain metastasis • In vivo • Mouse • Intracerebral • Immunohistochemistry

13.1 Introduction

Brain metastasis occurs in over 20 % of all cancer patients, which is more than tenfold greater than the incidence of primary brain tumours [1]. In particular, breast cancer incidence can lead to brain colonisation in up to 40 % of patients, depending on which type of primary tumour, and the median survival of untreated patients is 1–2 months only [2].

M.S. Soto • N.R. Sibson (✉)
Department of Oncology, Cancer Research UK and Medical Research Council
Oxford Institute for Radiation Oncology, University of Oxford, Oxford OX3 7LE, UK
e-mail: nicola.sibson@oncology.ox.ac.uk

C. Koumenis et al. (eds.), *Tumor Microenvironment*, Advances in Experimental Medicine and Biology 899, DOI 10.1007/978-3-319-26666-4_13

The process of metastasis to the brain is complex and depends on the success of several stages, including detachment and survival of tumour cells from the main tumour, escape from the immune-surveillance within the blood stream, transmigration across the natural barrier conferred by the blood–brain barrier (BBB) and secondary growth within the brain microenvironment [3]. In all of the above stages, cellular adhesion molecules are key molecules that facilitate the cross-talk between tumour cells and the brain environment.

Van de Hurk and colleagues [4] published a 30-year follow-up study with more than 33,000 patients, in which 60 % of breast cancer patients developed metastasis to distant organs with the central nervous system being one of the sites with higher incidence. Moreover, Patricia Steeg and colleagues [5] showed in a study of more than 1000 breast cancer patients that 15 % developed a single metastasis in the brain. These two studies together highlight the importance of developing in vivo models, such as the intracerebral model described here, to enable researchers to find new targets to impair tumour progression.

Preclinical metastatic mouse models are a fundamental tool to develop new therapies and approaches to treat the disease [6]. Several categories of in vivo cancer models exist; on the one hand, spontaneous metastatic models exist in which mice are genetically engineered, typically with oncogenes that have been either down- or up-regulated, to induce the disease. On the other hand, experimental metastasis models have been developed in which the researcher has more control over the number of cells delivered and the site to which the disease is targeted. The greater control over disease induction in the latter models, further enables longer time courses of progression within the brain to be studied by restricting or eliminating systemic dissemination [7]. If the tumour is genetically identical to the animal strain in which it was developed, it is termed a syngeneic model. In contrast, xenogeneic models involve introduction of human tumour cells into (immunocompromised) animals. With regards to the site of implantation, if the tumour is implanted into its natural environment, it is classified as an orthotopic model, whilst those models in which the tumour is injected into a different tissue or organ are heterotropic [8].

The use of in vivo models to examine brain metastasis is a powerful tool for understanding the interactions that occur between the infiltrating tumour cells and the resident brain cell population. Together with immunologic, molecular and microscopy techniques these models form a solid platform on which researchers can recapitulate the metastatic cascade. Following successful establishment of in vivo models of brain metastasis, the intricacies of cross-talk between tumour cells and host tissue can be elucidated at the molecular scale; to achieve this, one of the most common approaches used is immunohistochemistry [9, 10]. The use of antibodies against proteins specifically expressed either on the tumour cells or the brain parenchyma during tumour progression, enables researchers to determine their possible influence on disease progression and also to extrapolate the use of humanised antibodies into the clinic for either detection or treatment.

Over the last 7–8 years, with the use of experimental metastatic models and immunohistochemical analysis, we have demonstrated close association between brain metastases and the cerebral vasculature over the early stages of development [10–12], with up-regulation of multiple cellular adhesion molecules, including endothelial VCAM-1 [13]. Further, we have demonstrated an active role for cellular adhesion molecules in both the seeding and downstream colonisation stages of metastasis to the brain [10, 12, 13]. Taken together, these studies suggest the potential of cellular adhesion molecules as targets for both early detection and treatment of brain metastases.

13.2 Materials

13.2.1 Animal Models

13.2.1.1 Syngeneic Model

- Mouse mammary carcinoma cells (4T1) were transfected with green fluorescent protein (GFP) and injected into BALB/c mice.
- Cells were a kind gift from Ruth Muschel's Lab (Oxford, UK).
- Mice purchased from Charles Rivers Limited, UK.

13.2.1.2 Xenogeneic Model

- A sub-clone of the metastatic human breast carcinoma cell line MDA231 that preferentially metastasises to the brain (MDA231Br) were transfected with GFP and injected into severe combined immunodeficiency (SCID) mice.
- Cells were a kind gift from Patricia Steeg's Lab (Maryland, USA).
- Mice purchased from Charles Rivers Limited, UK.

13.2.2 Cell Culture

1. Seed cells onto 75 cm^2 flasks (Sarstedt AG & Co, Germany). **See Note 1**.
2. Growing Factors: Dulbecco´s Eagle modified medium (DMEM, Gibco) supplemented with 10 % foetal bovine serum (Sigma, UK) and 2 mM L-Glutamine (Sigma, UK).
3. Sterile PBS. Autoclave before use to maintain sterile conditions. Prepare 1 L of PBS mixing 8 g NaCl, 0.22 g KCl 1.44 g $Na_2HPO_4 \cdot 2H_2O$, 0.24 g KH_2PO_4 all in distilled water.
4. Scraper (Gibco, UK). **See Note 2**.

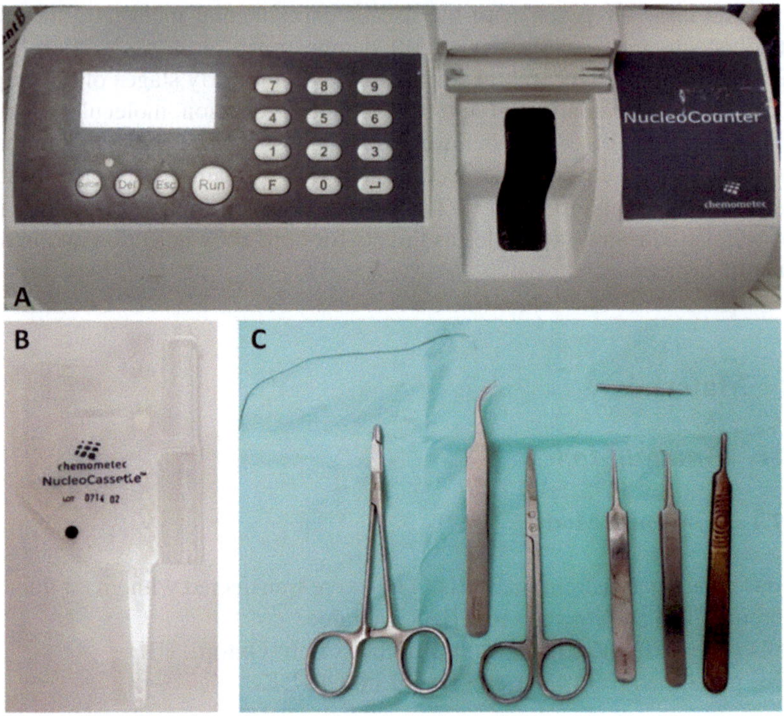

Fig. 13.1 Pictures showing the nucleocounter (**a**), in which the nucleo-cassette (**b**) is placed in order to quantify the correct number of cells. (**c**) Set of tools used for animal surgery: from *left* to *right*—Olsen-Hegar extra delicate needle holder 12 cm (with scissors built in), Dumont #7 biologie tip Dumoxel forceps 11.5 cm, Metzenbaum scissors curved blunt/blunt (14.4 cm), two Dumont #5/45 fine tipped forceps and Standard #3 scalpel handle suitable for #11 blades. At the top of (**c**) is shown the suture thread and the drill bit

13.2.3 Tools

13.2.3.1 Cell Quantitation

1. Nucleo counter (ChemoMetec AS, Denmark) (Fig. 13.1).
2. Nucleo counter SP-1 Cassette (ChemoMetec AS, Denmark). **See Note 3**.

13.2.3.2 Surgery Instruments

1. Scalpel and sterile blade, size 11. (InterFocus Ltd Cambridge, UK) (Fig. 13.1).
2. Forceps, tweezers and stainless steel burr. (InterFocus Ltd Cambridge, UK) (Fig. 13.1). **See Note 4**.
3. Suture tools. (InterFocus Ltd Cambridge, UK) (Fig. 13.1).

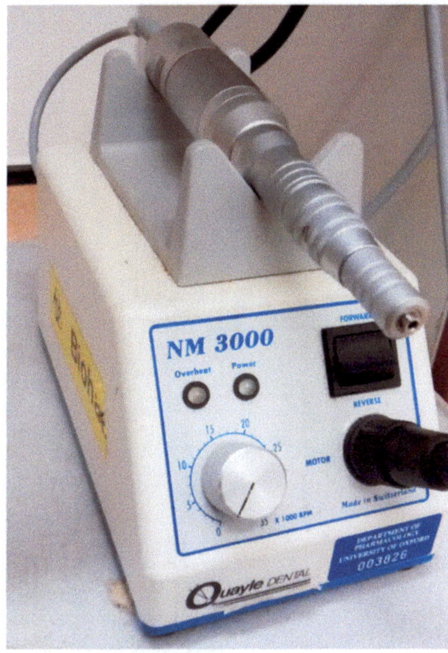

Fig. 13.2 Drill used to drill burr holes with stainless steel burr 0.9 mm diameter (Fig. 13.1c), prior to insertion of microcapillary

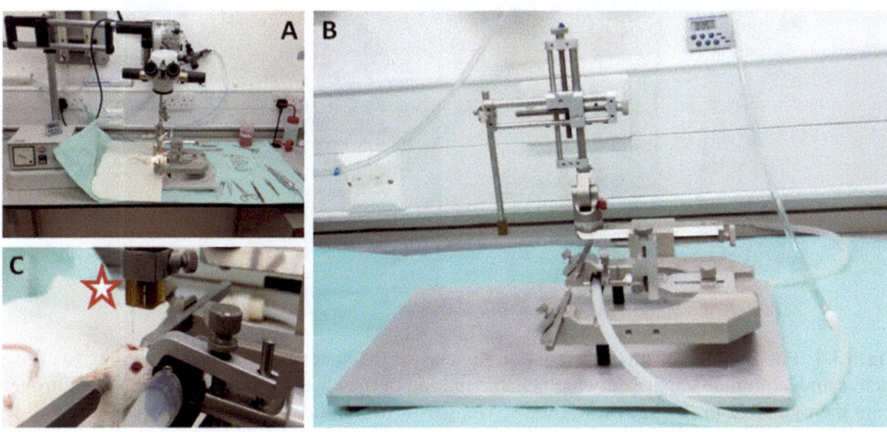

Fig. 13.3 (**a**) Sterile surgical set-up comprising the surgical tools (Fig. 13.1), the surgical microscope, and the mouse placed on top of the sterile surface. In more detail, (**b**) shows an example of the anaesthetic tubing arrangement and stereotaxic holder, whilst (**c**) shows in more detail the animal positioned on the stereotaxic frame and the adapter (*star*) for the capillary implanted into the left striatum through the burr hole

4. Drill (Quayle Dental Manufacturing (Export) Ltd). (Fig. 13.2). **See Note 5.**
5. Microscope and lens (Leica, Germany) (Fig. 13.3).
6. Stereotaxic frame (Kopf Instruments, USA). (Fig. 13.3) **See Note 6.**

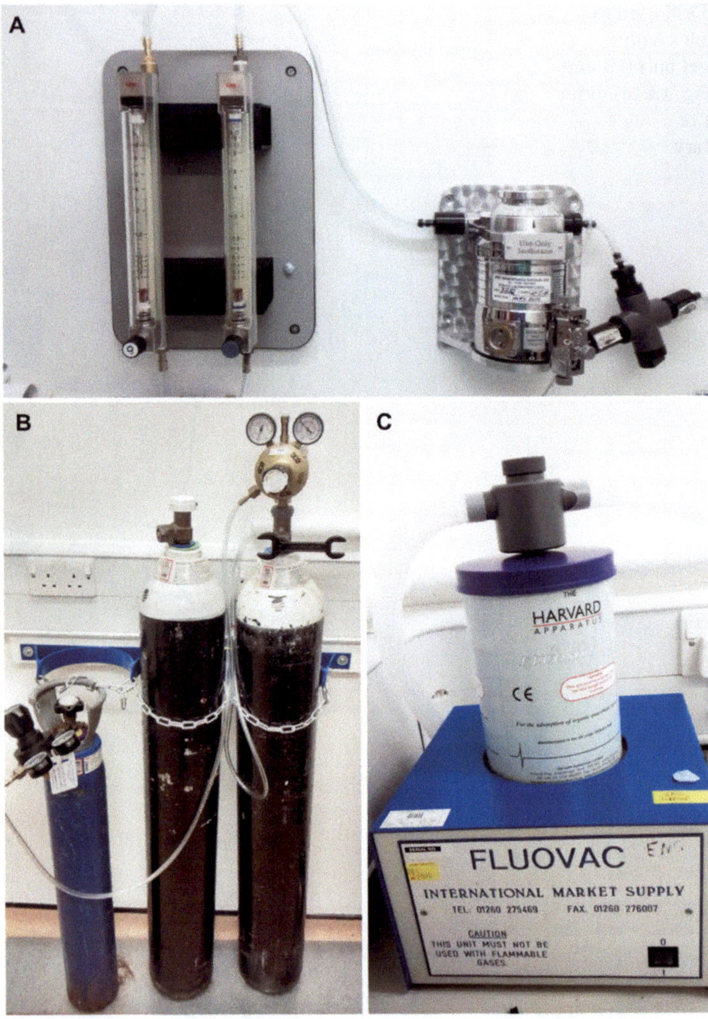

Fig. 13.4 Photographs of the different components of the anaesthetic set-up, including (**a**) flow-meters and isoflurane vaporiser, which enable mixing of the anaesthetic with oxygen and nitrogen from the cylinders in (**b**). (**c**) Shows the scavenger in which the excess anaesthetic agent will be collected

13.2.4 Surgery Room

1. Gas cylinders (British Oxygen Company, UK) for oxygen and nitrogen, with gas flow piped through appropriate flow meters (Cole-Parmer Instrument Co. Ltd. UK) (Fig. 13.4).
2. Isoflurane vaporiser (Abbott Laboratories, USA) (Fig. 13.4).
3. Fluovac Scavenger (VWR International LLC, USA).

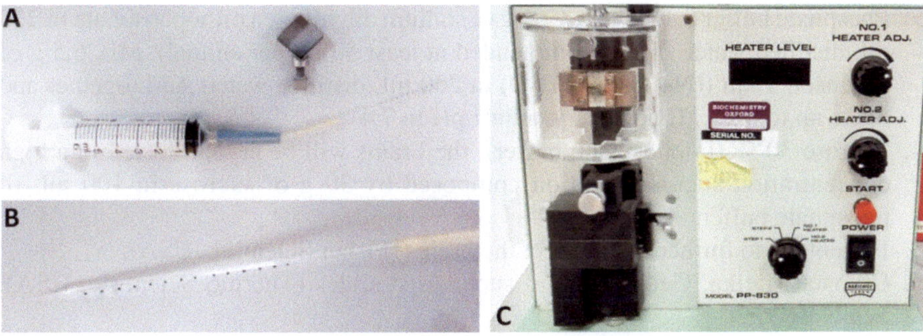

Fig. 13.5 Capillaries are a crucial component of the surgery. (**a**) Microcannula connected to a 5 ml syringe, which will be used to apply sufficient gentle pressure to inject the cells into the brain, and the holder that is used to hold capillary straight during injection (also Fig. 13.3c). (**b**) The capillary is marked every 2 mm, which equates to an injection volume of 0.5 μl. (**c**) Capillary puller, which is used to pull the capillaries to a finely drawn point

4. Anaesthetic chamber and tubing. **See Note 7**.
5. Heating blanket and rectal probe to keep animal core temperature at 37 °C. (Harvard Biosciences, Inc. USA).
6. Capillary puller (Narishige International, Ltd. Japan) and micro-capillaries (1 μm OD × 0.58 ID × 150 L mm, Harvard apparatus, USA) for intracerebral cell delivery (Fig. 13.5). **See Note 8**.
7. Suture needle (Ethicon, USA).
8. Recovery area (heating blanket).

13.2.5 Sample Processing

1. Heparinized sodium chloride (NaCl): Prepare 50 mL of 0.9 % sodium chloride per animal in distilled water and add 250 μl of sodium heparin (25,000 U/mL), WorckHardt, UK.
2. Paraformaldehyde 4 % or $PLP_{light.}$ (periodate lysine paraformaldehyde (PLP) containing only 0.025 % glutaraldehyde). For PLP_{light}, dissolve 3.4 g Lysine HCl in 94 mL distilled water. Dissolve 0.45 g di-sodium hydrogen orthophosphate dehydrate (Sorenson's salt) in 25 mL distilled water. Add this to lysine solution in order to adjust the pH to 7.4. Discard any remaining phosphate solution. Dissolve 5 g of paraformaldehyde in 50 mL of distilled water at 60 °C. Add paraformaldehyde slowly add a few drops of 1 M NaOH as a catalyst, while stirring until the solution clears. Leave to cool down. Prepare 0.53 g of sodium metaperiodate. Mix the lysine solution, paraformaldehyde solution and the sodium periodate together. Make up to 250 mL with 0.1 M phosphate buffer and adjust pH to 7.2 with NaOH. Finally add 0.25 mL of glutaraldehyde 0.01 % for fixing tissue.

3. Phosphate buffer 0.1 M: mix 1.65 g of sodium dihydrogen orthophosphate in 250 mL distilled water (It is recommended at least 50 ml per animal). Mix 6.5 g of Sorenson's salt $((Na_2HPO_4)2{\cdot}H_2O)$ in 200 mL distilled water. Add together and make up to 0.5 L. If necessary, adjust pH to 7.4.
4. Sucrose 30 % (in phosphate buffer); the brains will be cryoprotected in a high concentration sucrose solution composed by 30 g of sucrose in 100 mL of phosphate buffer.
5. Isopentane to further cryoprotect the brains (Fisher Scientific, USA).
6. Cryostat (Leika, Germany) and super-frost slides (Thermo Scientific, USA). **See Note 9.**

13.2.6 Immunohistochemistry

A number of cell adhesion molecules are involved in brain metastasis progression, but for the purposes of this chapter, we will focus on the staining of Vascular Cellular Adhesion Molecule-1 (VCAM-1) as an example.

1. PBS: see Step 3 of Sect. 13.2.2. **See Note 10**.
2. Quench solution: add 2.5 mL of hydrogen peroxide 30 % (Sigma-Aldrich, UK) to 250 mL of Methanol (Fisher Scientific, UK).
3. Blocking solution: endogenous streptavidin and biotin will be blocked using the streptavidin/biotin Kit (Vector Laboratories, USA).
4. Sections will be blocked with a specific animal serum (10 % in PBS) depending on the species in which the secondary antibody was raised (Vector Laboratories, UK).
5. Primary antibody against mouse VCAM-1 (Abcam, UK; 1:200 in PBST and 1 % Rabbit serum).
6. Secondary biotinylated antibody against rat (species where the primary antibody was raised; Vector Laboratories Inc, USA), 1:200 in PBS.
7. VECTASTAIN Elite ABC kit (Avidin-Biotin Complex kit, 1:1:100; Vector Laboratories).
8. 3, 3′-diaminobenzidine (DAB; Sigma-Aldrich) for peroxidase visualisation. **See Note 11**.
9. Cresyl violet for counterstaining (Sigma-Aldrich).
10. DPX mounting solution (Thermo Fisher Scientific, USA).
11. Coverslips (Fisher Scientific, UK).

13.3 Methods

The purpose of the intracerebral model is to mimic downstream growth of metastatic tumour cells within the brain parenchyma, once they have successfully extravasated from the brain vasculature. To minimise unwanted additional effects within the brain arising from the injection process itself, the mode of delivery of the tumour cells into the brain is critical. In the case of the intracerebral model, injection into the brain must be performed using a finely drawn microcannula (tip *ca.* 75 μm), at a slow and constant rate to avoid physical disruption of the brain tissue. For the same reason, it is not desirable to inject greater volumes than 0.5–1.0 μl into the mouse brain.

Mouse and human mammary carcinoma cells have a limited lifespan from the point of harvest. Once the cells are detached from the flask, the average duration of viability is 1.5–2.5 h, depending on the aggressiveness used during the detachment step. In order to determine the exact life expectancy for any new cell line, it is necessary to perform a time-course study in which cell viability is quantified at different time-points after detachment from the flask. Knowing this timeframe enables the researcher to circumscribe the time limit of surgery and the number of animals that can be injected from each batch of harvested cells. It is also highly recommended that the surgical room is prepared in advance and that the animals are ready for surgery (e.g. surface of head shaved) before the cells are harvested. In this case, both tumour cell lines used are viable for *ca.* 2 h post-harvest.

Sample processing is also a critical aspect of this experiment, and must be rigorous. It is important to preserve the "natural" state of the architecture and protein "network" of the brain before death. The fixation and following brain manipulation must be constant between all of the samples to ensure the consistency of the immunohistochemistry.

13.3.1 Cell Harvest

1. Seed cells onto the flasks and maintain in the growing conditions described above until they achieve 90 % confluence. **See Note 12.**
2. Harvest the cells by mechanical detachment using a plastic scraper. **See Note 13.**
3. Resuspend cells in DMEM and centrifuge for 5 min at 1200 rpm (300 × g).
4. Once the supernatant is discarded, resuspend cells again in sterile PBS. **See Note 14.**
5. Prior to injection, the time between cell quantitation, resuspension and the preparation of the animals for surgery is sufficient to allow the cells to sediment and potentially form clumps. To avoid clump formation, just prior to injection and once the burr hole has been drilled (see Step 4 of Sect. 13.3.2), resuspend cells using a wide calibre needle to minimise cell damage (gauge 23 or lower), and then loaded into the capillary using a 27 G needle that will perfectly fit into the capillary.

13.3.2 Surgery

1. Anaesthetise mouse using 2 % isoflurane and 70 %/30 % N_2/O_2 in an anaesthetic chamber.
2. Once deeply anaesthetised, position mouse on the stereotaxic frame.

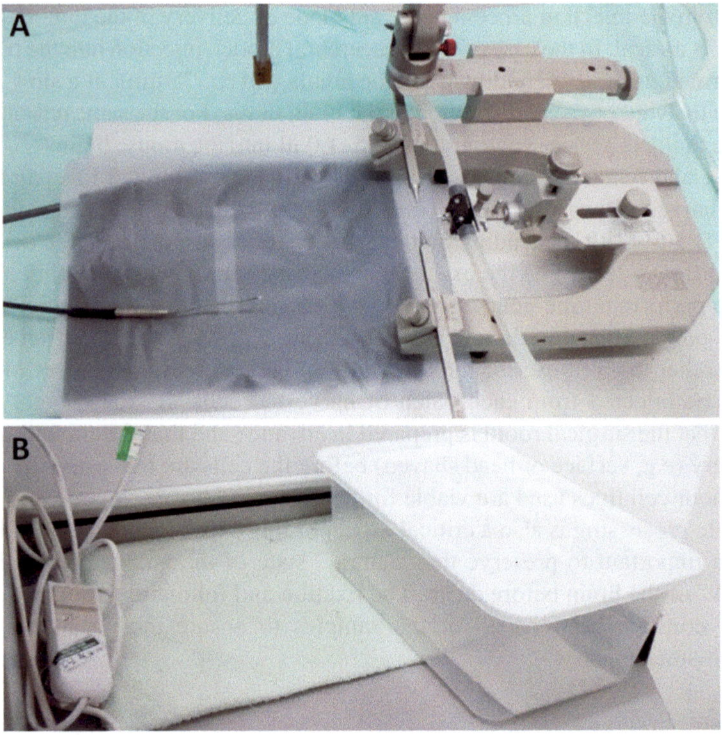

Fig. 13.6 Core temperature must be maintained during and after surgery. To achieve this, animals are placed onto a heating blanket (**a**) and a rectal probe is inserted into the rectum to monitor core body temperature; this is maintained at 37 °C by a feedback loop through the control unit. After surgery, animals are placed in the recovery cage, which is situated partly on a pre-warmed heating blanket (**b**)

3. Owing to the core temperature drop under anaesthesia, the mouse must be maintained at 37 °C using a suitable heating system. Then, turn down the isoflurane concentration to 1.5 % (Fig. 13.6).
4. Make a small incision in the scalp to expose the skull. Taking Bregma as a reference (0, 0), drill a burr hole centred at +0.5 antero/posterior and -2 lateral to Bregma [14].
5. After drilling, owing to possible overheating of the area, it is useful to wait for a couple of minutes before proceeding with the injection. Position the microcapillary, using the stereotactic frame at +0.5 antero/posterior, -2 lateral and -1.5 ventral relative to Bregma. Once the microcapillary is in place, inject the cells at 0.1 μl per minute through a 75 μm diameter microcapillary. **See Note 15**.
6. After injection, to avoid reflux of the tumour cells, wait for at least 5 min prior to retraction of the capillary. In the first instance, gently withdraw the capillary by a few micrometres only, and wait for a further minute or two before completely removing the microcapillary from the brain at a very slow speed.

7. Once the capillary is out of the brain, wipe the surface of the skull with 70 % ethanol in case of any reflux up the injection tract. Then, suture the scalp using the suture needle.
8. After suturing, place the animal in a pre-warmed recovery area until it has fully recovered from anaesthesia. **See Note 16.**

13.3.3 Brain Processing

1. The animal must be deeply anesthetised (sodium pentobarbital; 30 mg/kg i.p.) and the heart exposed by opening the chest wall with the small scissors (Fig. 13.1c). Then, perfuse into the left ventricle 50 mL of heparinized saline, followed by 50 mL of PLP_{light} at ~40 mL/min. As soon as transcardial perfusion begins, the right atrium of the heart must be cut to allow the saline to flush the blood out of the system. Once the fluid coming from the atrium runs clear, the perfusate can be switched to the fixative. The perfusion can be done manually or using a perfusion pump (Fisher Scientific, UK).
2. Following transcardial perfusion, cut the head off using strong scissors and then peel the skull off using strong tweezers (Fig. 13.3c). Remove the brain, using a spatula to gently leverage it out of the skull cavity, and post-fix it for 4 h at 4 °C in the same fixative previously used. After this, transfer the brain into 30 % sucrose until it has sunk (after 24–36 h at 4 °C), indicating that cryoprotection is complete.
3. Place the brain in isopentane at −20° for 30 min. Once frozen, wrap it in foil and transfer to −20 °C for long-term storage. **See Note 17.**
4. Place the brain in the cryostat at −20 °C, and cut sections at 10 μm thickness. Once cut, place the sections on the slides. **See Note 18.**

13.3.4 Immunohistochemistry

1. Place 10 μm sections onto the superfrost slides and hydrated for 5 min in PBS (see Step 3 of Sect. 13.2.2). **See Note 19.**
2. Quench sections in methanol with 1 % hydrogen peroxide for 20 min. (see Step 2 of Sect. 13.2.6).
3. After three washes in PBST, slides must be Streptavidin- and biotin-blocked in two segments of 15 min each, with a quick wash in PBST of 5 min in between (Vector Laboratories, USA).
4. Block the sections with the appropriate animal serum (10 % in PBS) for 1 h; in our case, normal rabbit serum was used.
5. Coat slides overnight with anti-VCAM-1 antibody (1:200; Abcam, UK; see Step 5 of Subheading 13.2.6.) at 4 °C in a humid chamber.
6. On the following day, after rinsing with PBS, incubate sections with biotinylated anti-rat secondary antibody (Step 6 of Sect. 13.2.6) for 1 h at room temperature.

7. Wash brain sections three times in PBS and incubate with ABC kit (see Step 7 of Sect. 13.2.6) in PBS for 45 min.
8. After three washes, place sections in DAB solution.
9. Finally, cover-slip slides using Vectashield mounting medium (see Step 10 of Sect. 13.2.6) with DAPI to stain nuclei. The slides are now ready to move to the microscope. See Fig. 13.6.

13.4 Notes

1. Cell lines or primary cancer cell cultures will exhibit different growth rates. It is important to know the optimal seeding concentration and flask size, prior to scheduling the experiment, for each individual cell line.
2. The material of the scraper should be as soft as possible to avoid damage to the transmembrane proteins of the tumour cells.
3. NucleoCounter is based on the quantitation of dead cells within the sample. The cell population can also be quantified in several other ways prior to injection: using a haemocytometer; by spectrophotometry; by electrical resistance, etc. It is critical to keep the cells under sterile conditions and, consequently, it is recommended that a small volume of working solution is collected for the cell quantitation, whilst the main volume of the sample is kept on ice.
4. The size of the drill bit must be appropriate for the animal species. In our case, the size of the head of the burr is 0.9 mm, enabling drilling of a suitable hole in the mouse skull. In case of other species, such as rat, the drill burr size may vary.
5. It is important to set the drill speed at an appropriate rate to avoid going through the skull too quickly and causing damage to the surface of the brain. If required, stop and wash the surface of the skull with sterile saline to cool during drilling. Use cotton buds to dry or stop possible bleeding.
6. The stereotaxic frame must contain a specific adapter for the mouse nose.
7. The animal must be permanently anaesthetised. The gas mix must go into the stereotaxic frame and the excess of anaesthetic should be collected via another tube connected directly to the scavenger. To enable all of this, the mouse adapter requires specific modifications; See Fig. 13.3.
8. The tip of the capillary should not exceed 75 μm to avoid undesired damage to the brain, and should be no smaller than this to prevent cell clumping within the microcapillary during injection. Once the capillary has been pulled, the tip should be cut under the microscope using a reference grid to measure the 75 μm diameter. Attach the capillary to a short length of catheter tubing (See Fig. 13.5); we find that the tubing from a butterfly needle works well and provides a suitable fitting at the end for syringe attachment (**See Note 15**).
9. Once the sections are cut in the cryostat, they must be placed on pre-treated slides and left to dry. In order to secure the section to the surface of the slides, these must be either pre-coated with gelatine or another substance that will electrostatically keep the sections adhered to the slide surface. Otherwise, the brain sections will detach from the slides after the first few washes.

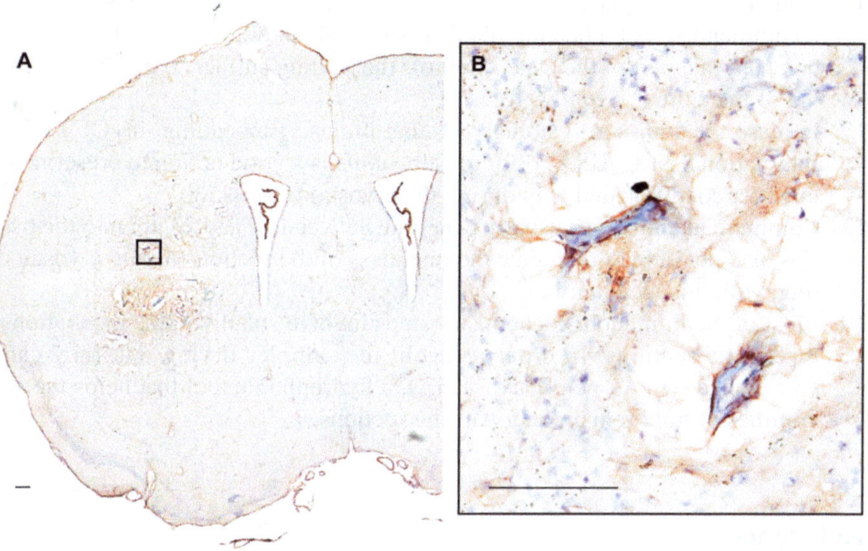

Fig. 13.7 (**a**) Photomicrograph of a coronal brain section from a mouse injected intracerebrally with MDA231Br-GFP cells. (**b**) VCAM-1 staining (*brown*) shows clear expression on cells at the margins of the tumour colonies (*dark blue*) and in the immediately surrounding tissue. Scale bars 300 μm (Colour figure online)

10. Depending on the degree of fixation, localisation of our target proteins or the specifications of the antibody, it is sometimes necessary to artificially permeabilise the samples. The use of PBS tween (PBS with 0.05 % Tween, Sigma, UK) or antigen retrieval [15] will give the antibody more access to the target protein.
11. 3,3′-diaminobezidine tetrahydrochloride is a powder that needs to be dissolved in phosphate buffer, filtered and stored at −20 °C away from light.
12. If different cell lines are used, it is important to read the specifications for that cell line. Concentrations of serum, nutrients (e.g. glutamine) or growth factors may vary between cell lines.
13. Trypsin is frequently applied to dissociate adhesive cells from the substratum. However, owing to the proteolytic activity of trypsin, cell surface proteins are often cleaved leading to deregulation of cell functions. Although most of the cellular adhesion molecules are very resistant to trypsin activity, mechanical detachment has been shown to be a preferable approach for harvesting the cells and provides an efficient and harmless method.
14. In the model described here, we inject 5000 cells in 0.5 μl of PBS; consequently, a concentration of at least 10,000,000 cells per ml is required. It is important to resuspend the cells in a larger volume enough (200 μl at least) to allow us to load the capillaries.
15. A 5 ml syringe will be attached to the capillary via the catheter tubing (See Fig. 13.5) to execute the right pressure to perfuse the cells into the striatum once the capillary is in place.

16. Animals must be placed onto a pre-warmed area for recovery after surgery. It is recommended that a heating blanket is placed underneath half of the recovery box, and that part of the cage is left off the heating surface to prevent overheating of the animal. See Fig. 13.6.
17. In case of long-term storage of the brains. Embedding in OCT (VWR International LLC, USA) prior to isopentane is a good option to preserve them in better condition and help during the cryostat processing.
18. Commercial antibodies usually penetrate between 10 and 20 μm into the tissue. It is also possible to modulate the thickness of the sections during cryostat cutting, with this idea in mind.
19. Most of the immunohistochemistry steps involve small volume incubations on top of the sections. In order to avoid the samples drying out, they can be surrounded by PAP pen (Dako, USA), a hydrophobic tool that helps the small volumes of fluid remain on top of the sections.

References

1. Gril B, Palmieri D, Qian Y, et al. Pazopanib reveals a role for tumor cell B-Raf in the prevention of HER2+ breast cancer brain metastasis. Clin Cancer Res. 2011;17:142–53.
2. Steeg PS. Tumor metastasis: mechanistic insights and clinical challenges. Nat Med. 2006;12:895–904.
3. Kienast Y, Von Baumgarten L, Fuhrmann M, et al. Real-time imaging reveals the single steps of brain metastasis formation. Nat Med. 2010;16:116–22.
4. Van Den Hurk CJ, Eckel R, Van De Poll-Franse LV, et al. Unfavourable pattern of metastases in M0 breast cancer patients during 1978-2008: a population-based analysis of the Munich Cancer Registry. Breast Cancer Res Treat. 2011;128:795–805.
5. Steeg PS, Theodorescu D. Metastasis: a therapeutic target for cancer. Nat Clin Pract Oncol. 2008;5:206–19.
6. Daphu I, Sundstrom T, Horn S, et al. In vivo animal models for studying brain metastasis: value and limitations. Clin Exp Metastasis. 2013;30:695–710.
7. Francia G, Cruz-Munoz W, Man S, et al. Mouse models of advanced spontaneous metastasis for experimental therapeutics. Nat Rev Cancer. 2011;11:135–41.
8. Khanna C, Hunter K. Modeling metastasis in vivo. Carcinogenesis. 2005;26:513–23.
9. Muller W, Burgart LJ, Krause-Paulus R, et al. The reliability of immunohistochemistry as a prescreening method for the diagnosis of hereditary nonpolyposis colorectal cancer (HNPCC) – results of an international collaborative study. Familial Cancer. 2001;1:87–92.
10. Soto MS, Serres S, Anthony DC, et al. Functional role of endothelial adhesion molecules in the early stages of brain metastasis. Neuro-Oncology. 2014;16:540–51.
11. Carbonell WS, Ansorge O, Sibson N, et al. The vascular basement membrane as "soil" in brain metastasis. PLoS One. 2009;4:e5857.
12. Connell JJ, Chatain G, Cornelissen B, et al. Selective permeabilization of the blood-brain barrier at sites of metastasis. J Natl Cancer Inst. 2013;105:1634–43.
13. Serres S, Soto MS, Hamilton A, et al. Molecular MRI enables early and sensitive detection of brain metastases. Proc Natl Acad Sci U S A. 2012;109:6674–9.
14. Paxinos G, Franklin K. The mouse brain in stereotaxic coordinates. Academic Press, 2008.
15. Shi SR, Cote RJ, Taylor CR. Antigen retrieval immunohistochemistry: past, present, and future. J Histochem Cytochem. 1997;45:327–43.

Chapter 14
Quantification of Lung Metastases from In Vivo Mouse Models

Joan Chang and Janine T. Erler

Abstract Cancer research has made significant progress in terms of understanding and targeting primary tumors; however, the challenge remains for the successful treatment of metastatic cancers. This highlights the importance to use in vivo models to study the metastatic process, as well as for preclinical testing of compounds that could inhibit metastasis. As a result, proper quantification of metastases from in vivo models is of the utmost significance. Here, we provide a detailed protocol for collecting and handling lung tissues from mice, and guidance for subsequent analysis of metastases, as well as interpretation of data.

Keywords Quantification • Metastasis • In vivo model • Tissue collection • ImageJ

14.1 Introduction

Metastasis, the spread of cancer cells from the primary site where they first arise, is responsible for more than 90 % of deaths amongst patients with solid tumors [1]; as such, it is important for researchers to utilize appropriate models to understand this process, in order to investigate and develop new therapeutics that can inhibit metastasis and improve patient survival.

Metastasis is a very complex process that includes multiple steps—in terms of solid tumors, cancer cells at the primary site need to first invade through the extracellular matrix, intravasate into the vasculature (blood and/or lymph), survive in circulation, extravasate out of the vasculature, and proliferate in the secondary site [2].

J. Chang
Biotech Research & Innovation Centre (BRIC), University of Copenhagen,
Ole Maaløes Vej 5, 2200 Copenhagen, Denmark

Department of Cell Biology and Physiology, University of North Carolina at Chapel Hill,
27599 Chapel Hill, NC, USA

J.T. Erler (✉)
Biotech Research & Innovation Centre (BRIC), University of Copenhagen,
Ole Maaløes Vej 5, 2200 Copenhagen, Denmark
e-mail: Janine.erler@bric.ku.dk

C. Koumenis et al. (eds.), *Tumor Microenvironment*, Advances in Experimental Medicine and Biology 899, DOI 10.1007/978-3-319-26666-4_14

Each of these steps may be targeted to inhibit the metastatic process; as such, when a new potential therapeutic target for metastasis is discovered, it is very important to understand where in the metastatic process it is targeting. This allows the possibility of combination therapy, where multiple steps of the metastatic process are inhibited and combined with cytotoxic or cytostatic agents to maximize effects against the disease.

In vivo mouse models are used for proof-of-concept demonstrations of new molecules that are involved in mediating metastasis; they are also used in preclinical testing of inhibitors or antibodies that may be qualified to enter clinical trials. The most common in vivo models used for metastasis research are (1) spontaneous metastasis models where metastases are derived from injection of an orthotopic/subcutaneous primary tumor or from spontaneously arising primary tumors in transgenic mice, or (2) experimental metastasis models, whereby cancer cells are injected into the circulation to study their colonization capabilities (e.g. tail-vein lung colonization, intrasplenic liver colonization, intracardiac bone colonization) [3]. The former provides a comprehensive study in the ability of the cancer cells to escape the primary tumor and metastasize, whereas the latter focuses on the later stages of metastasis only, specifically the ability of cancer cells to survive in circulation, extravasate and proliferate at the secondary site. Regardless of the metastatic model being used, correct quantification of tumor cells that successfully colonized the secondary site is of utmost importance. For example, if metastasis was only quantified as number of metastasis per tissue area, molecules that are involved in tumor cell proliferation in the secondary site but not extravasation may be overlooked. It is therefore the aim of this chapter to provide a comprehensive guide to this quantification process. Here, the focus is put on quantification of lung metastases, but the principle described is applicable to analyzing metastases in other organs.

14.2 Protocol

Reagents and Equipment

4 % paraformaldehyde solution (PFA) or 10 % buffered formalin solution (BFS)
70 % ethanol
Phosphate buffered solution (PBS)
Dissection tools
18G/27G needle with 1 ml syringe
15 ml polypropylene tubes
Paraffin or optimal cutting temperature (OCT)
OCT mixed with PBS (1:1)
Digital slide scanner and software, or microscope with camera-function
ImageJ Software

14.2.1 Collection of Tissues

Sacrifice the mouse as per protocol approved by your Institution. After sacrifice, pin the mouse onto a piece of paper towel (or any absorbent material) on top of a Styrofoam back, sterilize the mouse by spraying with 70 % ethanol, and cut open the rib cage carefully without disturbing the lungs and heart.

In order to aid visualization of the metastases in the lungs, it is very important to inflate the lungs with either 4 % PFA/10 % BFS, or OCT, depending on downstream applications. PFA/BFS are optimal for immunohistochemistry (IHC) or hematoxylin–eosin staining (H and E) analysis, and OCT is optimal for frozen tissue sectioning for immunofluorescence (IF) staining. For PFA fixation (Note 1), there are two ways to inflating the lungs:

1. Remove the majority of the rib cage, extend the cut up to the throat of the mouse, exposing the windpipe (Fig. 14.1, left panel). Using a 18G needle with syringe filled with PFA, insert the needle into the windpipe of the mouse and gently inject PFA until the lungs are slightly inflated (Fig. 14.1, right panel. Note 2). After inflation, using forceps, gently pull out the heart with the lungs still attached to it; remove the heart and trim off any lymph nodes attached to the lungs, and submerge the tissue in 5 ml of PFA solution in a 15 ml tube.

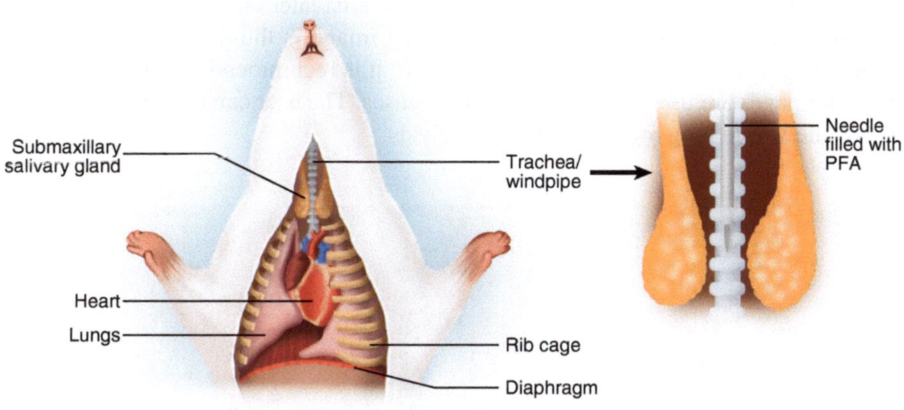

Fig. 14.1 Collection and inflation of lungs. *Left*—cut open the rib cage and expose the lungs and heart. Extend the cut up to the throat of the mouse to reveal trachea/windpipe. *Right*—enlarged view of the trachea/windpipe. Using an 18G needle filled with PFA, insert the needle into the windpipe and gently inject circa 100 µl of PFA until lungs are slightly inflated

2. Use this approach if only select lobes can be used for analysis; for example, other lobes needed for additional experiments such as flow cytometry analysis. After exposing the lungs and heart, gently pull the heart out with the lungs still attached. In a petri dish, remove the heart and any lymph nodes attached. Flip the lungs over so the bronchus is visible (Fig. 14.2a), and carefully insert a 27G needle with PFA in the syringe into the bronchus entry point of one of the lung nodules (Fig. 14.2b, left and right panels). Gently and slowly injected PFA into the lungs until the lungs are slightly inflated. Submerge tissue in 5 ml of PFA solution in a 15 ml tube.

Allow the tissue to be submerged in PFA for between 20 and 36 h (Note 3), then change to PBS. Prior to paraffin embedment, incubate the tissues with 70 % ethanol.

14.2.2 Visualization of Tissue Sections

Once the tissues are embedded, section and carry out H and E staining using whichever standard protocol available from your Institution. After the slides are mounted and dried, it is recommended that they are scanned using a digital slide scanner (e.g., Hamamatsu digital slide scanner), so that the whole tissue section is captured (Fig. 14.3, left panel). Software associated with your choice of digital slide scanner should have a function that allows for calculation of tissue area through freehand selection of the tissue border (Fig. 14.3, right panel). This parameter will allow for analysis of metastases corrected to the total lung area later on.

One advantage of using a digitally scanned image is the ease to zoom in to a higher magnification without losing resolution. It is recommended that 10× magnification images are used for analysis of metastases. The user can then export images across the whole lung area for detailed analysis.

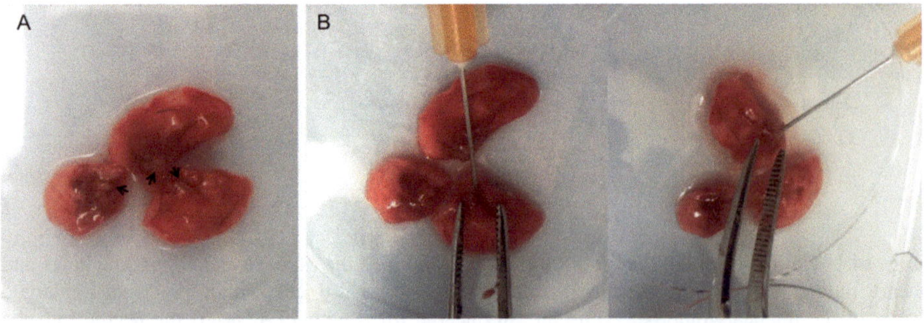

Fig. 14.2 Collection and inflation of lungs outside the mouse. (**a**). After lungs are pulled out of the body and the heart removed, arrange the lung nodules such that the entry points of the bronchioles (indicated by *arrows*) are visible. (**b**). Carefully insert a 27G needle filled with PFA into the entry point, and gently inject until the lungs slightly swell up

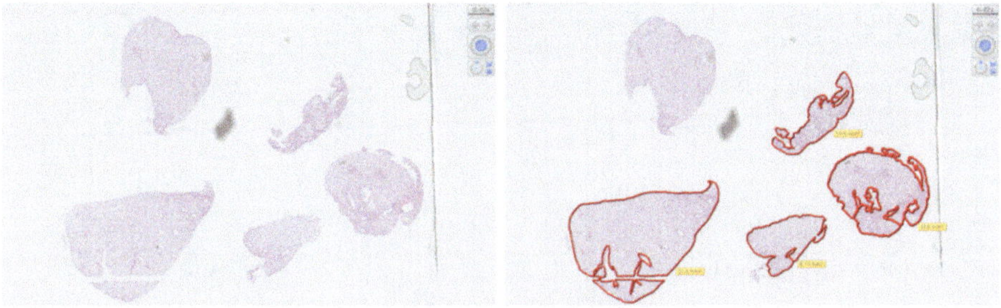

Fig. 14.3 Example of a scanned H and E stain of the lungs. *Left*—a digital image of the whole scanned slide. *Right*—using free hand selection tool the area of individual lung tissues can be determined

The first and foremost step of analysis of metastases is to first define what counts as a "metastasis". In our hands, we define metastasis as a cluster of four or more cells with abnormal-looking nuclei as tumor cells tend to have larger nuclei with irregular shapes, and are more packed together (Fig. 14.4a, indicated by arrows). However, sometimes tightly packed cells may be immune cells infiltration without tumor cells within (Fig. 14.4b, circled); additionally, areas around blood vessels and bronchioles also have packed cells as a result of normal lung structures and not metastasis (Fig. 14.4c). Another important rule to metastasis analysis is to keep your definition of metastasis consistent between different samples; a blinded analysis may also provide a better and unbiased analysis.

14.2.3 Analysis of Tissue Sections

Once the parameters are defined, the Image J software, which is free to download, can be used for quantification purposes. Open the exported high-magnification image in ImageJ. Go to Analyze → Tools → ROI Manager (Fig. 14.5, left panel). Once ROI Manager is opened, select both "Show All" and "Label" boxes, as this will allow the user to record which area they have highlighted as metastases.

On the ImageJ tool bar, select "Freehand selections", and start mapping out the area of metastasis in the image. After each metastasis area selection, either press the "t" key, or click the "Add" tab on the ROI Manager. Once all metastases area were selected, go to ROI Manager window, click on the "More>>" tab, and select "Multi Measure" (Fig. 14.5, right panel). Select "one row per slice", a results table will then pop up with the area of the selected areas measured in pixels (Note 4).

The figures can then copied into Excel spreadsheet. A few numbers derived from either the digital slidescanner software or ImageJ analysis are important: total lung area (pixels and/or mm^2, Note 5), total metastatic area (pixels), and number of metastases. The total metastatic area can be calculated using the "SUM" function of all the metastatic area measured in ImageJ, and the total number of metastasis from one measurement can be calculated using the "COUNTA" function.

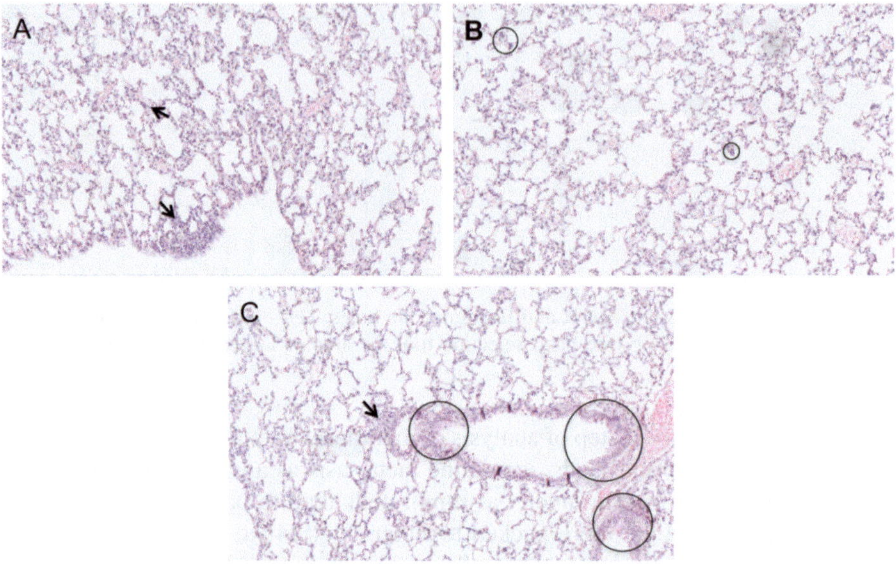

Fig. 14.4 Examples of lung metastases. Shown here are lungs collected from mice injected orthotopically with the human breast cancer cell line MDA-MB-231. (**a**) *Arrows* pointing towards metastases defined as a packed cluster of more than four cells with abnormal nuclei. (**b**) *Circles* indicate packed cells that are not tumor cells but are instead immune infiltration. (**c**) *Circles* indicate normal cells with packed appearance surrounding bronchioles. However, a cluster of metastasis is still observed next to the structures as indicated by the *arrow*

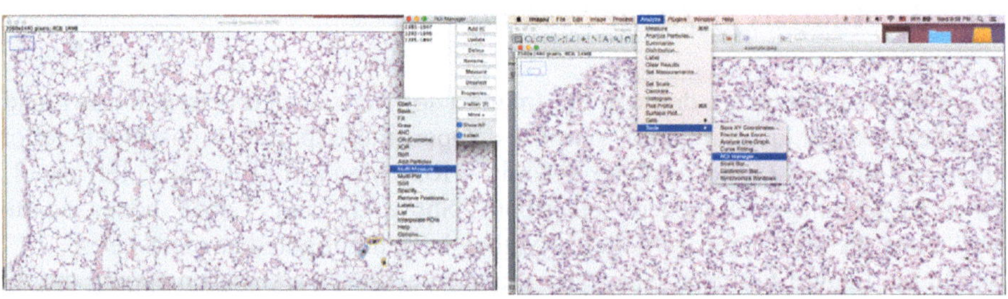

Fig. 14.5 ImageJ analysis of exported images of lung H and E sections. *Left*—location of the ROI Manager tool for analysis. *Right*—after selecting areas of metastasis in the lungs, the areas can be measured using the multi measure function

From the total metastatic area and number of metastasis, the average area of each metastasis can be calculated by dividing total area by the number. This gives the user an idea if the experimental setup had an effect on proliferation of metastatic tumor cells in the secondary site. Using the number of metastasis and the area of the lungs, the number of metastasis per pixel/mm2 of lung tissue can be calculated. This indicates whether the experimental setup is affecting extravasation of the tumor cells. Finally, % metastatic load can be calculated by dividing the total metastatic area with total lung area, then multiply by 100. This suggests if the experimental setup has an effect on metastatic burden.

14.3 Conclusions

Here we provided a detailed description for quantification of lung metastases. The basic theory, especially when interpreting the data, could be applied to analysis of other types of metastases. Regardless, with improved software development, it is possible that in the near future these kinds of analyses could be automated.

14.4 Notes

1. If you are using OCT as embedment, use an OCT/PBS mix for the inflation (1:1), and use process 2 for inflation, before placing the tissue in a cryomold with a small amount of OCT in the bottom. Put the cryomold on top of dry ice, fill up the mold and cover the tissue with OCT. Transfer to −80 °C freezer once the OCT is solidified.
2. Take care not to over-inflate the lungs as this may break up a metastasis into smaller portions, leading to inaccurate counts. In general, adequate inflation is achieved once the lungs are slightly plumped up.
3. For larger organs (e.g., liver), incubate in a larger volume of PFA for a longer period of time. Be careful not to over-fix the tissue in PFA to ensure minimal tissue damage. If prolonged period of time is required between fixation and paraffin embedding, it is advised to store the tissues in 70 % ethanol.
4. If the results window gives more than just the area of the metastasis, right-click on the results window, and select "Set Measurements". Check that only "Area" box is ticked, and then click "OK". You will need to close the window and remeasure the areas.
5. If there is no access to a digital slide scanner, or the area of the tissue could not be determined in a satisfactory manner, the user can calculate the total pixel area of the lungs using the freehand selection tool in ImageJ, and derive the various parameters of metastasis analysis using pixels instead of mm^2.

References

1. Sporn MB. The war on cancer. Lancet. 1996;347:1377–81.
2. Chang J, Erler J. Hypoxia-mediated metastasis. Adv Exp Med Biol. 2014;772:55–81
3. Khanna C, Hunter K. Modeling metastasis in vivo. Carcinogenesis. 2005;26:513–23.

Chapter 15
A Multimodal Data Analysis Approach for Targeted Drug Discovery Involving Topological Data Analysis (TDA)

Muthuraman Alagappan, Dadi Jiang, Nicholas Denko, and Albert C. Koong

Abstract In silico drug discovery refers to a combination of computational techniques that augment our ability to discover drug compounds from compound libraries. Many such techniques exist, including virtual high-throughput screening (vHTS), high-throughput screening (HTS), and mechanisms for data storage and querying. However, presently these tools are often used independent of one another. In this chapter, we describe a new multimodal in silico technique for the hit identification and lead generation phases of traditional drug discovery. Our technique leverages the benefits of three independent methods—virtual high-throughput screening, high-throughput screening, and structural fingerprint analysis—by using a fourth technique called topological data analysis (TDA). We describe how a compound library can be independently tested with vHTS, HTS, and fingerprint analysis, and how the results can be transformed into a topological data analysis network to identify compounds from a diverse group of structural families. This process of using TDA or similar clustering methods to identify drug leads is advantageous because it provides a mechanism for choosing structurally diverse compounds while maintaining the unique advantages of already established techniques such as vHTS and HTS.

Keywords In silico • Topological data analysis • Virtual screening • High-throughput screening • Fingerprint • Computer aided drug discovery

---

M. Alagappan, B.S. • D. Jiang, Ph.D. • A.C. Koong, M.D., Ph.D. (✉)
Department of Radiation Oncology, Stanford University School of Medicine, Stanford, CA 94305, USA
e-mail: muthuram@stanford.edu; jiangd@stanford.edu; akoong@stanford.edu

N. Denko, M.D., Ph.D.
Department of Radiation Oncology, Wexner Medical Center and Comprehensive Cancer Center, Ohio State University, Columbus, OH 43210, USA
e-mail: nicholas.denko@osumc.edu

C. Koumenis et al. (eds.), *Tumor Microenvironment*, Advances in Experimental Medicine and Biology 899, DOI 10.1007/978-3-319-26666-4_15

15.1 Introduction

In silico drug discovery refers to the use of computational technology to advance the process of drug discovery. More generally, in silico refers to a testing environment, in contrast to in vitro and in vivo, named after silicon-based computer chips. In silico drug discovery methods include basic processes such as database storage and querying and also technically advanced methods such as virtual ligand screening and topological data analysis [1]. These methods accelerate various steps in the drug discovery process, ranging from identification, 3D-reconstruction, and modeling of protein targets to identification of promising hits and lead drug compounds [2]. Empirically, in silico drug discovery, or as some refer to it, computer-aided drug design (CADD), has had numerous successes, such as aiding in the discovery of drugs against human immunodeficiency virus (HIV) including ritonavir and indinavir, as well as captopril, an angiotensin-converting enzyme (ACE) inhibitor for treating hypertension [3–5].

The rise in popularity of in silico drug discovery is correlated with the advent in computational power, the advancement of computational methods, and the failures of traditional drug discovery methods. Modern drug discovery on average requires 12.5 years and $1 billion for the launch of a technically successful drug, which is a highly prohibitive amount for most groups to pursue [6]. As a result, fewer entrants participate in drug discovery and those that do often necessitate exorbitant drug prices to recoup the costs of development. Fortunately, the improvement of computational speed and techniques has paved the way for in silico applications to lower the threshold and costs for participating in drug discovery and to accelerate the process of launching a successful drug. Modern processing power is constantly improving and current parallel processing systems can perform structure-based screening on more than 100,000 compounds per day [7]. We can only expect that as computational power and techniques continue to expand, the time and cost required to perform in silico drug discovery will be an even greater advantage when compared to traditional lead generation.

In this chapter, we describe a specific in silico approach to drug discovery that harnesses and combines the power of three popular techniques—virtual ligand screening, high-throughput screening (HTS), and fingerprint structural analysis—by using a fourth technique called topological data analysis (TDA), with the goal of identifying promising drug compounds from compound libraries, serving as a replacement to the hit identification stage and the subsequent lead generation stage of traditional drug discovery (Fig. 15.1). These methods will be employed once a

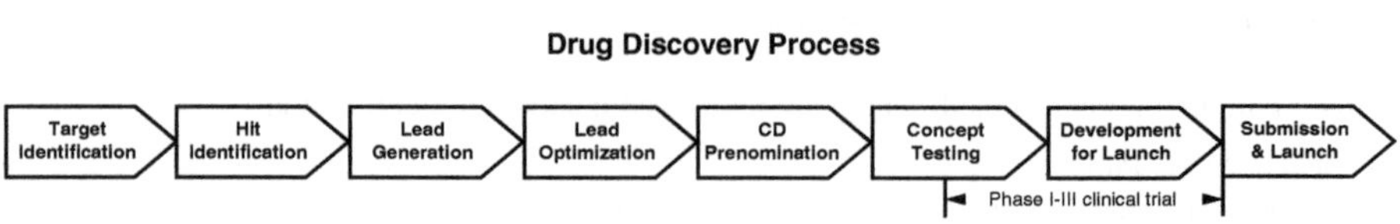

Fig.15.1 Steps in the traditional drug discovery pathway

biological target (receptor, enzyme, ion channel, etc.) has already been identified and validated.

The goal of the hit identification stage of drug discovery is to identify a subset of compounds from a much larger compound library that meet a success criterion against a certain target [8]. Hit identification is currently most often performed by high-throughput screening (HTS), a technique in which hundreds of thousands of compounds are assayed by robotics to determine which have the most significant activity against the target. The libraries that are screened include random libraries, thematic libraries (focused toward the biochemical function of the target), and knowledge-based libraries (focused toward compounds that possess characteristics known to be required of a lead) [8]. These HTS strategies have been extremely successful and adept at identifying potent leads and eventually successful drugs, and in fact, this process has initiated most approved drugs on the market. However, the current limitations of high-throughput screening for hit identification are cost, time required, and low hit rate. In a direct comparison of HTS to computer-aided drug discovery, researchers demonstrated a hit rate of 34.8 % (127 of 365 compounds) when using CADD versus only 0.021 % (81 of 400,000) when using HTS, representing a 1700-fold enrichment of the hit rate when using computational methods [9]. Our approach will offer a means of combining the unique advantages of HTS and virtual screening into a single workflow.

After hit identification, the next step in drug discovery is "hit-to-lead" (H2L) or lead generation. A lead is a hit that represents a compound series with the potential (signified by its potency, pharmacokinetic properties, selectivity, and low toxicity) to become a technically successful drug [8]. Lead generation takes into account practical aspects of the compound, such as its ability to be synthesized at large scales for low costs, availability of intellectual property, low cytotoxicity, favorable pharmacokinetics, and high selectivity amongst other characteristics.

This chapter focus on a novel approach to in silico drug discovery that aims to improve the two aforementioned stages: hit identification and lead generation, via the use of combined computational methods. The compounds that are identified must then undergo the later stages of drug discovery, which include lead optimization and concept testing (Fig. 15.1).

Our pathway for early stage lead generation will follow four stages: Stage 1 is virtual high throughput screening (vHTS), Stage 2 is traditional high throughput screening (HTS), Stage 3 is fingerprint analysis of small molecules, and Stage 4 will integrate the results with topological data analysis (TDA). Stage 1 and 2 are commonly used techniques for hit generation. In Stage 3, we will use PubChem's fingerprints to harvest complex, granular structural information about our compounds. Finally, in Stage 4 we will create a topological network of our compound library based on their structural similarities as derived from molecular fingerprints (Stage 3). The topological network will serve as a framework for more intelligent hit selection using the results from Stages 1 and 2 (Fig. 15.2).

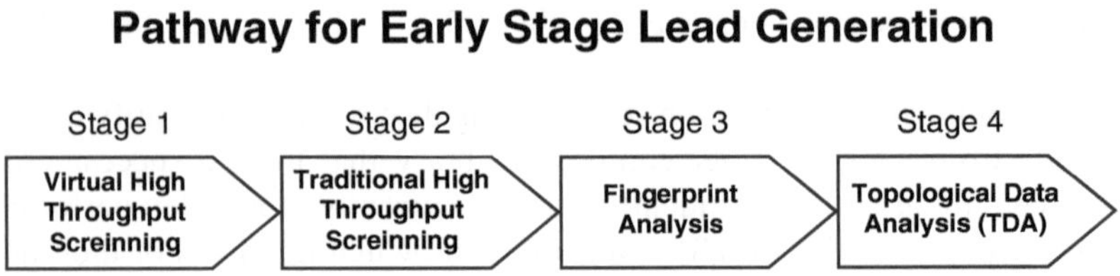

Fig. 15.2 A schematic view of our proposed multimodal technique for early stage lead generation

15.2 Drug Discovery Techniques

15.2.1 Virtual Ligand Screening

Virtual ligand screening or virtual high-throughput screening (vHTS) is an in silico approach to drug discovery which involves the computational simulation of compound-target binding to determine which compounds have the best binding potential.

15.2.2 High-throughput Screening (HTS)

High-throughput screening is a robotic approach for screening thousands of compounds in short time frames to obtain an initial sense of their viability.

15.2.3 Fingerprint Structural Analysis

Fingerprints are a collection of binary variables that describe structural features of a compound, which allow researchers to perform multivariable data analysis.

15.2.4 Topological Data Analysis (TDA)

Topological data analysis is a mathematical technique for studying relationships among data points in high dimensional datasets through the creation of similarity networks [10–13].

15.3 Choosing a Compound Library

The first step of this methodology requires the researcher to have access to a library of small molecule compounds, which will serve as the basis for the remainder of the techniques. The compound library can consist of any number of compounds, ranging from thousands to millions of small molecules. Although even a generic, broad library of millions of compounds from a publicly available sources, such as PubChem's entire compound library of more than 50 million compounds, is suitable, it is preferable to choose selective libraries that are enhanced toward the functions of the intended target or that are already proven to be pharmacologically successful, such as The Library of Pharmacologically Active Compounds (Sigma-Aldrich, St. Louis, MO) or the FDA Approved Drug Library (Enzo Life Sciences, Farmingdale, NY). The advantage to smaller, selective compound libraries is multifold: (a) they allow for marginally faster computational processing times, (b) they are sold in sets that allow them to be easily tested in HTS assays, and (c) some have been empirically validated as potentially successful compounds, thus eliminating the need to iterate through inherently unstable compounds. This final advantage allows the researcher to be more successful in hit-to-lead advancement, as the hits are likely to be high quality, high potential drug compounds.

15.4 Stage I: Virtual High Throughput Screening (vHTS)

Structure-based drug design (SBDD) is a general term for drug discovery techniques that utilize the 3-dimensional structure of a target to predict and optimize the activity of drug compounds. A specific method of SBDD is virtual screening or virtual high throughput screening (vHTS), which is a technique for computationally simulating the drug-target interactions of compounds to quantify their effect potential [14]. Its objective is to quickly identify "hits" or promising compounds within a larger library, which makes it comparable to traditional high throughput screening. However, its comparative advantage is that all of the simulations can be done computationally rather than experimentally, resulting in large savings in time and cost.

The primary distinction to be made within vHTS is between a ligand-based and receptor-based approach [15]. In the ligand-based approach, a particular ligand of interest is used to identify similar ligands, using techniques such as similarity searching, fingerprint analysis, and quantitative structure–activity relationships (QSAR). In this method, the objective is to start with a potentially promising ligand and find others that share similar qualities. In contrast, the receptor-based approach starts with a 3D target protein of interest and attempts to identify potential ligands based on their ability to successfully interact with the target, through computational docking and scoring algorithms. We suggest the receptor-based approach of vHTS because it allows one to discover a broad diversity of ligands, as the identification methods are based on their relationship to the target rather than their similarity to each other.

The first step in vHTS is to select a docking program to run the virtual screen. Several such programs are publicly available including AutoDock (Scripps Research Institute, San Diego, CA), DOCK (UCSF, San Francisco, CA), LigandFit [16], and FlexX (Universitat Hamburg, Hamburg, Germany). We have personally employed AutoDock Vina as it offers comprehensive tools and is freely available for academic purposes.

Once a docking program is chosen and installed, the next process is to prepare the protein target, which involves two sub-steps: (a) resolving the 3D structure, and (b) choosing a binding site for docking. Owing to the advances in experimental methods such as nuclear magnetic resonance (NMR) spectroscopy, X-ray crystallography, and electron microscopy (EM), we now know the 3D structures of thousands of protein targets [17]. The vast majority of these structures are deposited in the Protein Data Bank (PDB), which contains structures ranging from protein fragments to large macromolecules. As of 2007, the PDB included over 53,000 protein structures with more than 8000 new structures being added each year [17]. However, if the 3D structure of a protein of interest has not yet been resolved, there are comparative homology modeling techniques, which involve sequence alignment and construction of missing coordinates, to predict its 3D structure [3]. Although not perfect, these methods are well-described and empirically successful [18]. Once the 3D structure is available, the researcher must determine the optimal binding site on the target for the program to use in its docking simulations. Binding sites are usually chosen based on either known biological information about the mechanism of the protein or on cocrystal structures that have a known ligand [3]. However, computational programs, including POCKET and SURFNEt also exist to discover novel binding sites within a target using techniques such as locating concave invaginations and evaluating protein dynamics [3].

Now that a docking program, compound library, and protein target are all chosen and prepared, the remaining steps involve running the vHTS on your library of compounds. When operating on the docking software, there are a few prerequisite steps. First, the docking site (active site) of the target protein needs to be defined by an accurate "grid box" that encompasses the entire surface of the binding site (Fig. 15.3). Second, the structure files of the target protein and screening compounds need to be formatted according to the requirements of the docking software. Third, requisite information for both the target protein and the virtual compound library need to be appropriately recorded in the configuration file of the docking software. With these steps completed, the virtual screening should proceed without complication.

The output of the vHTS should be a list of the compounds and their respective scores (often presented as binding energies) as it relates to their binding efficacy. The compounds with the best scores represent the "hits" from the vHTS, and any number of them can be tested experimentally to verify their binding activity. Although it is sufficient to proceed with these hits to the "hit-to-lead" stage of drug discovery, we will instead save these scores as Column 1 in a datasheet, which we will use later when we integrate the results of the three stages of analysis.

15.5 Stage II: Traditional High-Throughput Screening (HTS)

The introduction of automated high-throughput screening in the 1990s represented a significant milestone in the field of drug discovery. For perhaps the first time, large compound libraries, containing hundreds of thousands of compounds, could

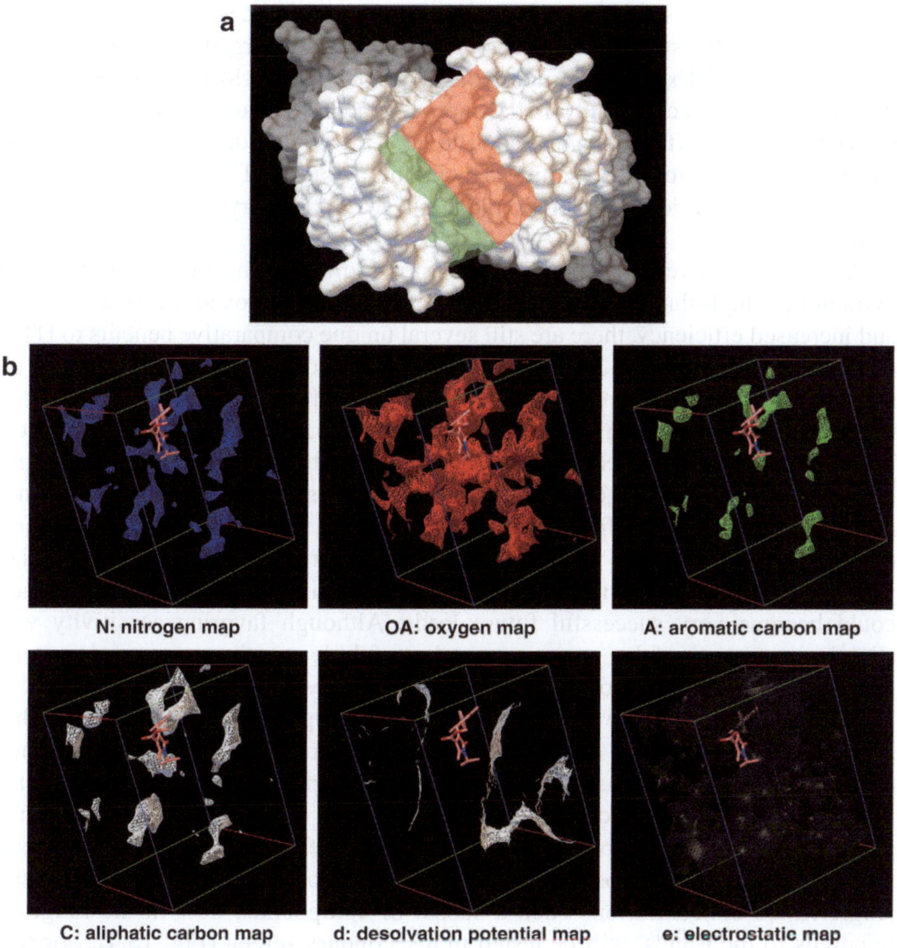

Fig. 15.3 A visual depiction of AutoDock's virtual screening software. (**a**) A grid box encompasses the ribonuclease domain of an IRE1α dimer. (**b**) Affinity grids are calculated for each atom of the compound

be quickly and efficiently screened by robots in the order of days to reveal a smaller subset of compounds with the highest potential for activity. By doing so, researchers could quickly identify a group of high-potential compounds to progress to the lead generation stage of discovery. This method further optimized the drug discovery process by eliminating the need for extensive "hit-to-lead" translation, as most of these compounds were already ready for large-scale pharmaceutical development [8]. These screenings were traditionally performed on large diversity-driven libraries, where the focus was on quantity of compounds rather than likelihood of activity. However, as discussed previously, researchers are currently trending toward using thematic libraries that are built with prior knowledge of the target using combinatorial chemistry.

High-throughput screening is the most empirically successful method of lead generation, as almost every new drug compound has emerged through a process involving HTS [8]. Examples are numerous and include Merck Research Laboratories' discovery of diketoacids, a novel HIV-suppressing class of compounds which block viral integration of HIV-1 integrase and Harvard University's discovery of monastrol, an anticancer agent that blocks mitosis by inhibiting kinesin Eg5, after screening the Diverset E (Chembridge Corporation, San Diego, CA) library of more than 16,000 compounds [8].

Although many researchers are now favoring virtual high-throughput screening to traditional high-throughput screening because of the improved speed, lower cost, and increased efficiency, there are still several unique comparative benefits to HTS, which help it remain as an important step in the drug discovery process. First, HTS allows you to identify compound hits without significant prior knowledge about the target, such as binding sites, compound affinities, or structural characteristics. This advantage allows researchers to identify hits for targets where the 3D structure is unresolved or for targets that are not mechanistically understood. Second, improvements in HTS efficiency and assay quality will improve the hit-finding ability of HTS compared to vHTS [19]. Newer assays are being developed to optimize sensitivity, thereby increasing the ability to detect weakly active compounds, which could become very successful future leads. Although favoring sensitivity will slightly increase the false positive rate, these falsely positive compounds can be discarded in future stages of the drug discovery process.

We briefly describe the steps of our high-throughput screens. We begin with a primary screen that tests our entire compound library. As there are thousands compounds to test at this stage, the screening is performed on the main reporter cell line at only one concentration per compound. Since the majority of compounds in the library will be negative hits, this step serves to quickly narrow down the library to only the most promising compounds based on their efficacy in the single tested concentration. Then a subset of compounds, now in the range of hundreds to thousands, will be tested in a secondary screen (Fig. 15.4). For this step, an approach called quantitative high throughput screening (qHTS) can be applied, in which each compound is tested at a series of concentrations on both the main reporter cell line and a counter-screen reporter cell line, usually used to control for undesired effects (e.g., cytotoxicity) [20]. The results of the secondary screen are a dose-activity curve for each compound at the various tested concentrations.

As before, these results can be independently used to advance certain compounds to the lead optimization stage. However, for our methodology, we will save the secondary screen assay results from one specific concentration as a "percent-inhibition" value into a new column (Column 2) in the same spreadsheet as before. These two columns will be utilized in the fourth stage of our drug discovery process, when we use topological data analysis to integrate the results.

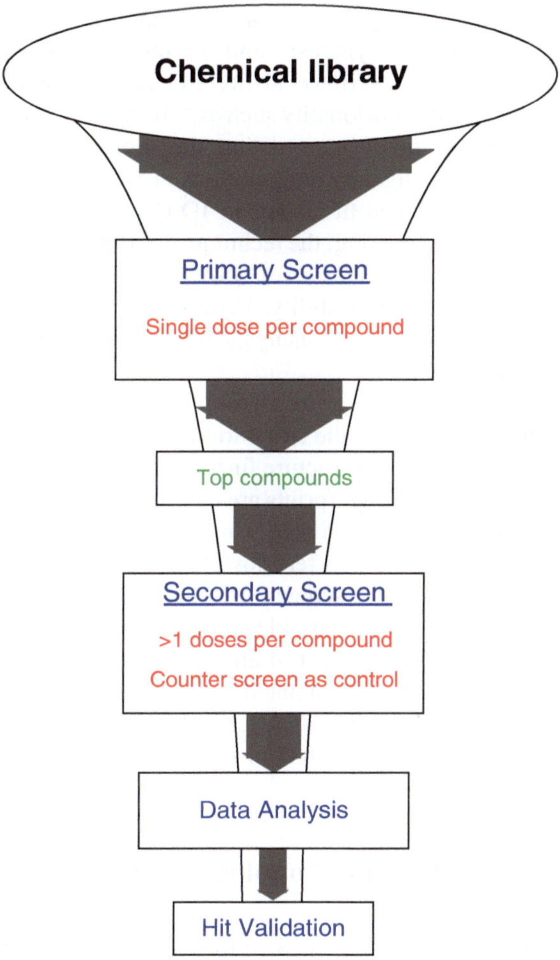

Fig. 15.4 The workflow of our high-throughput screening: a primary and secondary screen are performed on an initial compound library

15.6 Stage III: PubChem Fingerprint Analysis

In the final stage of this process, we use structural information about compounds to further enhance our ability to identify hits. The major advancement in the use of chemical and structural information to assist with drug discovery was quantitative structure–activity relationship (QSAR) models, which uses statistical models to predict how different physicochemical properties of chemical substances affect biological activity [21]. The earliest example of QSAR dates back to 1893, when Charles Richet described a novel relationship between the solubility of compounds and their toxicity [22]. From that starting point, QSAR has developed tremendously as a means of rapidly evaluating compounds for their predicted activity, prioritizing compounds for synthesis, and serving as a cheaper alternative to costly biological assays [21]. As Verma et al. describe in their book, new evolutions in QSAR include expanded dimensionality such as, "3D-QSAR correlating activity with non-covalent interaction fields surrounding the molecules, 4D-QSAR additionally including ensemble of ligand configurations in 3D-QSAR, 5D-QSAR explicitly representing different induced-fit models in 4D-QSAR" [21].

Virtual screening, the technique introduced in "Stage 1" of this chapter, is a natural, automated extension of QSAR, as it uses the structural properties of compounds to predict binding ability. However, in this stage, we want to introduce another technique, fingerprint analysis, which also incorporates structural information about compounds.

Fingerprints refer to a group of variables that are collectively used to convey information about the structural features of a compound. PubChem generates a list of 881 binary substructure fingerprints for every chemical compound in their database [23]. The fingerprints are distributed into broad structural categories, including element counts, atom pairs, ring characteristics, atom neighborhoods, and SMARTS patterns. PubChem offers download of fingerprint information for any compound in their database. Subsequent use of Base64 decoding can convert the fingerprint into a list of 881 binary variables for each compound (Fig. 15.5). We can then update our dataset to include a list of all of the compounds from the secondary screen (rows), which were each annotated with several variables: (1) the virtual binding score (from Stage 1) in Column 1, (2) the HTS "percent inhibition" score (from Stage 2) in Column 2, and (3) 881 binary fingerprint variables in Columns 3-883.

15.7 Stage IV: Topological Data Analysis

Using the results aggregated from the prior three stages, we now have a dataset that contains information about compounds with respect to their binding affinity to the target, their empirical HTS assay result, and their granular structural features. In this stage, we will employ topological data analysis (TDA), a mathematical technique for studying shapes and preserving high-dimensionality, to create a similarity network of our compounds. TDA will allow us to visualize our library of compounds in a two-dimensional network, whereby compounds (located in nodes) are connected to each other by a series of edges that reflects their level of shared similarity (Fig. 15.6). Therefore, two compounds that share several similar properties will appear closer together in the network, whereas two vastly different compounds will be farther apart. This network will make it simple to create subgroups or families of similar compounds, which can then be used to select the best compound leads.

We use Ayasdi Core (Ayasdi Inc., Menlo Park, CA) to create our TDA network of compounds. However, if access to Ayasdi Core is unavailable, alternative options include other TDA applications or employing weaker techniques such as K-means clustering to achieve somewhat similar results. We first discuss the methodology as

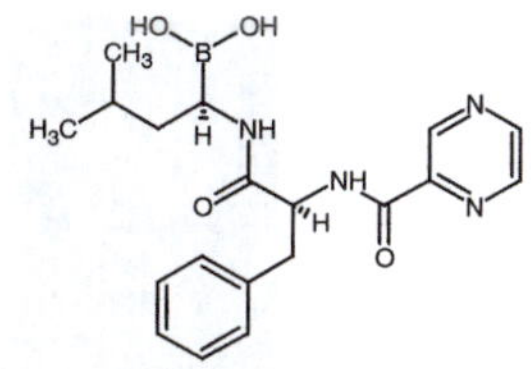

Bortezomib

156 bytes fingerprint:

AAADceJ7uAAAAAAAAAAAAAAAAAAAAAAA8QAAAAAAAAAABwAA
oHgAQCAAADSjBngQ+gJLIEACoAzV3VACCgCQ3EiAI2IG4dMgIYHrA0TG
UIlgglgDliMcYiICOAAAAAAAAAAAAAAAAAAAAAAAAAAAAA==

Binary	ASCII	Binary	ASCII	Binary	ASCII	Binary	ASCII
000000	A	010000	Q	100000	g	110000	w
000001	B	010001	R	100001	h	110001	x
000010	C	010010	S	100010	i	110010	y
000011	D	010011	T	100011	j	110011	z
000100	E	010100	U	100100	k	110100	0
000101	F	010101	V	100101	l	110101	1
000110	G	010110	W	100110	m	110110	2
000111	H	010111	X	100111	n	110111	3
001000	I	011000	Y	101000	o	111000	4
001001	J	011001	Z	101001	p	111001	5
001010	K	011010	a	101010	q	111010	6
001011	L	011011	b	101011	r	111011	7
001100	M	011100	c	101100	s	111100	8
001101	N	011101	d	101101	t	111101	9
001110	O	011110	e	101110	u	111110	+
001111	P	011111	f	101111	v	111111	/

881 binary substructure fingerprint:

Byte A A A D c e J 7 u ....
Bit 000000 000000 000000 000011 000010 000100 001001 111011 010100 ....
Bit position 0 6 12 18 24 30 36 42 48

Byte .... A A A A A A A = =
Bit 000000 000000 000000 000000 000000 000000 000000
Bit position 882 888 894 900 906 912 918

Fig. 15.5 Schematic diagram depicting the translation of a 156-byte PubChem fingerprint into an 881 variable binary output, which will be used to describe the structural features of each compound

it relates to TDA and then explain a parallel process that can be employed with clustering algorithms.

A topological analysis is created with two types of parameters: a metric and a lens. A metric is a mathematical function used to measure the similarity between two points in some space (usually between rows in the data). The choice of a metric

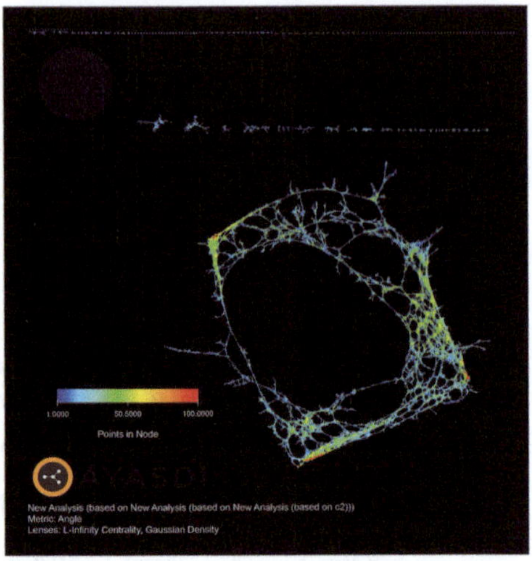

Fig. 15.6 An example network created by performing Topological Data Analysis (TDA) on sample biological data sets using the Ayasdi Core software platform (Ayasdi.com, Ayasdi Inc., Menlo Park, CA). Nodes in the network represent clusters of compounds and edges connect nodes that contain similar compounds. The color scheme in this graph is the average number of data points in each node

greatly influences how the similarity of data points is assessed. Lenses are real valued functions on the data points. Lenses are used to create overlapping bins in the data set, where the bins are preimages under the lens of an interval. Overlapping families of intervals are used to create overlapping bins in the data. Metrics are used with lenses to construct the Ayasdi Core output. Further, multiple lenses can be used in each analysis. There are two user-determined parameters that are important in defining the bins. The first is *resolution*, which determines the number of bins. Higher resolutions correspond to a greater number of bins and a fewer number of data points per bin. The second is *gain*, which determines the degree of overlap of the intervals. Increasing the gain increases the overlap between bins, such that they share more data points in common [10–13].

Once the bins are constructed, the software performs a clustering step within each bin. To do so, it uses single linkage clustering with a fixed heuristic for the choice of the scale parameter [11]. Finally, the network is formed by creating a node for each cluster and connecting nodes if the corresponding clusters contain at least one data point in common. TDA also allows the user to identify the important factors or variables that distinguish two groups of nodes. To do so, it employs a nonparametric statistical test (Kolmogorov–Smirnov) in combination with the p-value (t-test).

The metric we will select for our analysis is Angle, and the lenses are L-Infinity Centrality and Gaussian Density. The Angle metric computes the angle between two rows, by taking the inverse cosine of the dot product of the vectors. The L-infinity Centrality lens calculates for each point x the maximal distance from x to any other data point in the dataset. Therefore, this lens is strongly correlated with density in normally distributed variables, but not as much in bimodal distributions. The Gaussian Density lens applies a kernel Gaussian density estimator by treating each row in Euclidean data space to estimate the density of that point.

The next choice with TDA algorithms is which columns in the data set you want to use for creation of the similarity network. The columns you choose will dictate

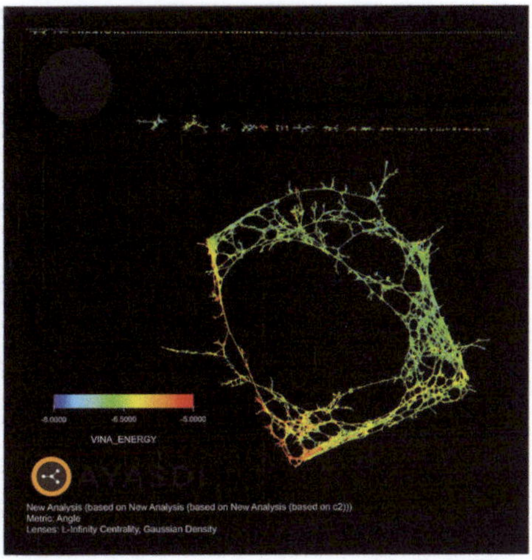

Fig. 15.7 The same network shown in Fig. 15.6 is now colored by virtual docking energy from Stage 1. For virtual docking energy ("VINA_ ENERGY"), more negative values indicate higher binding affinity. Thus, nodes in red contain compounds with the best binding affinities. A range of –8 to –5 kcal/mol is displayed

the nature of the similarities. For our methods, we will use only the 881 structural fingerprint variables to create our network. The resulting graph will contain every compound in our library, connected to one another based on their structural fingerprint similarities (Fig. 15.6). Therefore, compounds in the same section of the network will inherently share a large set of common structural features. Ayasdi Core allows for further analysis by coloring the network by our variables of interest. In our technique, we will color our network first by the vHTS score and then by the HTS score. The resulting pictures of the network provide a visual demonstration of which areas of the network contain compounds with the best binding energies and HTS results. Since we know the network was created based on structural fingerprint similarities, we can infer that those areas of the network must inherently contain certain structural features that may be related to their success.

After creating the network, we will first examine it to understand its shape. Distinct "shapes" within the network represent families of compounds that share common properties, in this case structural features. These two-dimensional shapes instruct us of hidden multidimensional meaning about the structural features they share [11, 12]. We will physically create these groups by drawing in boundaries between distinct shapes. Each enclosed group or family will then contain a set of compounds that we hypothesize shares similarities.

Next, we will annotate the network with the findings from Stages 1 and 2 to begin the process of picking lead compounds. First, we will annotate the network by virtual binding score (Fig. 15.7). Annotating refers to overlaying the network with a heat map (also referred to as "coloring") that reflects each compound's value for a selected variable, in this case the virtual binding score. The annotations will depict which compounds within each family have the best virtual binding affinity. We can then select the 3–5 best compounds by virtual affinity score within each family as our leads. Second, we will annotate the network by the HTS assay result (Fig. 15.8). Once again, we will select the 3–5 best compounds in each family, making note of which compounds were also chosen because of their virtual affinity score.

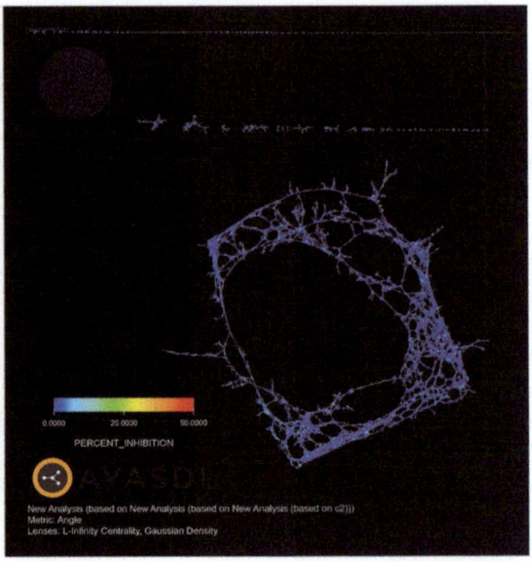

Fig. 15.8 The same network shown in Fig. 15.6 is now colored by "percent-inhibition" values by high-throughput screening from Stage 2. For HTS ("PERCENT_INHIBITION"), more positive values indicate a higher percent inhibition of our selected protein target. A range of 0–50 % inhibition is shown

This method of choosing lead compounds after stratifying by structural families is advantageous because it ensures that a diverse set of leads are chosen (as they come from a diverse collection of structural families) and it is also more forgiving to certain compounds that may not have great absolute virtual binding or HTS scores, but may still turn out to be excellent drug choices. If we had simply identified our hits by choosing the best 100 compounds by virtual binding score, we may unfairly bias ourselves towards one specific family of compounds that happen to be favored by that specific docking mechanism. As a result, we may overlook compounds with excellent in vivo potential that simply didn't have the features to make them successful in initial screens with virtual docking or in vitro HTS.

As a further refinement step, we can use the annotation results to determine which 1–2 families of compounds performed best in both the virtual screen and HTS. With this knowledge, we can recursively add more compounds from those families to our initial library, as we know those families may contain certain important features. This method of expanding compound libraries around the hit compounds is becoming more prevalent in the pharmaceutical industry [24].

If you do not have access to TDA, another process of lead identification can be accomplished using k-means clustering, whereby you separate your compounds into k clusters based on shared properties, in this case the 881 PubChem structural fingerprints. Once the clusters are chosen, you can rank the compounds within each cluster first by vHTS and next by HTS score. As was done above, select the 3–5 highest ranked compounds within each family for each scoring system. Instead of using a heat map or coloring mechanism to identify the best compounds, you will then numerically rank the compounds based on the value of their scores (vHTS and HTS).

To then accomplish the refinement step of adding new compounds, rank the entire compound library by these two scores to determine which 1–2 families demonstrate the most consistent success. Recursively add new compounds from these families to the initial compound library.

15.8 Conclusion

Our methodology described here combines virtual screening, high-throughput screening, structural fingerprints, and topological data analysis to more intelligently identify lead compounds from large compound libraries. Each of these individual techniques has several strengths but also shortcomings that can be mitigated by utilizing the techniques together. For example, virtual screening, although extremely fast and inexpensive, suffers from needing access to the 3D structure of the protein target and having some preexisting knowledge about its binding domains and tendencies. Conversely, HTS allows for comprehensive in vitro testing without any prior knowledge of the target, yet it often only tests the compound at one dose and in one type of assay, both of which are restrictions that could unfairly filter out otherwise excellent compounds. By combining both methods, we make use of their unique advantages without inheriting their shortcomings.

Researchers have already shown the benefit of combining multiple types of methods in their work. For example, prior research has shown that a machine-learning model trained on HTS and chemical fingerprints performed similar or better than a model trained on either subset alone [24]. But even such approaches suffer from the same problem of selectively favoring compounds that perform well in the tested assays. Although this seems like a logical choice, it misses the mark because the ability of HTS, virtual screening, or fingerprints to predict in vivo drug success is far from perfect. There are many compounds that demonstrate excellent in vitro success but fail to have an effect in vivo, and vice versa [25]. And most of these shortcomings are because of pharmacokinetic and metabolic properties that are potentially secondary to their chemical structures. In other words, there are many compounds that aren't structurally suited for vHTS or HTS success, which are eliminated at an early stage in the drug discovery processes, even though they may have been excellent drugs. Similarly, certain structural features may predispose a certain family of compounds to receive very high scores in vHTS and HTS, which would lead to a disproportionately large number of compounds from that family advancing through the drug discovery pipeline. Thus, by using topological data analysis to first create families of structural compounds, and then using our virtual screening and HTS results to choose the most promising compounds within each family, we ensure that a diversity of compounds are chosen for the next stage of the drug development cycle.

References

1. Ekins S, Mestres J, Testa B. In silico pharmacology for drug discovery: methods for virtual ligand screening and profiling. Br J Pharmacol. 2007;152(1):9–20. doi:10.1038/sj.bjp.0707305.
2. Drews J. Drug discovery: a historical perspective. Science. 2000;287(5460):1960–4.
3. Sliwoski G, Kothiwale S, Meiler J, Lowe EW. Computational methods in drug discovery. Pharmacol Rev. 2014;66(1):334–95. doi:10.1124/pr.112.007336.

4. Van Drie JH. Computer-aided drug design: the next 20 years. J Comput Aided Mol Des. 2007;21(10-11):591–601. doi:10.1007/s10822-007-9142-y.
5. Talele TT, Khedkar SA, Rigby AC. Successful applications of computer aided drug discovery: moving drugs from concept to the clinic. Curr Top Med Chem. 2010;10(1):127–41.
6. Bains W. Failure rates in drug discovery and development: will we ever get any better? 2004.
7. Agarwal AK, Fishwick CW. Structure-based design of anti-infectives. Ann N Y Acad Sci. 2010;1213:20–45. doi:10.1111/j.1749-6632.2010.05859.x.
8. Golebiowski A, Klopfenstein SR, Portlock DE. Lead compounds discovered from libraries. Curr Opin Chem Biol. 2001;5(3):273–84.
9. Doman TN, McGovern SL, Witherbee BJ, Kasten TP, Kurumbail R, Stallings WC, et al. Molecular docking and high-throughput screening for novel inhibitors of protein tyrosine phosphatase-1B. J Med Chem. 2002;45(11):2213–21.
10. Carlsson G. Topology and Data. Bull Amer Math Soc. 2009;46:255–308.
11. Singh G, Memoli F, Carlsson G. Topological methods for the analysis of high dimensional data sets and 3D object recognition. Eurograph Symp Point Based Graph. 2007.
12. Lum PY, Singh G, Lehman A, Ishkanov T, Vejdemo-Johansson M, Alagappan M, et al. Extracting insights from the shape of complex data using topology. Sci Rep. 2013;3:1236. doi:10.1038/srep01236.
13. Sarikonda G, Pettus J, Phatak S, Sachithanantham S, Miller JF, Wesley JD, et al. CD8 T-cell reactivity to islet antigens is unique to type 1 while CD4 T-cell reactivity exists in both type 1 and type 2 diabetes. J Autoimmun. 2014;50:77–82. doi:10.1016/j.jaut.2013.12.003.
14. Jain AN. Virtual screening in lead discovery and optimization. Curr Opin Drug Discov Devel. 2004;7(4):396–403.
15. Ghosh S, Nie A, An J, Huang Z. Structure-based virtual screening of chemical libraries for drug discovery. Curr Opin Chem Biol. 2006;10(3):194–202. doi:10.1016/j.cbpa.2006.04.002.
16. Adams PD, Afonine PV, Bunkóczi G, Chen VB, Davis IW, Echols N, et al. PHENIX: a comprehensive Python-based system for macromolecular structure solution. Acta Crystallogr D Biol Crystallogr. 2010;66(Pt 2):213–21. doi:10.1107/S0907444909052925.
17. Dutta S, Burkhardt K, Swaminathan GJ, Kosada T, Henrick K, Nakamura H, et al. Data deposition and annotation at the worldwide protein data bank. Methods Mol Biol. 2008;426:81–101. doi:10.1007/978-1-60327-058-8_5.
18. Evers A, Gohlke H, Klebe G. Ligand-supported homology modelling of protein binding-sites using knowledge-based potentials. J Mol Biol. 2003;334(2):327–45.
19. Mayr LM, Bojanic D. Novel trends in high-throughput screening. Curr Opin Pharmacol. 2009;9(5):580–8. doi:10.1016/j.coph.2009.08.004.
20. Inglese J, Auld DS, Jadhav A, Johnson RL, Simeonov A, Yasgar A, et al. Quantitative high-throughput screening: a titration-based approach that efficiently identifies biological activities in large chemical libraries. Proc Natl Acad Sci U S A. 2006;103(31):11473–8. doi:10.1073/pnas.0604348103.
21. Verma J, Khedkar VM, Coutinho EC. 3D-QSAR in drug design--a review. Curr Top Med Chem. 2010;10(1):95–115.
22. Kubinyi H. 3D QSAR in drug design. In: Theory methods and applications, vol 1. New York: Springer; 1993.
23. Bolton E, Wang Y, Thiessen P, Bryant S. PubChem: Integrated platform of small molecules and biological activities. Annual Reports in Computational Chemistry. 2008;4:217–241.
24. Riniker S, Wang Y, Jenkins JL, Landrum GA. Using information from historical high-throughput screens to predict active compounds. J Chem Inf Model. 2014;54(7):1880–91. doi:10.1021/ci500190p.
25. Lin JH, Lu AY. Role of pharmacokinetics and metabolism in drug discovery and development. Pharmacol Rev. 1997;49(4):403–49.

Chapter 16
Efficient Protocol for the Identification of Hypoxic Cell Radiosensitisers

Cho Rong Hong, Jingli Wang, Kevin O. Hicks, and Michael P. Hay

Abstract An evolution in radiotherapy practice is leading to greater use of stereotactic body radiotherapy (SBRT), raising the prospect of increased hypoxic cell radioresistance. New clinical interest in nitroimidazole radiosensitisers, combined with appropriate biomarkers, signals a revival for radiosensitisers in the context of SBRT. Our interest in modifiers of radiation therapy led us to revisit this area and we have identified a new class of nitroimidazole radiosensitiser. We have developed an abbreviated screening protocol suitable for an academic drug discovery laboratory which allows expeditious triage of compounds with poor physicochemical and in vitro properties and combines in vitro radiosensitisation data with tumour pharmacokinetic data to efficiently select candidates for further evaluation.

Keywords Hypoxia • Drug discovery • Radiosensitiser • Nitroimidazole

16.1 Introduction

16.1.1 Hypoxia Is Treatment Limiting

Hypoxia within solid tumours is a major component of the tumour microenvironment and, despite an on-going debate around the definitions, extent and heterogeneity of hypoxia [1], there is clear evidence that tumour hypoxia plays a significant role in shaping the microenvironment and development of the disease [2]. Hypoxia contributes to altered tumour metabolism [3], invasion [4], and metastasis [5] and is associated with poor prognosis and resistance to therapeutic agents [6–8]. This resistance to therapy has been most clearly catalogued in the context of radiation therapy [9]: in head and neck squamous cell carcinoma [10–13] and cervical carcinoma [14] where radiotherapy and, latterly, chemo-radiotherapy play definitive roles.

C.R. Hong • J. Wang, Ph.D. • K.O. Hicks, Ph.D. • M.P. Hay, Ph.D. (✉)
Auckland Cancer Society Research Centre, The University of Auckland,
Private Bag 92019, Auckland 1142, New Zealand
e-mail: c.hong@auckland.ac.nz; jingli.wang@auckland.ac.nz; k.hicks@auckland.ac.nz; m.hay@auckland.ac.nz

C. Koumenis et al. (eds.), *Tumor Microenvironment*, Advances in Experimental Medicine and Biology 899, DOI 10.1007/978-3-319-26666-4_16

The long history of hypoxia modification to improve treatment response has been reviewed extensively [8, 15–19]. Three main approaches to modify tumour hypoxia for therapeutic benefit were explored over several decades. Increased oxygen delivery to tumours was achieved with hyperbaric oxygen [20] or carbogen breathing [21]. Electron affinic nitroimidazoles were intended to mimic oxygen and "fix" radiation damage in hypoxic tumour cells [22–24]. These agents evolved into a third approach where hypoxic cell cytotoxins were designed to selectively kill hypoxic tumour cells [8, 25]. The clinical experience with these modalities has been less than stellar, beset by inadequate trial design and a lack of biomarkers to identify patients with hypoxic tumours. Nonetheless, when taken together in a retrospective analysis, these interventions have been shown to provide benefit [19].

16.1.2 Oxygen Mimetic Radiosensitisers

Oxygen mimetic radiosensitisers were most commonly nitroimidazoles where the electron affinic nitro group was designed to react with DNA radicals produced by ionising radiation in a manner similar to oxygen [24]. Formation of these adducts led to DNA strand breaks and cell death. The key factor driving the reaction of the nitroimidazole moiety with these initial DNA radicals is the electron affinity of the nitro group with the one-electron reduction potential [E(1)] being a surrogate measure of this affinity [26].

An early clinical trial of the 5-nitroimidazole antibiotic metronidazole with larger (3.3 Gy) doses of radiation in the treatment of gliobastoma multiforme demonstrated a significant increase in survival compared to radiation alone [27]. However, a second trial comparing this regimen with convention FRT and misonidazole (**1**, Fig. 16.1) failed to show any significant differences in survival time [28]. Misonidazole was extensively trialled in the clinic and, despite indications of clinical benefit [23], delayed peripheral neuropathy prevented treatment with an efficacious dose [29, 30]. Attempts to design more polar analogues with increased systemic clearance to minimise distribution to sensitive tissues were only partially successful with etanidazole (**2**) failing to provide benefit in head and neck cancer [31]. However, this hypothesis appears to have been somewhat more successful in the case of doranidazole (**3**) which underwent investigation in non-small-cell lung cancer [32] and pancreatic cancer [33] where doranidazole, in conjunction with intraoperative radiotherapy (25 Gy), demonstrated a survival advantage. Although nitroimidazole radiosensitisers were extensively investigated clinically, and a recent meta-analysis has confirmed their clinical activity [19], only nimorazole (**4**) [34] is in limited clinical use [18]. A recent development has seen a new European clinical trial to evaluate nimorazole (and a hypoxic gene signature) in combination with cisplatin-based chemoradiotherapy in patients with locally advanced, HPV-negative head and neck cancer (ClinialTrials.gov: NCT01880359).

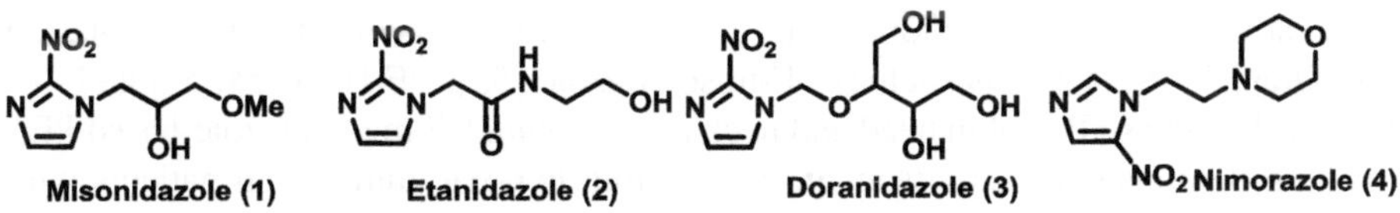

Fig. 16.1 Nitroimidazole radiosensitisers

16.1.3 Hypoxia Activated Prodrugs

Nitroimidazoles with higher electron affinity [E(1)>ca. –420 mV] were also observed to behave as hypoxia-selective cytotoxins [35–37] undergoing one electron reduction by cellular reductases [8]. The radical anion so formed may undergo oxidation in the presence of oxygen to regenerate the nitroimidazole, or further reduction to reactive species capable of attack on cellular macromolecules. This mechanism delivers selective cytotoxicity in the presence of hypoxia (and appropriate reductases) and was the basis for two decades of intense research on hypoxia-activated prodrugs (HAP) [8, 25]. The focus on HAPs continues today with TH-302 [38, 39], the leading candidate in the field, demonstrating activity in sarcoma [40] and pancreatic disease [41] in combination with chemotherapy; however TH-302 has recently failed to provide significant benefit compared to standard of care therapy in PIII trials (NCT01746979, NCT01440088). Another leading contender in the HAP space was the benzotriazine dioxide, tirapazamine (TPZ) [42]. In a pilot PII imaging study of patients with head and neck carcinoma in combination with chemo-radiotherapy TPZ showed benefit for patients with hypoxic tumours identified by ^{18}F-misonidazole PET imaging [43]. Unfortunately, this lesson and those of previous decades were ignored [44], and a PIII trial of TPZ in combination with platinum based chemo-radiotherapy was conducted without the benefit of imaging for hypoxia or the use of biomarkers such as p16 [45]. TPZ failed to show benefit [46] and further development appears unlikely. A second generation analogue of TPZ known as SN30000 is in preclinical development [47–49]. This compound has improved potency/solubility and extravascular transport, culminating in improved hypoxic cell killing in vivo [48]. Importantly, appropriate biomarkers for both hypoxia and activating reductases have been defined for SN30000 [49]. Other nitroimidazole based HAPs are in development, but few details have been published [8].

16.1.4 Need for Biomarkers

There is a growing understanding that to clinically develop agents that "target" hypoxia, it is necessary to identify this target prospectively in patients. The lack of a clear consensus on the most appropriate biomarkers has hindered the clinical development of numerous hypoxia targeted therapies [50, 51] and identification of suitable biomarkers matched to the investigational agent is a clear priority. Molecular tools for selection of patients with hypoxic tumours are now in clinical development [52].

Most advanced of these biomarkers are the 2-nitroimidazole positron emission tomography (PET) agents such as ^{18}F-misonidazole [53], ^{18}F-HX4 [54, 55] and ^{18}F-EF5 [56]. A Phase II trial in head and neck cancer using ^{18}F-misonidazole-based PET imaging demonstrated an advantage for treating hypoxic tumours in patients with TPZ compared to treatment with standard of care [43]. Another promising approach is the use of "hypoxia gene signatures" [57–61]. Micro-array analysis was used to identify a signature that, in a retrospective study, predicted the impact of hypoxic modification by nimorazole [62]. This study in head and neck tumours, not only shows the impact of hypoxic on radiotherapy outcome, but also the benefit of treating hypoxic patients with nimorazole in conjunction with radiotherapy [62]. This represents an exciting advance for further use of nitroimidazole radiosensitisers.

16.1.5 New Opportunities Presented by the Increasing Use of SBRT

Fractionated radiotherapy (FRT) is one of the main treatments for cancer patients with over 50 % of patients receiving FRT (typically 60–80 Gy delivered in 2–3 Gy fractions over 7–8 weeks), mostly with curative intent [63, 64]. FRT is a difficult regimen for both health delivery and patient compliance and often normal tissue toxicity precludes delivery of sufficient doses of radiation to achieve local control.

Stereotactic body radiotherapy (SBRT) uses hypofractionated (1–5 doses) high dose (25–60 Gy total dose) radiation to treat tumours [65]. This new approach leverages recent advances in the accuracy and precision of radiation delivery to allow dose intensification to small tumours while minimising the effects to adjacent normal tissue. Clinical trials using SBRT to treat various solid tumours have demonstrated comparable control, toxicity and efficacy profiles to FRT [65]. The reduced treatment time and number of patient visits, combined with emerging potential to replace surgery with an outpatient procedure, indicates substantial health, social and economic advantages for SBRT and is driving increasing use of SBRT for treating cancer.

16.1.6 Hypoxic Cell Radiosensitisers in Combination with SBRT

While the use of SBRT continues to grow, a debate has arisen around the role of hypoxia in radioresistance in SBRT. Evidence is emerging that SBRT accentuates hypoxia in radioresistance [15, 66] because the opportunity for reoxygenation that occurs between FRT doses is reduced [67]. While this may still be the subject of on-going debate [68], studies with radiosensitisers in conjunction with SBRT are warranted. The advance of SBRT, along with the development of suitable biomarkers, may herald a renaissance for radiosensitisers in general [69], and new oxygen mimetic nitroimidazoles in particular. Nimorazole is undergoing further evaluation (ClinialTrials.gov: NCT01880359) in combination with a microarray-based hypoxic gene signature. However, all other clinically evaluated nitroimidazoles have either limited or expired patent protection and their clinical development in a new setting is severely compromised as a result. Few examples of novel nitroimidazoles exist in the literature [70–72] and these do not appear to be in clinical development. We recently identified a novel class of nitroimidazole sulfonamide (NISA) radiosensitiser [73] and are currently exploring the activity of this class in order to identify a lead radiosensitiser for clinical development.

16.2 A Protocol for Radiosensitiser Evaluation

16.2.1 Why Develop a New Protocol?

Drug discovery within the academic laboratory is an increasingly difficult proposition with tight budgets and timelines and increasingly strict animal ethics constraints. Many earlier studies of radiosensitisers relied on extensive animal data to compare compounds [74, 75] and this approach is challenging in the current environment. While in vivo studies are critical to advance lead candidates it is no longer practical to screen a large number of candidates in vivo.

Our objective was to design and implement an in vitro-based protocol that could be used to identify (preclinical) leads in an efficient and cost effective manner (Fig. 16.2). We have used 96 well plate based clonogenic assays to improve throughput in radiosensitisation studies and in vitro evaluation of drug transport properties. When combined with tumour pharmacokinetics (PK) these methods accelerate the screening process to identify potential lead compounds and reduce the extent of in vivo studies required [48, 76].

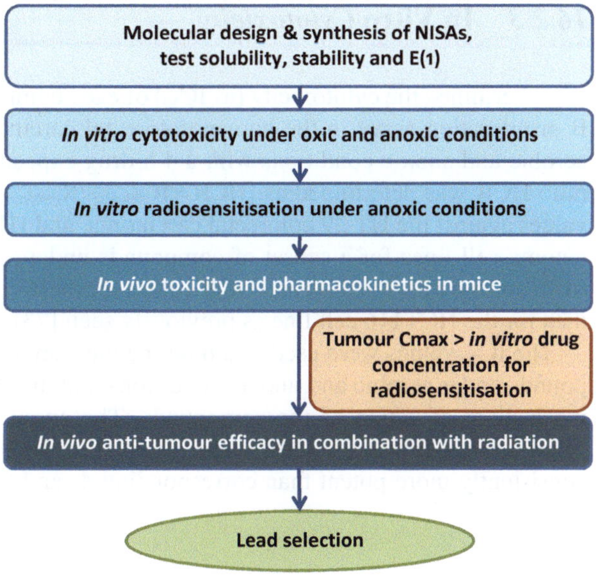

Fig. 16.2 Efficient screening protocol to identify lead radiosensitisers

16.2.2 *Drug Design*

A series of nitroimidazoles bearing sulfonamide, sulfoxide or sulfone linked side chains were prepared using novel chemistry established in our lab [73]. These sulfur-based side chains provide novelty and chemical versatility while exerting a strong electron withdrawing effect on the nitroimidazole unit. We have developed synthetic methodologies to access examples of each of the three possible 2-, 4- and 5-nitroimidazole regioisomers (Table 16.1). These regioisomers provide analogues that span the range of electron affinity for efficient reaction with DNA radicals (as defined by their E(1) values; −500 to −342 mV) [73]. Electron affinity dominates the in vitro structure–activity relationships for radiosensitisation [26] and toxicity [77]. Variations in the side chain also provide a range of solubility and lipophilicity. We use a trial set of 20 analogues, covering a range of these physicochemical properties to illustrate the implementation of this screening protocol.

Current oxygen mimetic radiosensitisers need to be present at relatively high (often mM) concentrations to be effective sensitisers and so aqueous solubility is an important prerequisite for a successful radiosensitiser. Solubility of the compounds was determined for solutions in αMEM medium with 5 % foetal bovine serum with assay by HPLC. (Table 16.1). The solubility of neutral nitroimidazole sulfonamides (e.g. **5–10** and **16–19**) is considerably less than either misonidazole (**1**) or etanidazole (**2**), but is still in the mM range. The use of basic amine side chains (e.g. **11**, **20–24**) provides a significant increase in solubility over similar neutral compounds. Removal of the amide unit also compromises aqueous solubility by some threefold (e.g. **6** vs **15**) and the presence of aryl side chains (**7**, **12–14**) reduces aqueous solubility below the mM range.

16.2.3 In Vitro *Cytotoxicity*

We determined the cytotoxicity (as IC_{50}) of each compound using a sulforhodamine B proliferation assay in the human colorectal carcinoma cell line HCT116 under aerobic and anoxic conditions with a 4 h drug exposure. The hypoxic cytotoxicity ratio HCR was determined as [$HCR = IC_{50(oxic)}/IC_{50(anoxic)}$]. We also determined IC_{50} values against the HT-29 colorectal carcinoma, and H1299 non-small-cell lung carcinoma cell lines for a subset of compounds under aerobic and anoxic conditions (data not shown). The IC_{50} and HCR values for these compounds closely tracked the data for the HCT116 cell line as previously seen [73].

The IC_{50} values were used as a baseline measure of the cytotoxicity of the compounds under aerobic and anoxic conditions and the HCR was used to indicate the mechanism of action of the compounds. The anoxic potency of the compounds spans a range from ca. 19 μM to ca. 3 mM (Fig. 16.3a). The 2-nitroimidazoles are consistently more potent than corresponding 4- and 5-nitroimidazoles as expected

Table 16.1 Nitroimidazole sulfonamide radiosensitisers

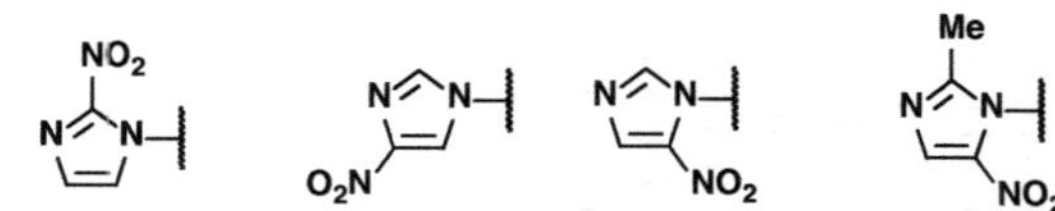

2-NI 4-NI 5-NI 2-Me-5-NI

No.	Structure	Sol.[a] (mM)	No.	Structure	Sol.[a] (mM)
1	2-NI-$CH_2CH(OH)CH_2OMe$	>100	**14**	2-NI-CH_2SO_2Ph	0.50
2	2-NI-$CH_2CONHCH_2CH_2OH$	>200	**15**	2-NI-$CH_2SO_2CH_2CH_2OH$	14.8
5	2-NI-$CH_2SO_2NHCH_2CH_2OMe$	6.2	**16**	4-NI-$CH_2SO_2NHCH_2CH_2OMe$	23.5
6	2-NI-$CH_2SO_2NHCH_2CH_2OH$	42.6	**17**	5-NI-$CH_2SO_2NHCH_2CH_2OMe$	>49
7	2-NI-$CH_2SO_2NHCH_2Ph$	0.04	**18**	2-Me-5-NI-$CH_2CH_2SO_2NHCH_2CH_2OMe$	29.6
8	2-NI-CH_2SO_2NMorpholine	1.08	**19**	2-Me-5-NI-$CH_2CH_2SO_2NHCH_2CH_2OH$	>49
9	2-NI-$CH_2CH_2SO_2NHCH_2CH_2OMe$	59.4	**20**	2-Me-5-NI-$CH_2CH_2SO_2NHCH_2CH_2$NPyrrolidine	61.7
10	2-NI-$CH_2CH_2SO_2NHCH_2CH_2OH$	75.3	**21**	2-Me-5-NI-$CH_2CH_2SO_2NHCH_2CH_2NMe_2$	46.8
11	2-NI-$CH_2CH_2SO_2NHCH_2CH_2$NMorpholine	>163	**22**	2-Me-5-NI-$CH_2CH_2SO_2NHCH_2CH_2$NPiperidine	>51
12	2-NI-CH_2SOCH_2Ph-4-OMe	0.63	**23**	2-Me-5-NI-$CH_2CH_2SO_2NHCH_2CH_2CH_2$NMorpholine	>55
13	2-NI-$CH_2SO_2CH_2$Ph-4-OMe	0.10	**24**	2-Me-5-NI-$CH_2CH_2SO_2$NPiperidine-4-NMe_2	14.5

[a]Solubility in αMEM + 5 %foetal calf serum

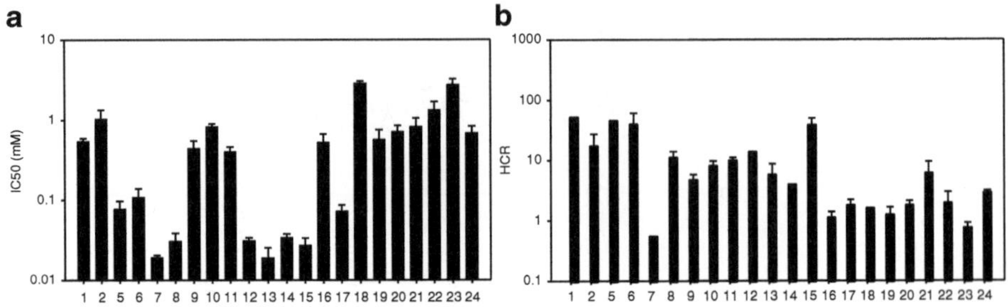

Fig. 16.3 (**a**) Anoxic IC_{50} values for compounds in HCT116 colorectal carcinoma cells. (**b**) Hypoxic selectivity as hypoxic cytotoxicity ratio [HCR = IC_{50}(normoxic)/IC_{50}(anoxic)]. Error bars represent the SEM for 2–3 independent experiments

on the basis of greater electron affinity. The compounds broadly fall into two categories: those that have modest (ca. 4–45 fold) hypoxia selective cytotoxicity and those that show no hypoxic selectivity (ca. 1–2) (Fig. 16.3b). The 2-nitroimidazole analogues (**5**–**15**) with reduction potentials higher than ca. –420 mV display hypoxic selectivity (with the exception of **7**) and this is also seen for misonidazole and etanidazole. These compounds have potential to have a dual mechanism of action; both radiosensitisation and bioreductive enzyme-mediated cytotoxicity against hypoxic cells. In contrast, analogues with *E*(1) values below ca –420 mV (4- and 5-nitroimidazoles) show little hypoxic selectivity, i.e. their HCR ~ 1 and are expected to be pure radiosensitisers, similarly to nimorazole.

16.2.4 In Vitro *Radiosensitisation*

16.2.4.1 Survival Ratios

We made a preliminary evaluation of radiosensitisation by compounds using clonogenic assay in HCT116 cells under anoxic conditions. Cells were treated with nitroimidazoles at a single non-toxic drug concentration and a single radiation dose in a custom-designed metal anoxic chamber apparatus [73, 78]. The anoxic IC_{50} was used as the drug concentration in this assay and was non-toxic due to the shorter drug exposure time (1 h) and the exposure at room temperature (21 °C). HCT116 cells were exposed to drug, irradiated in 96-well plates and plated for clonogenic survival (Fig. 16.4a). Survival Ratios (SR) were calculated as survival ratio (SR) = (cell survival with radiation)/(cell survival with drug + radiation).

SR is a measure of the efficacy of the radiosensitiser at a single high dose of radiation and provides a simple assessment of hypoxic cell radiosensitisation and allows triage of compounds at this stage. The radiation dose was determined empirically for HCT116 cells at 15 Gy, but we faced a dilemma in defining a drug concentration to evaluate. We elected to use the hypoxic IC_{50} value to compare the

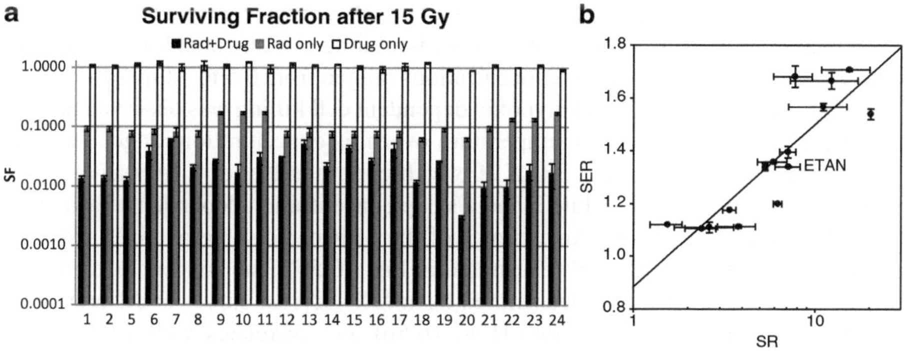

Fig. 16.4 (**a**) Surviving fractions after radiation with and without drug used in calculation of SR at 15 Gy. Drug only surviving fractions indicate no drug-only cytotoxicity at the chosen concentrations. (**b**) Correlation between the Survival ratios (SR) from (a) calculated as SF(radiation)/SF(drug+radiation) and Sensitiser Enhancement Ratios (SER) calculated as (radiation dose for 1 % survival—compound)/(radiation dose for 1 % survival+compound) for compounds under anoxia with misonidazole (**1**) in each experiment for quality control. Both SR and SER were determined at the hypoxic IC_{50} for each drug in independent experiments. Error bars for all compounds represent the SEM for 2–3 independent experiments

compounds at an equitoxic drug concentration rather than try to compare compounds at an equimolar concentration. No significant drug-alone toxicity was observed across the SR testing programme ($p=0.65$, one-way ANOVA) at these drug concentrations. This approach allowed us to compare compounds with widely varying solubility and hypoxic cytotoxicity.

Compounds demonstrating SR values of >2.5 and sufficient aqueous solubility and stability could then advance to a full clonogenic assay across a range of radiation doses. For the purposes of this study we elected to advance a larger set of compounds to examine the relationship between SR and Sensitiser Enhancement Ratio (SER).

16.2.4.2 Sensitiser Enhancement Ratios

We determined radiosensitisation for compounds at the IC_{50} drug concentration across a range of radiation doses in the same apparatus using a lead wedge [78] to cover the 96 well plate in an anoxic chamber. HCT116 cells were exposed to drug, dissociated and plated for clonogenic survival. Sensitiser Enhancement Ratios (SER) were calculated as the ratio of (radiation dose for 1 % survival) with or without drug.

SER correlated well with the SR at 15 Gy ($R^2=0.75$, $p<0.001$, Fig. 16.4b). This correlation could be improved using multiple regression to normalise for the effects cell kill by radiation alone, since SR is radiation dose dependent whereas the SER is usually considered constant. The correlation is also improved by the addition of IC_{50} to the multiple regression allowing prediction of the SER at the IC_{50} drug concentration, from data collected in the screening process, with an R^2 of 0.91.

The concentration dependence of SR can be efficiently determined directly from clonogenic assay data at 15Gy with and without drug as illustrated for ETAN and **5** and **20** (Fig. 16.5a) where drug concentrations ranged from 0.5 to 5 times the anoxic 4-hr IC_{50}. Again, no significant hypoxia dependent cell killing was observed at these short exposure times at room temperature over this concentration range. The concentration dependence of the SR of **20** was higher than that of ETAN as expected from its initial SR screen, while **5** had a steep concentration dependence as a result of its high electron affinity. An estimate of the SER can also be obtained from the data used to determine the SR (illustrated in Fig. 16.5b). The concentration dependence of the SER for **5** was determined from full survival curves at different concentrations using the lead wedge (Fig. 16.5b) and correlates well with the SR estimated at 15 Gy (Fig. 16.5c).

16.2.5 Evaluation of Drug Transport

We have identified that extravascular transport (EVT) is often limiting for the delivery of HAPs and that limited transport reduces the efficacy of these agents [76, 79]. We evaluated EVT using a multicellular layer (MCL) culture model in a dual chamber apparatus to measure drug flux through a slab of tumour tissue and determine a diffusion coefficient, D_{MCL} [80–82]. These structures grow to a thickness of 100–200 μm over 2–3 days in culture with tissue-like cell densities and an oxygen gradient forms that can lead to anoxia and subsequent necrosis in the centre of the MCL, similar to real tumours. D_{MCL} can be related to molecular properties such as molecular weight, lipophilicity and the presence of hydrogen bond donors and acceptors [81, 82].

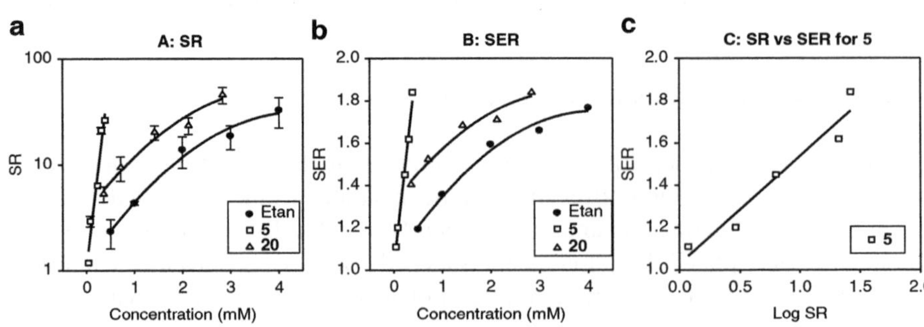

Fig. 16.5 Concentration dependence of radiosensitisation by etanidazole, **5** and **20**. (**a**) The 15 Gy SR was measured in three separate experiments at 15 Gy using radiosensitiser concentrations of 0.5, 1,2,3,4-fold the IC_{50} (etanidazole, **20**) or estimated from interpolation of radiation survival curves used to determine the SER of **5** at 0.5, 1, 3, 4, 5-fold the IC_{50} (see panel B). (**b**) Concentration dependence of the SER of **5** using full survival curves and estimates of the SER of etanidazole or **20** based on their SR shown in A. (**c**) Correlation of estimates SR and SER for **5** for a range of concentrations in one experiment (redrawn from A and B)

The diffusion coefficients of ETAN, **5**, **18** and **20** were determined under well oxygenated (95 % O_2) conditions to suppress bioreductive metabolism [79]. Diffusion coefficients for the compounds were fitted to the flux data obtained from both the donor and receiver compartments (Table 16.2). Under these conditions there was no substantial reaction (cell uptake or metabolism) as evidenced by mass balance using the donor and receiver concentration data. The data indicates that the experimental compounds have similar diffusion coefficients to etanidazole under oxic conditions, which result in typical equilibration times of 5–10 min at 100 μm into a planar tissue region such as a MCL, in good agreement with peak concentrations seen in tumour PK studies.

16.2.6 In Vivo *Radiosensitisation*

We have identified that PK differences between bioreductive compounds are a major limitation in identifying lead candidates. Approximately 60 % of the compounds in a recent HAP campaign with favourable in vitro PK/PD properties were triaged because of poor PK or predicted poor PK based on low MTD [48, 83]. Determination of plasma and tumour PK using HPLC or LCMS and reference to in vitro radiosensitisation data allows further triage of compounds and determines the optimal treatment times for therapy experiments (Fig. 16.6) (Table 16.3).

Table 16.2 Extravascular transport parameters

No.	Oxic $D_{MCL} \times 10^{-7}$ cm^{2}s^{-1} (mean ± SE; $N = 3$)	Diffusion time (min)[a]
ETAN	2.04 ± 0.10	8.2
5	1.95 ± 0.05	8.5
18	2.85 ± 0.17	5.8
20	1.62 ± 0.17	10.3

[a]Calculated as the characteristic diffusion time (x^2/D) for a distance of 100 μm in a plane tissue section found in MCLs

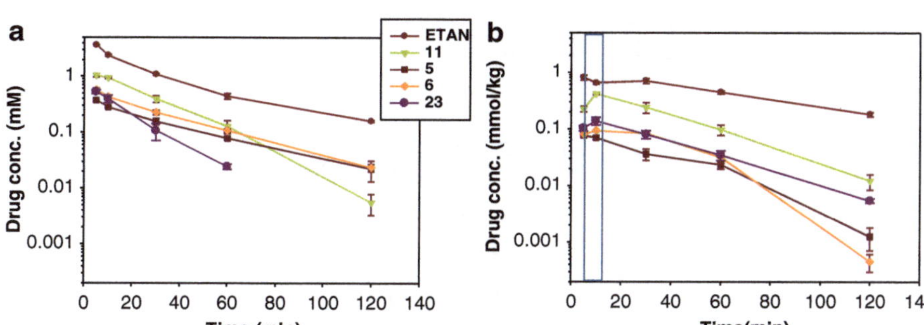

Fig. 16.6 (**a**) Plasma drug concentrations after i.v. injection in HCT116 tumour bearing NIH-III nude mice at MTD or MAD (see Table 16.3). (**b**) Tumour drug concentrations after i.v. injection; *box* shows approximate time of irradiation for subsequent radiosensitisation experiments (Section 16.2.6). ($n = 3$ at each time point)

Table 16.3 Selection parameters for compound decision making

No.	Structure	Aq solubility mM	OXIC IC_{50} mM	ANOXIC IC_{50} mM	HCR	SR	SER	MTD* or MAD mmol/kg	Plasma C_{max} mM	Tumour C_{max} mmol/kg	Tumour C_{max}/ in vitro [drug] for SER	Advance to in vivo evaluation?	In vivo SR
ETAN 2	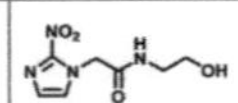	>200	13.50	1.03	13.1	7.2	1.34	2.33	3.64	0.8	0.78	Yes	4.04
5	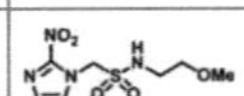	6.2	4.93	0.08	45.8	6.3	1.20	0.42*	0.37	0.077	1.01	No, formulation problem	
6	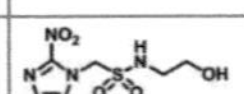	42.6	3.32	0.11	39.6	2.6	1.11	0.6	0.57	0.094	0.87	Yes	2.37
11	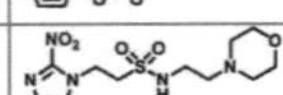	>163	3.94	0.40	10.0	5.9	1.36	1.12	1.04	0.41	1.03	Yes	1.24
20	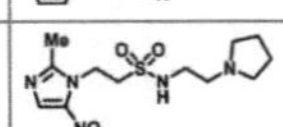	61.7	1.17	0.71	1.8	20.3	1.54	0.75*	ND	ND	ND	No, predicted tumour [drug] too low	
23	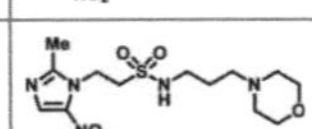	>55	1.62	2.76	0.8	7.8	1.68	0.55	0.53	0.28	0.10	No, tumour [drug] too low	
24	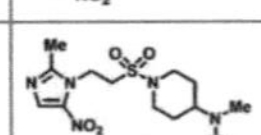	14.5	1.99	0.68	2.9	12.3	1.67	0.35*	ND	ND	ND	No, predicted tumour [drug] too low	

16.2.6.1 In Vivo Toxicity

A maximum tolerated dose (MTD) was determined for each of the compounds in non-tumour bearing mice. The MTD was defined as the highest dose causing no drug-related deaths, body weight loss of more than 15 %, or severe morbidity in a group of three to six animals, with an observation time of up to 14 days. In those cases where an MTD could not be determined because of solubility limitations a maximum administered dose (MAD) was defined as the maximum dose able to be dissolved in the injection volume.

16.2.6.2 Plasma and Tumour Pharmacokinetics

Plasma and tumour drug concentration-time profiles were determined for single i.v. doses to determine achievable drug concentrations and the optimal time for irradiation.

16.2.6.3 In Vivo Radiosensitisation

Candidates were compared with etanidazole for in vivo radiosensitisation of hypoxic cells in HCT116 human tumour xenografts using clonogenic survival as an end-point. NIH-III nude mice bearing HCT116 tumours treated with: (A) vehicle control; (B) 12.5 Gy RAD only; (C) sensitizer only; (D) sensitizer given as a single i.v. dose at the MAD or 75 % of the MTD before 12.5 Gy RAD. Radiosensitisation was determined as the difference in log surviving fraction (SF) (in vivo SR) after radiation with and without radiosensitiser present.

16.3 Discussion

The evolution in radiotherapy practice, combined with renewed interest in the use of radiosensitisers to overcome hypoxic cell radioresistance, offers a renaissance for the use of nitroimidazole-based radiosensitisers in the context of SBRT. We have explored an abbreviated screening protocol, suitable for an academic drug discovery laboratory, with a test set of 20 novel nitroimidazoles (Table 16.1) that cover a range of aqueous solubility, lipophilicity and electron affinity.

Given that existing nitroimidazole radiosensitisers are required to be present in high concentrations within the tumour cell to effect radiosensitisation, we quickly eliminated those analogues with aqueous solubility less than 1 mM. On this basis, compounds **7**, **8**, **12–14** could be triaged because of low aqueous solubility. Extensive literature has demonstrated that compounds with low electron affinity require relatively high drug concentrations to effectively radiosensitise cells. Metronidazole marks the practical bottom limit of electron affinity [E(1) –480 mV]

[84] and the 4-nitroimidazole analogue **16** has a lower E(1) value [73]. The 5-nitroimidazole analogue **18** also falls below metronidazole in terms of electron affinity, but related analogues (e.g. **20**) with strongly basic side chains are more electron affinic [73] and more soluble.

The aerobic cytotoxicity also provides a first screen with compounds having very low IC_{50} values likely to lead to normal tissue toxicity (e.g. **7**, **8**, **12–14**, **17**, **19**). The hypoxic selectivity allows partitioning of the compounds into two groups based on likely mechanism of action: those compounds with an HCR ~ 1 which are likely to act as pure radiosensitisers. However, the lower electron affinity of these analogues does mean that higher drug concentrations are required for effective sensitisation. On the other hand, those compounds with HCR > 5 have the potential for dual mechanism of action: radiosensitisation and hypoxic cell cytotoxicity. These compounds are more potent and may not require as high tumour drug concentrations for hypoxic cell killing.

We have compared the SR with the SER and find good agreement between the two methods (Fig. 16.4b). We suggest the SR can be used to efficiently identify effective radiosensitisers and rank these compounds for further evaluation. Depending on resources and compound numbers several strategies may be followed. While it would be simple to limit advancement to in vivo studies to only those compounds with a SR > etanidazole (7.2) this may preclude compounds with a steep dose response or high potency. This approach would have left only two structural groups: compound **10** and the very close analogues **20–25** for evaluation. Alternatively, a more liberal approach may be followed by setting the cut-off at a relatively low threshold and evaluating representative analogues from structural clusters of compounds. By setting a lower cut-off (SR > 2.5) a broader range of compounds would remain in contention (e.g. **5**, **6**, **9–11**, **18–24**). At this stage compounds can be evaluated further by determining the concentration dependence of the SR, which is particularly important for potent compounds which may have low SRs in the initial screen at the IC_{50}. An advantage of the SR is that clonogenic data can be directly compared a predetermined radiation dose and does not require interpolation of full survival curves as in the case of the SER.

Our MCL studies showed that the nitroimidazole sulfonamides diffuse similarly to etanidazole and EVT is unlikely to be limiting for this class. However, we would advise that each new class under investigation should undergo diffusion studies.

We elected to advance a matrix of six compounds (**5**, **6**, **11**, **20**, **23**, **24**) with a range of physicochemical and in vitro properties along with etanidazole to in vivo study (Table 16.3). These compounds have a broad range of hypoxic potencies and HCR values and a representative range of SR values. We determined the MTD or MAD for these compounds, and the plasma and tumour maximal drug concentrations (C_{max}) and the corresponding times for irradiation at the C_{max} for four analogues. This allowed comparison of the tumour C_{max} with the in vitro drug concentration used to determine the SR and provided an estimate of in vivo radiosensitisation based on intra-tumoural drug concentration for each compound.

Etanidazole achieved a high intra-tumoural drug concentration (0.8 mmol/kg) (Table 16.3) and this is comparable to the drug concentration required for in vitro radiosensitisation (anoxic IC_{50}). Thus we predicted significant in vivo radiosensitisation and indeed this was observed with an in vivo SR of 4.04 ($p<0.001$). In contrast, both **5** and **6** achieved ca. 10-fold lower plasma and tumour C_{max} values. However, based on the high potency of these compounds for in vitro radiosensitisation we predicted in vivo activity. We did not advance **5** because of difficulties with drug formulation caused by relatively low solubility, but were able to see significant radiosensitisation for **6** with a SR of 2.37 ($p=0.026$). The increased aqueous solubility of **11** enabled a higher MAD and, consequently, higher plasma and intra-tumoural C_{max} values than for **6**. Although **11** is approximately four-fold less potent than **5** or **6**, it was expected to provide radiosensitisation in vivo, but failed to achieve this with a SR of 1.24 ($p=0.096$). A similar situation was observed for the 5-nitroimidazole **23** where a relatively high intra-tumoural C_{max} was compromised by low potency; radiosensitisation was unlikely and the compound was halted at this stage. The related analogues **20** and **24** were triaged because their MTD values were unlikely to provide sufficiently high tumour drug concentrations for activity.

This preliminary study has explored a protocol to expeditiously screen potential radiosensitisers using an efficient in vitro/in vivo approach. We were able to triage compounds with poor physicochemical and in vitro properties at an early stage. The combination of in vitro radiosensitisation data with tumour PK data allows selection of likely candidates for further evaluation. Although this method does not have perfect predictive capability it does remove compounds with little chance of significant in vivo radiosensitisation and enriches the potential of in vivo candidates carried though to activity experiments.

16.4 Experimental Protocol

16.4.1 Chemical Design and Synthesis

Nitroimidazoles were prepared as previously described [73]. All compounds were assayed by HPLC with diode array detection for purity. A simplified measure of aqueous solubility was adopted; determining solubility by HPLC for solutions of compounds diluted from a DMSO stock solution to <1 % DMSO with culture medium containing foetal calf serum (FCS).

16.4.2 In Vitro *Cytotoxicity Testing*

HCT116 cells were authenticated in-house by short tandem repeat profiling. Cells were grown in αMEM medium with 5 % foetal bovine serum, without antibiotics, and were confirmed mycoplasma-free using a PCR-ELISA method (Roche Diagnostics). Log phase cells were seeded into 96-well plates at 700 cells/well, allowed to attach for 2 h, then test compounds were added by dilution from DMSO stocks to give a top concentration of <1 % DMSO before serial threefold dilution in the plates. After 4 h, cultures were washed three times with fresh medium and grown for a further 5 days before staining with sulforhodamine B to determine IC_{50} values as previously [85]. For hypoxic exposure to compounds, cells were pelleted by centrifugation, transferred to a Pd-catalyst anaerobic chamber (Bactron-II, Shel Lab), resuspended in anoxic medium and exposed to drugs as above but using medium and plates that had been equilibrated in the chamber for at least 3 days. After drug washout, cells were grown and stained as for the aerobic IC_{50} assays. The absorbance of aerobic and hypoxic controls (8 wells/plate) had a mean of 0.28 (CV 33 %) and 0.23 (CV 37 %) for aerobic and hypoxic exposures respectively, across all assays.

The hypoxic cytotoxicity ratio HCR was determined as [$HCR = IC_{50(oxic)}/IC_{50(anoxic)}$].

16.4.3 Radiosensitisation Studies

Cells were seeded onto 96-well plates at 10^5 cells per well and allowed to attach for 2 h. Replicates were treated with compound at the respective anoxic IC_{50} compound concentration 30 min prior to irradiation. For anoxic irradiation, plates were transferred to a custom-built, air-tight, stainless steel, portable box (13×16.5×3 cm) within the anaerobic chamber, then sealed and transported to the radiation machine. The plates were irradiated (Eldorado 78 ^{60}Co teletherapy unit, ~3 Gy/min) with 15 Gy under anoxia at room temperature for SR experiments or with a metal wedge on the top of the metal chamber to achieve a graduated radiation dose across the plate varying from 7.1 to 27.1 Gy, calibrated by Fricke dosimetry with ammonium thiocyanate as previously described [78] for SER experiments. The control plate (compound alone, no radiation) was left inside the anaerobic chamber at room temperature during the irradiation period. After treatment the cells were trypsinised and suspended in αMEM + 5 % FCS + 1 % PS, and tenfold serial dilutions were plated for clonogenic survival. After 10 days plates were stained with methylene blue (2 g/L in EtOH:H_2O, 1:1 v/v) and colonies with more than 50 cells were counted. The surviving fraction (SF) was determined as: $SF = PE_{(irradiated)}/PE_{(control)}$ where the plating efficiency (PE) = (No. of colonies)/(No. of cells plated). SF was plotted against radiation dose and either Survival Ratios (SR) were calculated as survival ratio (SR) = (cell survival with radiation)/(cell survival with drug + radiation), or Sensitiser Enhancement Ratios (SER) were calculated as (radiation dose for 1 % survival without compound)/(radiation dose for 1 % survival with compound). Misonidazole at its hypoxic IC_{50} (0.5 mM) was used as an intra-experiment control.

16.4.4 Multicellular Layer Studies

HCT116 MCL cultures were grown in αMEM with 10 % FBS and penicillin/streptomycin as described [79, 82]. Briefly, 10^6 cells were seeded onto collagen coated Teflon support membranes in Millicell-CM culture inserts (Millipore Corp.,

Bedford, MA), allowed to attach for 4 h, submerged in a reservoir of stirred medium, and grown for 3 days before use in diffusion experiments. Kinetics of diffusion across MCLs were determined using a customised diffusion chamber in which MCLs separate two well-stirred compartments containing medium without serum and gassed with 95 % O_2/5 % CO_2 to determine diffusion without bioreductive metabolism. Compounds were added to the donor compartment along with internal standards (^{14}C-urea for determination of MCL thickness and ^{3}H-mannitol to mark the paracellular route), and 100 μL of medium was sampled from each compartment at time zero and then half-hourly for 3 h. Radioactivity was determined by scintillation counting 25 μL of the sampled medium in 3 mL of Emulsifier-Safe scintillant using a Tricarb 2910TR Liquid Scintillation Analyzer (PerkinElmer), and the balance stored at −80 °C for HPLC analysis. The transport model for MCL is based of Fick's second law as described previously [82, 86, 87]. The diffusion equation was solved numerically for the drug concentrations (C) with initial conditions as the measured time zero (t_0) concentrations, and no-flux boundary conditions in the donor and receiver compartments to fit the transport parameters (diffusion coefficients) as previously [76,79].

16.4.5 In Vivo *Toxicity*

A MTD was determined for each compound in non-tumour bearing pathogen-free NIH-III nude female mice (~20 g). Freshly prepared solutions of compounds were given i.v. to mice at 10 mL/kg body weight, using 1.33-fold dose increments. The MTD was defined as the highest dose causing no drug-related deaths, body weight loss of more than 15 %, or severe morbidity in a group of three to six animals, with an observation time of up to 14 days. A MAD was defined as the maximum dose able to be dissolved in the injection volume (10 mL/kg). Drugs were administered as solutions in 0.9 % saline containing 1 % DMSO, with the exception of **5** which was dissolved in 5 %DMSO/5 % propylene glycol/14%PEG400 in saline.

16.4.6 Pharmacokinetics

HCT116 tumour bearing NIH-III female mice were injected with single i.v. doses at the MAD or 75 % of the MTD for each compound, with sampling by cardiac puncture and tumour excision under terminal CO_2 anaesthesia. Blood was immediately centrifuged (3000 × g, 3 min), and plasma and tumour stored at −80 °C for HPLC. Tumour samples were prepared and analysed by HPLC using standard protocols established in our laboratory [88, 89]. Noncompartmental PK parameters were determined by Phoenix WinNonLin v 6.2 (Pharsight Corp.).

16.4.7 In Vivo *Radiosensitisation*

Candidates were compared with etanidazole for in vivo radiosensitisation of hypoxic cells in HCT116 human tumour xenografts using clonogenic survival as an endpoint. HCT116 tumours were grown subcutaneously on the flanks of NIH-III nude mice by injecting 10^7 cells. When tumours reach a volume of approximately 300 mm^3 mice were randomly assigned to four treatment groups and treated with: (A) vehicle control; (B) 12.5 Gy RAD only; (C) sensitiser only; (D) sensitiser given before 12.5 Gy RAD. Drugs were administered as a single i.v. dose at the MAD or 75 % of the MTD. Tumours were excised 18 h after treatment, and tumour cells were dissociated enzymatically and plated to determine the number of surviving (clonogenic) cells per gram of tumour tissue [79]. Surviving fractions (SF) were calculated and the radiosensitisation determined as the difference in log SF after radiation with and without radiosensitiser present. Statistical significance of drug effects was tested using one-way ANOVA with Holm-Sidak test for multiple comparisons.

Acknowledgements The authors would like to thank Dr Thorsten Melcher (J&J Innovation) and Professor Bill Wilson for helpful discussions and thank Dr Adrian Blaser, Ms Karen Tan and Mr Sisira Kumara for technical assistance. The authors acknowledge support from the University of Auckland's Biopharma Thematic Research Initiative, UniServices Investment/Ministry of Business, Innovation and Employment Pre-Seed Accelerator Fund and the Cancer Society of New Zealand.

References

1. Koch CJ, Evans SM. Optimizing hypoxia detection and treatment strategies. Semin Nucl Med. 2015;45:163–76.
2. Dhani N, Fyles A, Hedley D, et al. The clinical significance of hypoxia in human cancers. Semin Nucl Med. 2015;45:110–21.
3. Cairns RA, Harris IS, Mak TW. Regulation of cancer cell metabolism. Nat Rev Cancer. 2011;11:85–95.
4. Pennacchietti S, Michieli P, Galluzzo M, et al. Hypoxia promotes invasive growth by transcriptional activation of the met protooncogene. Cancer Cell. 2003;3:347–61.
5. Chang Q, Jurisica I, Do T, et al. Hypoxia predicts aggressive growth and spontaneous metastasis formation from orthotopically grown primary xenografts of human pancreatic cancer. Cancer Res. 2011;71:3110–20.
6. Rohwer N, Cramer T. Hypoxia-mediated drug resistance: novel insights on the functional interaction of HIFs and cell death pathways. Drug Resist Updat. 2011;14:191–201.
7. Vaupel P, Mayer A. Hypoxia in cancer: significance and impact on clinical outcome. Cancer Metastasis Rev. 2007;26:225–39.
8. Wilson WR, Hay MP. Targeting hypoxia in cancer therapy. Nat Rev Cancer. 2011;11: 393–410.
9. Gray LH, Conger AD, Ebert M, et al. Concentration of oxygen dissolved in tissues at the time of irradiation as a factor in radiotherapy. Br J Radiol. 1953;26:638–48.
10. Evans SM, Du KL, Chalian AA, et al. Patterns and levels of hypoxia in head and neck squamous cell carcinomas and their relationship to patient outcome. Int J Radiat Oncol Biol Phys. 2007;69:1024–31.

11. Koukourakis MI, Bentzen SM, Giatromanolaki A, et al. Endogenous markers of two separate hypoxia response pathways (hypoxia inducible factor 2 alpha and carbonic anhydrase 9) are associated with radiotherapy failure in head and neck cancer patients recruited in the CHART randomized trial. J Clin Oncol. 2006;24:727–35.
12. Nordsmark M, Bentzen SM, Rudat V, et al. Prognostic value of tumor oxygenation in 397 head and neck tumors after primary radiation therapy. An international multi-center study. Radiother Oncol. 2005;77:18–24.
13. Overgaard J, Eriksen JG, Nordsmark M, et al. Plasma osteopontin, hypoxia, and response to the hypoxia sensitiser nimorazole in radiotherapy of head and neck cancer: results from the DAHANCA 5 randomised double-blind placebo-controlled trial. Lancet Oncol. 2005;6:757–64.
14. Fyles A, Milosevic M, Hedley D, et al. Tumor hypoxia has independent predictor impact only in patients with node-negative cervix cancer. J Clin Oncol. 2002;20:680–7.
15. Brown JM, Diehn M, Loo BW. Stereotactic ablative radiotherapy should be combined with a hypoxic cell radiosensitizer. Int J Radiat Oncol Biol Phys. 2010;78:323–7.
16. Hoogsteen IJ, Marres HA, van der Kogel AJ, et al. The hypoxic tumour microenvironment, patient selection and hypoxia-modifying treatments. Clin Oncol (R Coll Radiol). 2007;19:385–96.
17. Moeller BJ, Richarson RA, Dewhirst MW. Hypoxia and radiotherapy: opportunities for improved outcomes in cancer treatment. Cancer Metastasis Rev. 2007;26:241–8.
18. Overgaard J. Hypoxic radiosensitization: adored and ignored. J Clin Oncol. 2007;25:4066–74.
19. Overgaard J. Hypoxic modification of radiotherapy in squamous cell carcinoma of the head and neck-a systematic review and meta-analysis. Radiother Oncol. 2011;100:22–32.
20. Bennett MH, Feldmeier J, Smee R, et al. Hyperbaric oxygenation for tumour sensitisation to radiotherapy. Cochrane Database Syst Rev. 2012;4:CD005007. doi:10.1002/14651858.CD005007.pub3.
21. Kaanders JH, Bussink J, van der Kogel AJ. ARCON: a novel biology-based approach in radiotherapy. Lancet Oncol. 2002;3:728–37.
22. Dische S. Chemical sensitisers for hypoxic cells: a decade of experience in clinical radiotherapy. Radiother Oncol. 1985;3:97–115.
23. Overgaard J. Clinical evaluation of nitroimidazoles as modifiers of hypoxia in solid tumors. Oncol Res. 1994;6:509–18.
24. Wardman P. Chemical radiosensitizers for use in radiotherapy. Clin Oncol. 2007;19:397–417.
25. Brown JM, Wilson WR. Exploiting tumor hypoxia in cancer treatment. Nat Rev Cancer. 2004;4:437–47.
26. Adams GE, Clarke ED, Flockhart IR, et al. Structure-activity relationships in the development of hypoxic cell radiosensitizers. I. Sensitization efficiency. Int J Radiat Biol Relat Stud Phys Chem Med. 1979;35:133–50.
27. Urtasun RC, Band P, Chapman JD, et al. Radiation and high dose metronidazole in supratentorial glioblastomas. N Engl J Med. 1976;294:1364–7.
28. Urtasun R, Feldstein ML, Partington J, et al. Radiation and nitroimidazoles in supratentorial high grade gliomas: a second clinical trial. Br J Cancer. 1982;46:101–8.
29. Grigsby PW, Winter K, Wasserman TH, et al. Irradiation with or without misonidazole for patients with stages IIIB and IVA carcinoma of the cervix: final results of RTOG 80–05. Radiation Therapy Oncology Group. Int J Radiat Oncol Biol Phys. 1999;44:513–7.
30. Saunders M, Dische S. Clinical results of hypoxic cell radiosensitisation from hyperbaric oxygen to accelerated radiotherapy, carbogen and nicotinamide. Br J Cancer. 1996;27:S271–8.
31. Lee DJ, Cosmatos D, Marcial VA, et al. Results of an RTOG phase III trial (RTOG 85–27) comparing radiotherapy plus etanidazole with radiotherapy alone for locally advanced head and neck carcinomas. Int J Radiat Oncol Biol Phys. 1995;32:567–76.
32. Nishimura Y, Nakagawa K, Takeda K, et al. Phase I/II trial of sequential chemoradiotherapy using a novel hypoxic cell radiosensitizer, doranidazole (PR-350), in patients with locally

advanced non-small-cell lung Cancer (WJTOG-0002). Int J Radiat Oncol Biol Phys. 2007;69:786–92.
33. Karasawa K, Sunamura M, Okamoto A, et al. Efficacy of novel hypoxic cell sensitiser doranidazole in the treatment of locally advanced pancreatic cancer: long-term results of a placebo-controlled randomised study. Radiother Oncol. 2008;87:326–30.
34. Overgaard J, Hansen HS, Overgaard M, et al. A randomized double-blind phase III study of nimorazole as a hypoxic radiosensitizer of primary radiotherapy in supraglottic larynx and pharynx carcinoma. Results of the Danish Head and Neck Cancer Study (DAHANCA) Protocol 5–85. Radiother Oncol. 1998;46:135–46.
35. Cole S, Stratford IJ, Adams GE, et al. Dual-function 2-nitroimidazoles as hypoxic cell radiosensitizers and bioreductive cytotoxins: in vivo evaluation in KHT murine sarcomas. Radiat Res. 1990;124:S38–43.
36. Cole S, Stratford IJ, Fielden EM, et al. Dual function nitroimidazoles less toxic than RSU 1069: selection of candidate drugs for clinical trial (RB 6145 and/or PD 130908. Int J Radiat Oncol Biol Phys. 1992;22:545–8.
37. Jenkins TC, Naylor MA, O'Neill P, et al. Synthesis and evaluation of alpha-[[(2-haloethyl) amino]methyl]-2-nitro-1H-imidazole-1-ethanols as prodrugs of alpha-[(1-aziridinyl)methyl]-2-nitro-1H-imidazole-1-ethanol (RSU-1069) and its analogues which are radiosensitizers and bioreductively activated cytotoxins. J Med Chem. 1990;33:2603–10.
38. Duan JX, Jiao H, Kaizerman J, et al. Potent and highly selective hypoxia-activated achiral phosphoramidate mustards as anticancer drugs. J Med Chem. 2008;51:2412–20.
39. Sun JD, Liu Q, Wang J, et al. Selective tumor hypoxia targeting by hypoxia-activated prodrug TH-302 inhibits tumor growth in preclinical models of cancer. Clin Cancer Res. 2012;18:758–70.
40. Chawla SP, Cranmer LD, Van Tine BA, et al. Phase II study of the safety and antitumor activity of the hypoxia-activated prodrug TH-302 in combination with doxorubicin in patients with advanced soft tissue sarcoma. J Clin Oncol. 2014;32:3299–306.
41. Borad MJ, Reddy SG, Bahary N, et al. Randomized phase II trial of gemcitabine plus TH-302 versus gemcitabine in patients with advanced pancreatic cancer. J Clin Oncol. 2015;33:1475–81.
42. Brown JM. SR 4233 (tirapazamine): a new anticancer drug exploiting hypoxia in solid tumours. Br J Cancer. 1993;67:1163–70.
43. Rischin D, Hicks RJ, Fisher R, et al. Prognostic significance of [18F]-misonidazole positron emission tomography-detected tumor hypoxia in patients with advanced head and neck cancer randomly assigned to chemoradiation with or without tirapazamine: a substudy of Trans-Tasman Radiation Oncology Group Study 98.02. J Clin Oncol. 2006;24:2098–104.
44. Peters LJ, O'Sullivan B, Giralt J, et al. Critical impact of radiotherapy protocol compliance and quality in the treatment of advanced head and neck cancer: results from TROG 02.02. J Clin Oncol. 2010;28:2996–3001.
45. Trinkaus ME, Hicks RJ, Young RJ, et al. Correlation of p16 status, hypoxic imaging using [18F]-misonidazole positron emission tomography and outcome in patients with loco-regionally advanced head and neck cancer. J Med Imaging Radiat Oncol. 2014;58:89–97.
46. Rischin D, Peters LJ, O'Sullivan B, et al. Tirapazamine, cisplatin, and radiation versus cisplatin and radiation for advanced squamous cell carcinoma of the head and neck (TROG 02.02, HeadSTART): a phase III trial of the Trans-Tasman Radiation Oncology Group. J Clin Oncol. 2010;28:2989–95.
47. Hay MP, Hicks KO, Pchalek K, et al. Tricyclic [1,2,4]triazine 1,4-dioxides as hypoxia selective cytotoxins. J Med Chem. 2008;51:6853–65.
48. Hicks KO, Siim BG, Jaiswal JK, et al. Pharmacokinetic/pharmacodynamic modeling identifies SN30000 and SN29751 as tirapazamine analogues with improved tissue penetration and hypoxic cell killing in tumors. Clin Cancer Res. 2010;16:4946–57.
49. Wang J, Foehrenbacher A, Su J, et al. The 2-nitroimidazole EF5 is a biomarker for oxidoreductases that activate bioreductive prodrug CEN-209 under hypoxia. Clin Cancer Res. 2012;18:1684–95.

50. Le QT, Fisher R, Oliner KS, et al. Prognostic and predictive significance of plasma HGF and IL-8 in a phase III trial of chemoradiation with or without tirapazamine in locoregionally advanced head and neck cancer. Clin Cancer Res. 2012;18:1798–807.
51. Lim AM, Rischin D, Fisher R, et al. Prognostic significance of plasma osteopontin in patients with locoregionally advanced head and neck squamous cell carcinoma treated on TROG 02.02 phase III trial. Clin Cancer Res. 2012;18:301–7.
52. Horsman MR, Mortensen LS, Petersen JB, et al. Imaging hypoxia to improve radiotherapy outcome. Nat Rev Clin Oncol. 2012;9:674–87.
53. Lee N, Nehmeh S, Schoder H, et al. Prospective trial incorporating pre-/mid-treatment [(18) F]-misonidazole positron emission tomography for head-and-neck cancer patients undergoing concurrent chemoradiotherapy. Int J Radiat Oncol Biol Phys. 2009;75:101–8.
54. Dubois LJ, Lieuwes NG, Janssen MH, et al. Preclinical evaluation and validation of [18F] HX4, a promising hypoxia marker for PET imaging. Proc Natl Acad Sci U S A. 2011; 108:14620–5.
55. van Loon J, Janssen MHM, Ollers M, et al. PET imaging of hypoxia using [18F]HX4: a phase I trial. Eur J Nucl Med Mol Imaging. 2010;37:1663–8.
56. Komar G, Seppanen M, Eskola O, et al. 18F-EF5: a new PET tracer for imaging hypoxia in head and neck cancer. J Nucl Med. 2008;49:1944–51.
57. Buffa FM, Harris AL, West CM, et al. Large meta-analysis of multiple cancers reveals a common, compact and highly prognostic hypoxia metagene. Br J Cancer. 2010;102:428–35.
58. Chi JT, Wang Z, Nuyten DS, et al. Gene expression programs in response to hypoxia: cell type specificity and prognostic significance in human cancers. PLoS Med. 2006;3:e47.
59. Toustrup K, Sorensen BS, Alsner J, et al. Hypoxia gene expression signatures as prognostic and predictive markers in head and neck radiotherapy. Semin Radiat Oncol. 2012;22:119–27.
60. Toustrup K, Sorensen BS, Nordsmark M, et al. Development of a hypoxia gene expression classifier with predictive impact for hypoxic modification of radiotherapy in head and neck cancer. Cancer Res. 2011;71:5923–31.
61. Winter SC, Buffa FM, Silva P, et al. Relation of a hypoxia metagene derived from head and neck cancer to prognosis of multiple cancers. Cancer Res. 2007;67:3441–9.
62. Toustrup K, Sorensen BS, Lassen P, et al. Gene expression classifier predicts for hypoxic modification of radiotherapy with nimorazole in squamous cell carcinomas of the head and neck. Radiother Oncol. 2012;102:122–9.
63. Barton MB, Jacob S, Shafiq J, et al. Estimating the demand for radiotherapy from the evidence: a review of changes from 2003 to 2012. Radiother Oncol. 2014;112:140–4.
64. Moding EJ, Kastan MB, Kirsch DG. Strategies for optimizing the response of cancer and normal tissues to radiation. Nat Rev Drug Discov. 2013;12:526–42.
65. Lo SS, Fakiris AJ, Chang EL, et al. Stereotactic body radiation therapy: a novel treatment modality. Nat Rev Clin Oncol. 2010;7:44–54.
66. Carlson DJ, Keall PJ, Loo Jr BW, et al. Hypofractionation results in reduced tumor cell kill compared to conventional fractionation for tumors with regions of hypoxia. Int J Radiat Oncol Biol Phys. 2011;79:1188–95.
67. Adams GE. Hypoxia-mediated drugs for radiation and chemotherapy. Cancer. 1981; 48:696–707.
68. Nahum AE. The radiobiology of hypofractionation. Clin Oncol (R Coll Radiol). 2015; 27:260–9.
69. Harrington KJ, Billingham LJ, Brunner TB, et al. Guidelines for preclinical and early phase clinical assessment of novel radiosensitisers. Br J Cancer. 2011;105:628–39.
70. Kumar P, Shustov G, Liang H, et al. Design, synthesis, and preliminary biological evaluation of 6-O-glucose-azomycin adducts for diagnosis and therapy of hypoxic tumors. J Med Chem. 2012;55:6033–46.
71. Nakae T, Uto Y, Tanaka M, et al. Design, synthesis, and radiosensitizing activities of sugar-hybrid hypoxic cell radiosensitizers. Bioorg Med Chem. 2008;16:675–82.
72. Uto Y, Nagasawa H, Jin CZ, et al. Design of antiangiogenic hypoxic cell radiosensitizers: 2-nitroimidazoles containing a 2-aminomethylene-4-cyclopentene-1,3-dione moiety. Bioorg Med Chem. 2008;16:6042–53.

73. Bonnet M, Hong CR, Gu Y, et al. Novel nitroimidazole alkylsulfonamides as hypoxic cell radiosensitisers. Bioorg Med Chem. 2014;22:2123–32.
74. Honess DJ, Wasserman TH, Workman P, et al. Additivity of radiosensitization by the combination of SR 2508 (etanidazole) and Ro 03–8799 (pimonidazole) in a murine tumor system. Int J Radiat Oncol Biol Phys. 1988;15:671–5.
75. Stone HB, Hirst VK, Cribbs R, et al. A comparison of radiosensitization by etanidazole and pimonidazole in mouse tumors. Int J Radiat Oncol Biol Phys. 1991;20:987–95.
76. Hicks KO, Pruijn FB, Secomb TW, et al. Use of three-dimensional tissue cultures to model extravascular transport and predict in vivo activity of hypoxia-targeted anticancer drugs. J Natl Cancer Inst. 2006;98:1118–28.
77. Adams GE, Clarke ED, Gray P, et al. Structure-activity relationships in the development of hypoxic cell radiosensitizers. II. Cytotoxicity and therapeutic ratio. Int J Radiat Biol Relat Stud Phys Chem Med. 1979;35:151–60.
78. Cross P, Marshall ES, Baguley BC, et al. Proliferative assays for the assessment of radiosensitivity of tumor cell lines using 96-well microcultures. Radiat Oncol Investig. 1994;1:261–9.
79. Hicks KO, Pruijn FB, Sturman JR, et al. Multicellular resistance to tirapazamine is due to restricted extravascular transport: a pharmacokinetic/pharmacodynamic study in HT29 multicellular layer cultures. Cancer Res. 2003;63:5970–7.
80. Hicks KO, Pruijn FB, Baguley BC, et al. Extravascular transport of the DNA intercalator and topoisomerase poison *N*-[2-(dimethylamino)ethyl]acridine-4-carboxamide (DACA): diffusion and metabolism in multicellular layers of tumor cells. J Pharmacol Exp Ther. 2001;297:1088–98.
81. Pruijn FB, Patel K, Hay MP, et al. Prediction of tumour tissue diffusion coefficients of hypoxia-activated prodrugs from physicochemical parameters. Aust J Chem. 2008;61:687–93.
82. Pruijn FB, Sturman JR, Liyanage HDS, et al. Extravascular transport of drugs in tumor tissue: Effect of lipophilicity on diffusion of tirapazamine analogs in multicellular layer cultures. J Med Chem. 2005;48:1079–87.
83. Hicks KO. Introducing drug transport early in the design of hypoxia selective anticancer agents using a mathematical modelling approach. In: D'Onofrio A, Cerrai P, Gandolfi A, editors. New challenges for cancer systems biomedicine. Italy: Springer; 2012. p. 337–54.
84. Wardman P. Reduction potentials of one-electron couples involving free radicals in aqueous solution. J Phys Chem Ref Data. 1989;18:1637–755.
85. Hunter FW, Wang J, Patel R, et al. Homologous recombination repair-dependent cytotoxicity of the benzotriazine di-N-oxide CEN-209: Comparison with other hypoxia-activated prodrugs. Biochem Pharmacol. 2012;83:574–85.
86. Hicks KO, Fleming Y, Siim BG, et al. Extravascular diffusion of tirapazamine: effect of metabolic consumption assessed using the multicellular layer model. Int J Radiat Oncol Biol Phys. 1998;42:641–9.
87. Hicks KO, Ohms SJ, van Zijl PL, et al. An experimental and mathematical model for the extravascular transport of a DNA intercalator in tumours. Br J Cancer. 1997;76:894–903.
88. Gu Y, Wilson WR. Rapid and sensitive ultra-high-pressure liquid chromatography-tandem mass spectrometry analysis of the novel anticancer agent PR-104 and its major metabolites in human plasma: application to a pharmacokinetic study. J Chromatogr B Analyt Technol Biomed Life Sci. 2009;877:3181–6.
89. Patel K, Lewiston D, Gu Y, et al. Analysis of the hypoxia-activated dinitrobenzamide mustard phosphate prodrug PR-104 and its alcohol metabolite PR-104A in plasma and tissues by liquid chromatography-mass spectrometry. J Chromatogr B Analyt Technol Biomed Life Sci. 2007;856:302–11.

Index

C. Koumenis et al. (eds.), *Tumor Microenvironment*, Advances in Experimental Medicine and Biology 899, DOI 10.1007/978-3-319-26666-4

M

N

O

P

MIX
Papier aus verantwortungsvollen Quellen
Paper from responsible sources
FSC® C105338

If you have any concerns about our products,
you can contact us on
ProductSafety@springernature.com

In case Publisher is established outside the EU,
the EU authorized representative is:
Springer Nature Customer Service Center GmbH
Europaplatz 3, 69115 Heidelberg, Germany

Printed by Libri Plureos GmbH
in Hamburg, Germany